D. FLOYD

# Dimensions

## A Changing Concept of Health

**Canfield Press**   ΦP   **San Francisco**

**A Department of Harper & Row, Publishers, Inc.**

# Dimensions

## A Changing Concept of Health

### Second Edition

Kenneth L.
Jones

Louis W.
Shainberg

Curtis O.
Byer

Cover and interior photographs by John Pearson
Cover, section, and chapter opening design by
Jaren Dahlstrom

For information address

Harper & Row, Publishers, Inc.
10 East 53rd Street
New York, N.Y. 10022


Library of Congress Cataloging in Publication Data

Jones, Kenneth Lamar, 1931–
    Dimensions: a changing concept of health.

    Includes bibliographies.
    1.  Hygiene.   I.  Shainberg, Louis W., joint author.
II.   Byer, Curtis O., joint author.   III.   Title.
IV.   Title: A changing concept of health.
[DNLM: 1.  Health.   2.  Medicine—Popular works.
WB120 J77d 1974]
QP36.J79  1974      613          74-1085
ISBN 0-06-384371-4


74 75 76  10 9 8 7 6 5 4 3 2

# to Malvina Hindus
## who made it all happen

# A Note
# From the Authors

The college health course has assumed a new importance in recent years. As a result of pressures from government, student interests, and society in general, this course must now come to terms with some of the most important aspects of man and his condition on this planet. Many of the major problems confronting the world today find their roots in the physical, emotional, and social health of people. This is a very unstable era—in which all phases of life are changing at the fastest pace in the history of man. The condition of the environment, the use of drugs, the quality of health care, the freedom in sexual behavior, and indeed many other aspects of interpersonal relationships are now subject to pressures which can only be considered revolutionary. The most pressing problem has become survival—the survival of the individual spirit as well as that of the human species as a whole. It may well be that the youth of the world will have to take the responsibility of insuring their own legacy.

At the focal point of this phenomenon is the changing definition of health. As our understanding of the environment, chemistry and pharmacology, mental health, interpersonal and societal relationships has gone through expansive changes, it is to be expected that our concept of health itself has changed. The interdependence of a wide variety of factors in the determination of a healthful way of life is now generally acknowledged.

As the concept of health has become more complex, it has perhaps become more difficult for each person to be well-informed, and to make personally valid decisions. Appropriate action on any matter must be based on accurate information.

We are constantly subjected to information about health from governmental commissions, private hospital groups, our casual and close friends, our families, and television and radio advertisements. It is essential to one's development as a human being and to his relationships with others that he find a way of sorting out all of this information and advice. Today's health courses are designed to help you accomplish just that, and we hope that this book will make an important contribution to their success.

*Dimensions* is intended as a basic text for college health courses, to provide a broad background and, we hope, a stimulus for enlightened classroom discussion. We do not expect every reader to agree with everything he finds here, since some of the material is, by its very nature, controversial. There are a few areas where not even all of us agree, though our friendship remains intact.

In order to emphasize our view of health science today as a multidimensional subject, we have made some major departures from the traditional approaches. For example, there is a decided shift away from the anatomical and physiological, toward the behavioral and sociological aspects of health, although biological material is introduced in some areas to provide a basis for understanding contemporary health issues, many of which have a biological foundation.

Further, we have tried a new approach in the organization of this book, moving along a continuum from the broadest to the most personal of health concerns. We start with a discussion of environmental quality, since all health—physical, mental, social, and personal—is dependent on a healthful environment. We then move to a discussion of emotional health, because a person's mental outlook influences his relationship with other people. We continue with material on drugs, alcohol, and tobacco; these substances being part of the general health picture as well as representing one aspect of the individual's response to his environment and his image of himself.

These first three sections of the book are followed by a discussion of those aspects which affect the health of the individual as a consumer. The choice of health care programs, health products, foods, and other dietary materials is a crucial one and should be made with care.

We then continue with material on sex and sexuality, an aspect of the human experience which focuses on yet a more personal area of feeling and responsibility than the chapters preceding it. The book concludes with a discussion of diseases, both those which involve transmission through the community via pathogens, and those which impinge on single individuals and probably result from as-yet-unknown threats from the environment and our life styles.

This revision of *Dimensions* is in line with our concept of health science as a dynamic, rapidly changing field, and with our goal of supplying students information that is as current as possible. In this edition, we have added extensive material on fitness, updated the discussions on drug laws and abortion to reflect new legal changes, expanded the section on venereal diseases, and updated all statistics throughout the book.

In addition to these relatively broad changes, we have incorporated throughout the book numerous suggestions from students and teachers. To these people and to all of the instructors and teachers who have used the first edition of *Dimensions,* we would like to express our appreciation for their gratifying acceptance of its concept.

We also want to thank the many people who helped in the preparation of the manuscript and the production of this book. We are particularly grateful to the following people for their thorough and constructive readings of the manuscript: Jack Brennecke, Mount San Antonio College; Barbara Combs, City College of San Francisco; Janet Faurot, Long Beach City College; Kenneth Hurst, Merritt College; Allure Jefcoat, Diablo Valley College; Alfred Mathews, California State College at Hayward; James Pryde, American River College.

We also appreciate the efficiency and cooperation of the outstanding staff of Canfield Press, especially Jack Jennings, publisher; Ted Ricks, editor; Mal Hindus, assistant developmental editor; and Gracia A. Alkema, production editor.

*January 1974*                                        K.L.J.
                                                      L.W.S.
                                                      C.O.B.

# Contents

SECTION 3

# Drugs, Alcohol, and Tobacco

SECTION 4

# Good Health in the Marketplace

SECTION 5

# Human Sexuality and Reproduction

SECTION 6

# Disease

# Dimensions

## A Changing Concept of Health

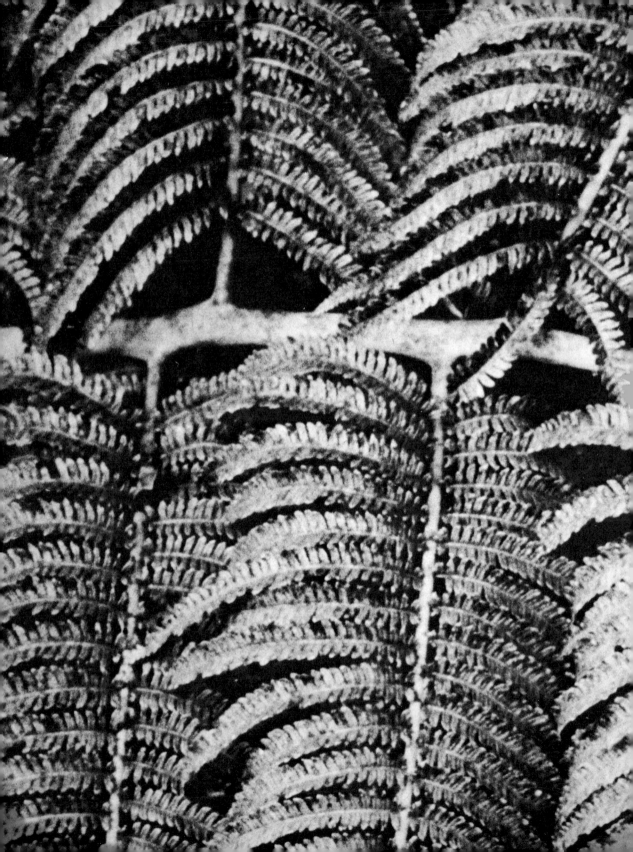

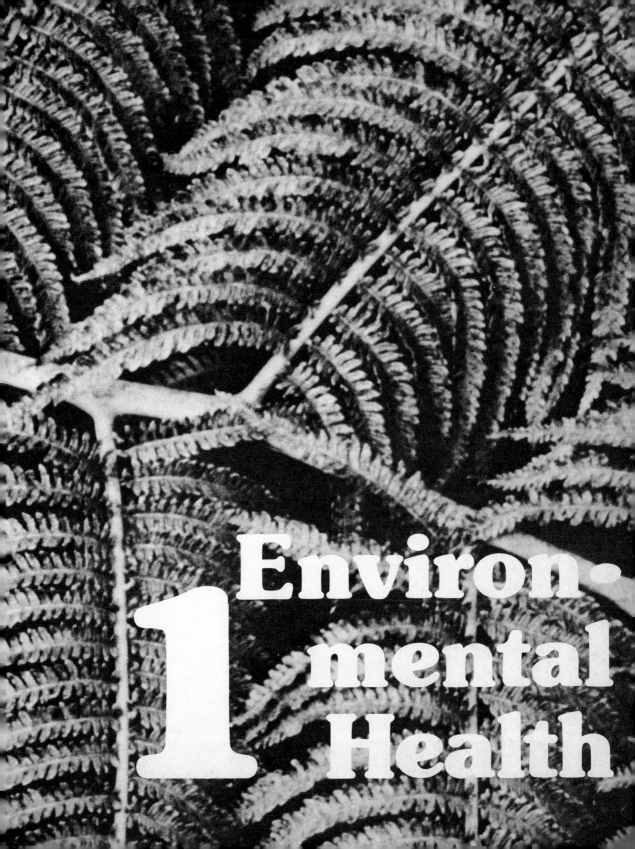

# 1 Environmental Health

# 1 The Threat to the Environment
The Quality of Life • Pollution • The Urban Environment

# 2 Population Dynamics
The Mechanism of Population Increase • The Boundaries of Population Growth

# 1
# The Threat to the Environment

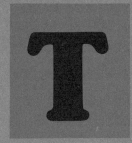

The most critical issue facing man today in his struggle for a long, healthful, and fulfilling life is the rapidly declining quality of his environment. Thus, an examination of the relationships between man and his environment is an important part of the contemporary health course. Because everyone is dependent on the environment for his survival, the environment is everyone's concern.

Several major, current trends, if projected forward for only a few decades, place mankind on a collision course with disaster. Some of these trends include *the rapid growth of world population, the acceleration of world industrialization,* and *the increasing per-capita consumption of resources—all resulting in increased pollution and other forms of environmental deterioration.*

## THE QUALITY OF LIFE

An essential first step in our study of ecological relationships is to consider the general nature of our surroundings. The concept of environment includes much more than just the physical side—land, air, water, and so forth. It encompasses every living and non-living thing that in any way influences the form, quality, or length of our lives. Thus, even social and cultural conditions are included in the concept of environment.

Thinking first about the physical aspects of our environment, the idea we would hope to convey is of the very finite or limited nature of the land, air, and water. While the continents once seemed vast and the air and water unlimited, we are increasingly aware of the really restricted nature of these resources. Most of the earth's surface that is really suitable for living or raising food is already being put to one of those uses. The remaining unexploited land masses are mostly too hot, cold, wet, dry, or otherwise unsuitable for use without tremendous expenditures of already scarce resources and further disruption of the world's physical balance. The atmosphere is actually made up of a very thin layer of gases, which cannot always tolerate the quantities of pollutants that are dumped into it. The oceans are important living systems in which small amounts of various pollutants can upset vital life cycles. The entire environment is not just a passive sink that can tolerate everything poured into it. It is a dynamic system, reacting to every abuse heaped upon it.

We must think of the healthful environment not only as one that is devoid of harmful substances, but as one that includes a wide variety of favorable factors as well. We must not be content with an environment that merely makes life possible, but must concentrate on maintaining or developing an environment that makes life worth living. A healthful environment allows the individual to achieve his full physical, emotional, and social potential. It contributes to emotional well-being through beautiful scenery, clean and orderly communities, and quiet surroundings for the enjoyment of leisure time. It provides for the needs of families and individuals, including adequate housing and educational and economic opportunities. It offers a variety of life styles and the opportunity to choose among them. It provides a social and technological environment within human adaptive capacity.

Thus, the concept of a healthful environment involves much more than the mere absence of pollutants. It raises basic questions about the design and size of metropolitan areas and about the effectiveness of social, economic, and political systems.

## POLLUTION

Foremost among the environmental health hazards today is pollution, the introduction into the environment of substances and forms of energy which unfavorably alter our environment. They are the by-products of man's activities—the residues of things he makes, uses, and throws away. They include the excretory wastes from humans and domestic animals, industrial sewage and gases, pesticides, automobile exhausts, empty cans and bottles, radiation, and even heat and noise.

Since most of these wastes have been with us for many years, one might wonder why pollution has only recently emerged as a major problem. One important reason is the recent increase in human population. An environment that could easily assimilate the wastes and by-products from a lesser population can be completely befouled by the proportionately increased pollutants from a larger population. In addition, new pollutants are constantly being introduced into our environment as a result of continuing technical advancement. An estimated 400 to 500 new chemical substances are being created for our use each year. The long-term effects of these new chemicals upon our environment and us are virtually unknown.

It must be remembered that many pollutants are the unavoidable consequences of man's nature as a biological organism and as a creative social being. These are the wastes from man's metabolic processes and from his efforts to feed, house, clothe, and transport himself. Some pollutants will always be with us. They will increase in abundance as our population increases and as the world standard of living (hopefully) rises. They will become more concentrated as urbanization continues and more people live in less space.

It is obvious, then, that we cannot eliminate all pollutants. Therefore, our goal must be to minimize the production of pollutants, particularly those with serious environmental consequences, and to manage the disposal of pollutants so that they can be effectively assimilated into the environment.

### Air Pollution

A man can live without food for weeks and without water for days, but he can live without air for only a few minutes. Accordingly, air is the most immediately vital resource.

For many years people have been treating the atmosphere as if it were a sewer, exhausting different kinds of waste products into it—gases, dusts, fumes, vapors, and smoke. Since the amount of contamination, until recent years was small in relation to the vastness of the atmosphere, little trouble resulted. In the last few decades, however, continuing contamination is producing concentrations that are harmful to man, animals, and plants.

Air pollution is produced by different air contaminants in different areas. By general definition, air pollution is the introduction of hazardous materials into the atmosphere as the result of man's activities. This definition would exclude air contaminants produced by such natural phenomena as volcanoes, hot springs, and dust storms. Some pollutants, such as smoke from forest fires, may stem from either natural or human causes. Pollution, as discussed here, will imply the possibility of control.

In order to understand the problem of air pollution more fully, let us briefly examine the nature and size of our atmosphere. "Pure" air is, of course, a mixture of many kinds of gases, including about 78 percent nitrogen, 21 percent oxygen, less than 1 percent argon, 0.03 percent carbon dioxide, traces of several other gases, and varying amounts of water vapor. So far, contrary to popular belief, the percentage of oxygen in the air has not been reduced significantly with the advent of air pollution. However, man's activities are reducing the world supply of green plants (our only sources of oxygen) at an alarming rate. An acre of food-crop plants produces far less oxygen than the acre of forest it may have replaced. An acre of pavement produces no oxygen at all. Thus, some authorities feel we may eventually run into oxygen depletion problems with the elimination of green plants, though other air problems are more pressing at this time.

About 95 percent of the earth's air mass is concentrated in a layer about twelve miles thick around the earth's crust. This represents an area no deeper, proportionately, than the skin of an apple to the apple itself. Thus, it is indeed necessary to regard the earth's air supply as limited.

The problem of air pollution is further complicated by the existence of inversion layers over many of the world's major cities. An inversion layer is a layer of warmer air over a cooler surface layer of air, and results from an area's topographical character and proximity to water. This inversion layer acts as an air trap, preventing air pollutants from mixing with upper layers of air. Thus, instead of pollutants being diluted through twelve miles of atmosphere, they may be held within several hundred feet of the ground. In some western cities, such as Los Angeles, inversion layers may be present on as many as 340 days of the year.

*Sources of Air Pollutants.* The majority of the thousands of air-contaminating activities of man can be grouped into three general categories: attrition, vaporization, and combustion.

*Attrition* means the wearing or grinding down by friction. Have you ever wondered what becomes of the tread rubber from the millions of tires that are worn out each year? And the asbestos from millions of brake shoes? Much of this worn-off material drifts into the air as microscopic dustlike particles. Additional sources of particulate pollutants include sanding, sand blasting, drilling, grinding, and a multitude of other industrial processes.

*Vaporization* is the change of a substance from the liquid to the gaseous state. Vaporization is a major source of air pollution. Such materials as gasoline and many industrial solvents vaporize freely at normal air temperatures and are troublesome air polluters. Other materials will vaporize only under the less common conditions of increased heat and pressure. Some of the most noxious pollutants result from vaporization of industrial chemicals.

*Combustion* is the process of burning. Combustion is never complete or perfect, regardless of where it takes place. The fuel may not be a pure hydrocarbon; there may be too much or too little air; or the temperature may be too low or too high. The by-products of combustion may include unburned bits of carbon, carbon monoxide gas, and products from impurities in the fuel. When sulfur is present, it is converted into sulfur dioxide and sulfur trioxide. In addition to being undesirable by themselves, these gases can combine with water vapor to form sulfuric acid.

Another pollutant results from what might be considered perfect combustion conditions—very high temperatures and an air supply beyond that needed for complete combustion. Under such conditions, the high temperature causes the nitrogen and oxygen of the air to combine into nitric oxide which further oxidizes to form nitrogen dioxide, one of the most troublesome components of air pollution. Nitrogen dioxide irritates the eyes and mucous membranes, damages vegetation, and contributes to *photochemical smog.*

*Photochemical Smog.* Smog is a coined word, combining "smoke" and "fog." It is a phenomenon common to many metropolitan areas, particularly those along sea coasts. Photochemical smog results when air pollutants trapped beneath an inversion layer are changed to more noxious chemicals by the action of sunlight.

The basic ingredients of photochemical smog include nitrogen dioxide and incompletely burned hydrocarbons from auto exhausts. Carbon monoxide is not involved.

When nitrogen dioxide ($NO_2$) absorbs energy from sunlight, it separates into nitric oxide (NO). and atomic oxygen (O). The normal atmospheric oxygen is in the form of molecular oxygen ($O_2$). The atomic oxygen unites with the molecular oxygen to form ozone ($O_3$). Ozone induces much eye irritation and is also thought to cause lung damage (pulmonary fibrosis) after long exposure. Ozone also reacts with other air pollutants (especially hydrocarbons) to form literally hundreds of undesirable compounds. Among the worst offenders of photochemical smog are PAN (peroxyacetylnitrate) and various aldehydes. Both PAN and the aldehydes are highly irritating to the eyes and respiratory tract and are harmful to vegetation as well. In the mountain ranges of Southern California, thousands of acres of prime forest are currently being killed by photochemical smog.

*The Effects of Air Pollution.* Some of the effects of air pollution are immediately obvious to even the most casual observer. His eyes sting, his throat burns, the view is spoiled, he may suffer from a vague state of emotional depression. But the more serious effects of air pollution are insidious. Occurring over a period of years, they often go unnoticed until permanent damage has been done. In the following paragraphs we will survey some of these more serious effects of air pollution.

Smog damage to vegetation is creating an alarming situation. At a time when the world food supply is growing ever more scarce, many important food plants are showing increasing damage—and subsequent reduction in yield—due to air pollution. In addition, the world's only oxygen supply—photosynthesis in green plants—is being impaired by air pollution. However, though it may not be much comfort, most authorities say that if air pollution goes uncontrolled, we will starve to death before we run out of oxygen.

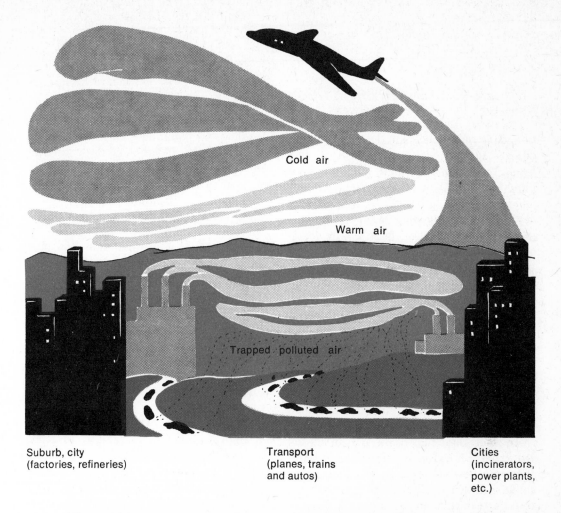

Cold air

Warm air

Trapped polluted air

Suburb, city
(factories, refineries)

Transport
(planes, trains
and autos)

Cities
(incinerators,
power plants,
etc.)

The activities of modern urban and suburban communities include many practices which produce air pollution; when natural phenomena, such as temperature inversions, are added to this a situation like that shown above can result.
This is particularly dangerous for living things because the pollutants emitted
into the lower atmosphere will stay close to their sources until the temperature
pattern is altered by weather changes.

The effect of air pollution on animals is
of double concern: in addition to the illness
and death of the animals themselves, there
is the ominous portent that the same fate

lies ahead for man. Among the many alarming examples of the effects of air pollution
on animals are cases where arsenic from
smelting operations has settled on vegetation

and poisoned grazing animals; where fluorides from aluminum and fertilizer plants have so crippled grazing animals that they had to be killed; and where cattle grazing several miles from lead and zinc foundries have been poisoned.

The economic loss from damage to various materials is almost incalculable. Few, if any, materials are totally impervious to air pollution. Materials that commonly show smog damage are such metals as steel, iron, zinc, brass, copper, nickel, lead, tin; and such building materials as marble, slate, mortar, and paint. Particularly susceptible to damage are such organic materials as rubber, leather, paper, and both natural and synthetic fibers.

When man lives day-in and day-out in a pall of air pollution, it is only the rare clear day that reminds him what he is missing. In addition to the obvious problems of reduced visibility for driving or flying, there are the subtle psychological results of foul air. Every mountain view blocked by air pollution, every flower soiled by smog, and every expanse of blue sky turned gray destroys a portion of man's identity with nature and leaves the quality of his life diminished by the loss.

The most disastrous result of air pollution is its effect on human health. In addition to the more obvious effects, such as eye and throat irritation, air pollution is believed to cause more serious harm to the respiratory system and heart. Air pollution levels have been correlated to chronic bronchitis, asthma, emphysema, lung cancer, and, through impaired lung function, to heart disease. Initially there is an acute inflammation of the lungs, with fluid partially filling the tiny air sacs, or alveoli, of the lungs. The normal breathing reflex is affected. Breathing becomes shallow, and the usual rate of oxygen consumption is decreased. Over the long-term, an irreversible disease known as *emphysema* may result. Asthma or heavy cigarette smoking can cause emphysema. Toxic air pollutants, sulfur dioxide, and ozone are other known causes. The walls between the alveoli break down. The walls of the respiratory tubes become fibrous and constricted, and breathing becomes harder and harder. Other long-term or chronic effects are suspected but as yet have not been conclusively identified. Air pollution is particularly harmful to infants, the elderly, and those suffering from chronic respiratory disorders. Some scientists warn that residue from the internal combustion engine results in high levels of lead capable of affecting human behavior.

Because so much definite evidence of the harmful effects of air pollution has been compiled, many public health authorities now recommend curtailing vigorous outdoor activities during intense smog attacks. In Los Angeles County, ozone levels are monitored daily as indicators of photochemical smog levels, and schools are advised to keep pupils indoors during recess and lunch periods when ozone levels exceed 0.35 part per million—a condition occurring several times each year in parts of the county.

Many people hold exaggerated ideas about the ability of humans to "adjust" to a poisoned environment, feeling that so long as pollution levels increase gradually, we will be able to accommodate to almost any level of pollution. During the 1971 "mercury scare," a representative of the fishing industry was quoted as stating that the American public might have developed such a level of tolerance to mercury-contaminated fish that it might be dangerous to discontinue eating such fish, perhaps resulting in some kind of "withdrawal" symptoms. Needless to say, his fears were unfounded and just might have been influenced by his concern for the "health" of the fishing industry.

Obviously, the human species must have

some ability to adapt to adverse environmental conditions or we would not have survived this long. But our ability to tolerate any particular poison is definitely limited and regardless of how gradually its level in the environment increases, a point would be reached at which continued human life would be impossible. Unfortunately, it seems that for certain poisons in certain areas this level is approached from time to time, or even exceeded.

Suppose that in your city the level of some air pollutant reached the point where medical authorities agreed that it had become hazardous to engage in any outdoor activities—ever! This hypothetical situation is probably already an unrecognized reality in many cities today. Imagine what life would be like if all outdoor activities were forbidden. Children would rush from sealed, air-filtered homes to sealed, air-filtered schools, perhaps wearing gas masks while in transit. Adults similarly would live in fear of the unfiltered air. This joyless situation could become a reality if air pollution is not effectively controlled.

*Control of Air Pollution.* The control or prevention of air contamination is a complex, and often expensive, problem. Some authorities believe it is now possible to eliminate such pollution almost entirely, but each locality must decide how clean its air should be and how much it is willing to pay for smog control. At the present time, toleration levels can be determined for only a few contaminants. Ideally, pollution should be eliminated at the source.

In some places the answer is to reduce the source of pollution by using cleaner-burning home-heating fuels, such as switching from coal to oil, or better, to natural gas or electricity. In other cases, for example, motor vehicles, the problem requires reduction of private auto use by developing better rapid transit systems and by stricter control of auto emissions. The reduction of car size and horsepower also contributes to cleaner air, as will the development of a replacement for the internal combustion engine.

Also involved are the legal and regulatory aspects of pollution control. A person must be free to use his property, yet at the same time, he must be prevented from doing harm to others. The atmosphere must be kept clean enough for humans to breathe safely and to insure the growth of food crops. Conflicts of interest must be overcome. The "right" to discharge waste products into the atmosphere must be made subordinate to the "right" to breathe safe air. Such priorities must be established and they will require the modification of certain practices by both corporations and individuals. Does anyone really have the "right" to pollute the air that others must breathe in order to live?

*Government Controls.* Traditionally, the regulation of pollution has been left to state and local governments. But it has become increasingly clear that such regulation is not always adequate. State and local agencies hesitate to enact or enforce regulations that would restrict the activities of corporations which contribute significantly to the employment and tax rolls within their jurisdiction. These same corporations may make sizeable contributions for the election of "reliable" candidates. The citizens within an area are reluctant to push for pollution control when it might affect their "bread and butter."

Pollution obviously does not confine itself to the political jurisdiction in which it originates. Polluted air drifts freely from county to county. Polluted rivers may flow through many states. Untreated refuse dumped into the ocean by one city may easily wash up on the beaches of another. Thus, the control of pollution rightfully becomes an interstate problem, subject to federal control.

Federal control of pollution has evolved slowly, over a span of several decades. Until recently, federal efforts were often ineffective, as responsibilities were fragmented among many different agencies and departments of the government. There have even been instances where the policies of two federal agencies were directly contradictory—one agency actively polluting the environment with the same pollutant another agency has sought to control.

In a move to coordinate and strengthen the environmental control activities of the federal government, President Nixon in 1970 authorized the formation of the Environmental Protection Agency (E.P.A.). This agency consists of units transferred from other federal agencies, including the Departments of the Interior, Agriculture, Health, Education, and Welfare, and the Atomic Energy Commission. Thus, the federal agencies dealing with air and water pollution, the regulation of pesticides, atomic radiation, and solid waste control were brought under one roof. The E.P.A. operates with a budget in excess of $2 billion per year. Among the specific activities and powers of E.P.A. are the setting of air-quality standards for all sources of air pollutants, with authority to assess penalties up to $25,000 per day for first violations, and up to $50,000 per day and up to 2 years in prison for second offenses.

Other E.P.A. activities include control over all industrial waste discharges into bodies of water, though the elimination of such discharges will be a gradual process. Local government agencies are being given financial and technical aid in the construction of sewage treatment facilities. Another goal is the closing down of 5000 open dumps scattered across the country.

## Water Pollution

Water, in its natural state, is never 100 percent pure. As soon as it condenses as rain, water begins gathering impurities which it carries until purified or until it evaporates. Much of this impurity is not sufficient to spoil the usefulness of water; some materials and substances, however, do limit its usefulness.

By definition, "water pollution" means the presence in water of any substance that interferes with any of its legitimate uses—for public water supplies, recreation, agriculture, industry, the preservation of fish and wildlife, and esthetic purposes.

The principal forms of water pollution are domestic, industrial, and agricultural wastes, and silt. Domestic wastes include sewage, detergents, and everything else going down the drains of a city into its sewer system—used water from toilets, bathtubs, sinks, and washings from restaurants, laundries, hospitals, hotels, and other businesses. Industrial wastes are the acids, oils, greases, other chemicals, and animal and vegetable matter discharged by factories. These wastes are discharged either through some sewer system or through separate outlets directly into waterways. Agricultural wastes include pesticides (insecticides, fungicides, and herbicides), fertilizers (mainly nitrates and phosphates), and animal wastes. Silt includes the soil that is washed into streams that muddies waters and fills up reservoirs and waterways. In addition to these principal forms, other pollutants, such as heat and radioactive substances, can contribute to water pollution.

Pollution in a body of water can be measured several ways. Most common pollutants are organic. Bacteria break them down into simpler compounds, and in doing so, need oxygen. With more organic material, the bacteria population increases, and a greater demand is placed on oxygen in the water.

The demand for oxygen by bacteria is called *biological oxygen demand* (BOD). BOD is an indicator of organic pollution. It also determines which forms of life can best survive in the stream. Large water animals need more oxygen and therefore have a higher BOD than invertebrate animals and bacteria, which have a much lower BOD. In fact, certain invertebrate animals living in bottom mud of freshwater streams occur in inverse proportion to the oxygen content of the water. One, a small worm, *Tubifex,* has an occurrence as high as 20,000 individuals per square foot in badly polluted water, but may be absent altogether in clean water. Not all water pollutants are broken down by bacteria. Radioactive substances, silt, pesticides, detergents, and certain oil products are more difficult to clean up.

*Wide-Range Effects of Polluted Water.* Not only is clean water needed for domestic uses, but water is also the most extensively used of all raw materials in industry. Since the availability of good-quality water determines the location of many industries, having good water becomes an economic asset for most communities. Correspondingly, lack of good water may turn into an economic liability.

There are other economic considerations. Crops irrigated with polluted water may transmit disease. Certain forms of industrial pollution in irrigation waters may damage crops. Heavy metals such as mercury and arsenic and certain hydrocarbons such as DDT are particularly difficult to keep out of water resources. As natural sediments flow into a body of water, nitrate and phosphate concentrations begin to build up. Algae and other plants flourish. While algae is an oxygen-producer during daylight hours, it is an oxygen-consumer during the nighttime. With great "blooms" of algae, the oxygen level of the water may fall below the level required for respiration of higher forms of animal life.

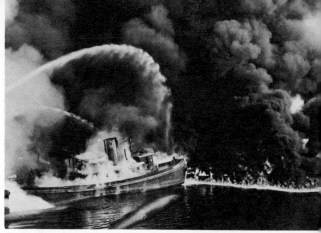

As a result of years of use as a dumping ground for the major industries of Cleveland, Ohio, the once-beautiful Cuyahoga River is now designated a fire hazard. A single match can set off the type of blaze shown here. *Photo by The Cleveland Plain Dealer.*

As increased bacterial action depletes the supply of dissolved oxygen, the water no longer supports animals requiring high levels of dissolved oxygen. Trout and salmon disappear, and are replaced by carp. Eventually, these coarser fish disappear and are replaced by worms or other animals requiring low levels of oxygen. Decay progresses. Hydrogen sulfide and other odorous gases are produced. The water tastes bad, and is unfit for swimming. "Polluted Water" and "Beach Closed" signs appear. Boating becomes undesirable, and outdoor water recreation limited. As lakeside businesses are affected, the economy of polluted localities is depressed.

Future demands on our country's water may well outstrip the supply. Many experts believe that only through increased reuse of water will future needs be supplied. Reuse cannot occur, however, if the water has been irreversibly damaged. Thus, it is of the utmost importance we find answers to deal with the present pollution problems.

*Purification Processes.* There are two primary methods of purifying water—either by natural processes or by specific treatment of domestic and industrial sewage.

*Natural processes.* Water can purify itself by natural means up to specific points of capacity. The time required for self-purification will depend on the degree of pollution and the character of the water.

Since the infiltration of sunlight is minimized in polluted water, few water plants will grow in it; thus the oxygen supply is reduced. This reduction leads to fewer bacteria that can break down organic wastes, which increases the pollution problem. The result is foul-smelling, unattractive water that cannot support fish or other aquatic life. The solution to such instances is to reduce incoming wastes sufficiently so that the stream can handle them through self-purification. The amount of reduction necessary differs from stream to stream depending on its specific characteristics.

(*Sewage treatment.*) Sewage treatment is designed to reduce the polluting effect of wastes before they are discharged into public waterways. Such treatment may be carried out by industries or by municipalities. Industrial treatment may be an in-plant process where the water is treated for reuse.

In municipal sewage treatment, the process may involve either a primary treatment or a primary-secondary treatment. In the primary process, about 35 percent of the pollution is removed. The organic material is first settled out; the water is then chlorinated to kill bacteria and discharged into a stream. The settled sludge is removed or dried, made harmless by heating, and then used for fertilizer, soil conditioners, or land fill.

Further purification is necessary when the water is to be reused by humans. In such instances, a further settling-filtering process is involved. The amount of pollution reduction required determines the intensity of this secondary treatment. However, even secondary treatment fails to remove dissolved minerals, such as nitrates and phosphates which cause excessive growth of algae in lakes and other bodies of water.

In addition to their stimulation of the growth of algae, nitrates can be detrimental to human beings. Damage results when nitrates, themselves relatively nontoxic, are converted to the more toxic compounds (nitrites). These nitrites combine with the blood's oxygen carrier, hemoglobin, in the red blood cells to form methemoglobin, a compound incapable of carrying oxygen. Thus, the oxygen-carrying ability of the blood is reduced. This condition is especially dangerous to infants, elderly people, and those with heart or respiratory disorders.

Phosphate levels are the determining factor in the growth of algae in most bodies of fresh water. (Nitrate levels are the critical factor in marine environments.) In recent years, we have seen a great increase in the phosphate levels of most American surface waters. The principal sources of these phosphates are agricultural runoff, domestic wastes, and industrial wastes. The major source of phosphates in domestic wastes comes from household detergents, which have contributed hundreds of millions of pounds per year. Fortunately, beginning in 1970, consumers became increasingly aware of the significance of phosphates in detergents and many began selecting products on the basis of phosphate levels. In response, the detergent manufacturers were forced to alter the composition of many cleaning products. Some localities even passed ordinances banning the sale of high phosphate detergents, because to remove them from the sewage would require entirely new treatment processes.

*Oil Spills.* Oil spills are, in the public mind, a particularly alarming form of water pollu-

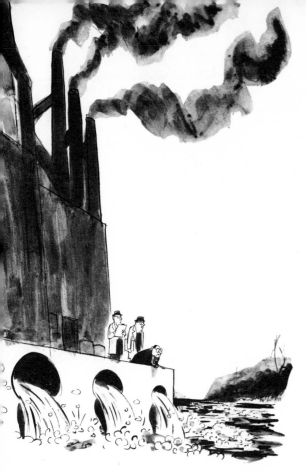

"So *that's* where it goes! Well, I'd like to thank you fellows for bringing this to my attention." *Drawing by Stevenson.* © *1970 The New Yorker Magazine, Inc.*

tion. They are highly visible, and they foul beaches for recreational use. Thus, even people of limited environmental awareness become disturbed when oil coats their favorite beach. There are many sources of oil spills. They may be accidents, as in collisions of oil tankers, or incidents involving offshore drilling rigs. Even more distressing are intentional discharges of oil when oil tankers dump a mixture of ballast water and residual oil from their tanks before reloading.

All oils contain some volatile substances that evaporate readily. As much as 25 percent of the volume of spilled oil evaporates during the first several days. Bacteria work to decompose the remaining mass. After three months on the surface of the sea, only about 15 percent of the original volume of spilled oil remains. This is a thick, asphaltlike lump of tar that often washes up on beaches. If the spill is close to shore, there isn't time for this breakdown process to occur, and a thick layer of oil is deposited onto any object coming into contact with it.

Oil covers swimming and diving birds. Their buoyancy is reduced and they cannot fly. The feathers no longer insulate and the birds die of exposure. Some believe, aside from damage to seabirds, that oil spills are more of an aesthetic pollutant than a biological one.

In any case, oil spills are undesirable and every effort must be made to reduce their frequency. Due to its visibility, oil was one of the first pollutants to receive governmental attention. The Oil Pollution Control Act of 1924 was designed to regulate the discharge of oil from ships in coastal waters. Since then, progressively more stringent laws have been passed. In 1970 a law was passed that imposes absolute financial responsibility on those guilty of causing oil spills in United States waters. The law also provides for fines that could run into millions of dollars for the polluters, and for prison sentences for officers of violating corporations. With today's increased awareness of pollution problems, we can expect to see even more effective anti-pollution legislation passed.

### The Subtle Pollutants— Radiation and Toxic Chemicals

If anything positive can be said for the problems of air and water pollution, it is that they are, at least in most cases, obvious. Their impact on our senses of sight, smell, and taste tells us that something is drastically wrong. In contrast, radiation and toxic chemicals may be entirely unnoticeable to the unequipped observer, even at extremely dangerous levels. They are detectable and measurable only with sophisticated instruments.

In addition, the effects of radiation and toxic chemicals may take years, or even generations, to become noticeable. While large doses of either will result in rapid death, the dosages more commonly encountered in the environment produce subtle damage, such as mutations which may not become apparent for several generations, or cancers which appear after many years.

Not only may the effects of radiation and toxic chemicals be remote in time, but in distance as well. Either of these factors may be carried thousands of miles from their source by air or water currents.

### Radiation in the Environment

Since the beginning of the "atomic age" over 25 years ago, there has been considerable concern about the effects of excessive radiation in our environment. Actually, there has always been some radiation present, referred to as natural background radiation. All forms of life have been subjected to low levels of radiation from natural sources throughout their evolution. In fact, such natural radiation is believed to be important in producing the mutations upon which evolution is based. Natural background radiation comes from radioactive substances in the ground, air, and water, as well as from space in the form of cosmic radiation.

In recent decades, however, man has also been subjected to his own man-made radiation. The intensity of man-made radiation ranges from high doses, such as result from a nuclear weapon, reactor accident, or from radiotherapy, down to low doses comparable to natural background radiation. Some of the major man-made radiation sources are outlined below.

*Radiotherapy.* This is the use of radiation (usually x- and gamma-radiation) as a means of diagnosis and treatment in medicine and dentistry. This is the major source of man-made radiation in the world today, and its value, in each case, should be weighed against its potential hazards.

*Radioactive isotopes.* These are atoms of radioactive elements used in research, in medical diagnosis and treatment, and in industry.

*Industrial x-rays.* These are x-rays used in industry for radiography of welds, castings, and products where flaws could impair the usefulness of the product.

*Radioactive fallout.* This is the result of the explosion of nuclear devices, as in the testing or use of nuclear weapons.

*Radioactive wastes.* These are produced from the use and processing of radioactive materials, fission products, and the possible accidental release of radioactive substances. Some of these affect only individuals who are subjected to radiation because of their occupation. But there are also radioactive wastes which constitute a hazard to the whole population through pollution of the environment.

*Effects of Radiation on the Body Tissues.* Large doses of all types of radiation will kill cells. With smaller doses of radiation, recovery is possible, and cells can continue to function. However, recovery may not be complete, causing malignant changes later. In general, certain cells are more readily affected by radiation than are others. Tissues that are actively regenerating with constant cell division and multiplication—such as embryonic tissue, intestinal mucosa, blood-forming tissue, gonadal germ cells, and skin—are more vulnerable. These various types of tissue damage may be simplified into two main classes: somatic tissue effects and genetic effects.

*Somatic tissue effects.* Somatic cells compose all body tissue, except for the eggs in the ovaries and the sperm in the testes. Large doses of radiation destroy somatic tissue, leading to the death of the individual. Lesser doses of radiation may show no immediate effect, but they will accumulate until cell function may be altered, possibly producing leukemia or another form of cancer.

*Genetic effects.* Genetic effects are the changes produced in the germ or reproductive cells. No damage will appear in the individual exposed to the radiation, but the effects will show up in his descendents as abnormalities of form and function. Such genetic effects may be caused by small doses of radiation; therefore, all radiation must be considered deleterious to one degree or another.

*Radioactive Fallout.* Fallout is the return to earth of radioactive material that has been carried up into the atmosphere by the detonation of a nuclear device or as a result of a nuclear accident. It also refers to any resulting contamination of food, drink, soil, air, or building materials caused by such fallout. Environmental contamination produced by the worldwide dispersion of radioactivity from nuclear weapon tests has been a source of both internal and external radiation.

Distribution of a fallout pattern is determined by yield, height, and location of the detonation, and by meteorological conditions. The dose rate (the amount of radiation absorbed by an individual) and the accumulated dose from fallout depend not only on the amount of radioactive fallout but also on the ionization effects of the radiation products.

For every megaton of fission involved in the detonation of a nuclear device, yield will be about 100 pounds of intensely radioactive substances. Fortunately, many of the substances formed have extremely short half-lives (period of time during which one-half of a substance's radioactivity decays) and thus have little significance other than in

## FADING RADIATION HAZARD

| CONTAMINATION IN CURIES OF RADIO-ACTIVE MATERIAL | TIME AFTER FORMATION OF FISSION PRODUCTS | RADIATION INTENSITY FROM FISSION PRODUCTS (ROENTGENS PER HOUR) |
|---|---|---|
| 1000 | 1 hour | 10,000 |
| 100 | 7 hours | 1000 |
| 10 | 49 hours (2 days) | 100 |
| 1 | 14 days (2 weeks) | 10 |
| 0.1 | 14 weeks (3 months) | 1 |

SOURCE: Adapted from C. W. Shilling, *Atomic Energy Encyclopedia*, Philadelphia, W. B. Saunders, 1964.

terms of local fallout. The isotopes remaining 1 hour after detonation decay approximately by a factor of 10 for every sevenfold increase in time after detonation time plus 1 hour. Thus, as is shown in the table on fading radiation hazard, 7 hours after a nuclear explosion, the radioactivity has decreased to one-tenth of what it was at 1 hour. In 49 hours, the radioactivity is only one one-hundredth of what it was at 1 hour, and so on.

It has been shown that the total dose to bone marrow from artificial sources of radiation in technically advanced countries is approximately equal to the typical natural background dose. In children under 5, fallout probably accounts for some 5 to 10 percent of the artificial dose to bone marrow. With the advent of a test ban treaty, the dosage will decrease in younger children. Fallout during atmospheric testing periods has been responsible for about one-fifth of the total artificial dose.

*Disposal of Radioactive Waste.* Radioactive wastes from industry vary so much that there is no single preferred method of management and disposal. The solution depends on such factors as the specific nature (radioactive half-life or type of radiation), concentration (quantity of radioactive material involved), and the environment in which disposal is being considered. The problem of disposal of radioactive wastes stems from the fact that there is no way to destroy the radioactivity immediately. Time alone renders the waste stable and harmless or at least reduces the level of radioactivity to the point that it is nontoxic.

The magnitude of the waste disposal problem far outweighs the problem of fallout or the operation of a reactor. Waste disposal is potentially the greatest hazard to public safety. And the time for concern is now! Many reactors are not currently in use, or are being run at reduced capacity, because

of the many tons of high-level radioactive waste already stored. Yet, no satisfactory method for disposal has been developed. As the nuclear power program builds up, the disposal of fission products in a manner that will not be injurious to health must have particular attention.

Spent fuel elements are now removed from reactors and shipped to one of the major United States Atomic Energy Commission processing sites. Here they are "cooled" for 90 days to allow decay of radioactive isotopes with short half-lives. They are classified as having high, medium, or low energy levels and are disposed of accordingly.

High-energy radioactive wastes must be handled by containment in tank storage to allow time for radioactive decay. Suggestions for final disposal of high-level wastes include conversion of liquid wastes to solids and permanent storage in geological strata, with salt beds serving as major sites. Or, liquids could be put directly into geological strata, either in deep wells or salt beds. Or, both solids and liquids could be disposed of in the sea.

Medium-energy radioactive wastes are usually held in trenches, in artificial ponds, or in tanks to allow radioactive wastes to decay to a level where they may be discharged into the environment. Some wastes with radioisotopes of reasonably short half-lives (weeks to months) are discharged directly into the ground. Some medium-energy wastes have been incorporated into concrete, poured into steel drums, and buried in trenches or dumped at sea.

Low-energy radioactive wastes are defined as having a radioactivity concentration in the range of one-millionth of a curie (a unit of measure of radioactive decay) per gallon. They are disposed of by dilution with water and released directly into the environment—into air, land, or sea. These wastes

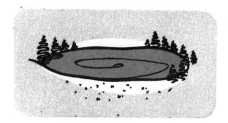

Lake "safe level" of DDT
used to kill pests

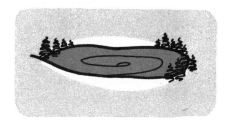

"Kill" successful; no
apparent ill effects

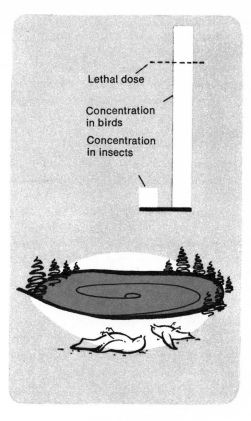

Lethal dose

Concentration
in birds

Concentration
in insects

Dead birds later found
near site of spraying

One of the "hidden" dangers of poorly planned pesticide use. The natural food
web, connecting insects with the birds that feed on them, multiplies the amount
of DDT in the birds' diet, and can have the lethal effect shown here. The birds
are killed by a concentration of the pesticide far greater than that which was
first used to clear the lake of insects.

include the reactor cooling water used in
nuclear-powered ships and submarines.

Various other forms of waste processing,
including chemical treatments, are being used
or experimented with in an attempt to find
a more economical and satisfactory method
of waste disposal.

### Pesticides in the Environment

The era of the synthetic organic pesticides
dawned in May, 1943 with the opening of
the first commerical plant for the production
of DDT. Production was soon measured in
millions of pounds per year. For centuries

before this, pesticides had been in use, but they were of entirely different types. Earlier pesticides consisted mainly of inorganic compounds, such as arsenicals, fluorides, and compounds of copper, sulfur, and mercury; or botanically derived, natural organic compounds, such as nicotine, pyrethrum, and rotenone.

The synthetic organic pesticides met with a tremendous reception. They offered a toxicity to insects far surpassing that of the older chemicals, and they were available in unlimited quantities at relatively low costs. They arrived on the scene at a time when rising populations demanded every possible means of increased food production. For several years it seemed that our insect control problems had been solved.

Then some unsettling problems began to arise. Many insect species began showing resistance to the effects of the new insecticides, stubbornly refusing to die. This situation was met by the development of more powerful poisons. Then traces of pesticides were found to remain in food products after harvest. Of course, this was not really a new problem; it was known that arsenic, for example, also had this unfortunate tendency. The pesticide residue problem resulted in a proliferation of government regulations limiting the quantity of a given pesticide in a given food product. Of course, it was not known for certain what the long-range effects of these "legal" residues would be, but at least no one was going to be poisoned outright.

Another unnerving problem was that a crop often showed evidence, exceeding the legal quantity, of some chemical with which that crop had never even been treated. Perhaps the only previous use of that chemical had been miles away. It became apparent that pesticides were drifting rather freely through the environment. Not too long after

that, traces of pesticides were detected on islands thousands of miles from the nearest site of pesticide application.

One of the original major selling points of certain pesticides was their persistence—or resistance to being broken down. They could control insects months or even years after their application. Less apparent was the fact that these persistent pesticides were gradually building up throughout the environment to levels where not only insects were killed but where many other kinds of organisms were being affected as well.

Widespread public attention was first drawn to this problem in 1962 with the publication of the now-classic *Silent Spring* by the late Rachel Carson. Even though Miss Carson was initially laughed off by agricultural and agrichemical interests as a "crank" or "sensationalist," her observations on the effects of pesticides on birds, fishes, and other wildlife have been largely substantiated.

Among the proven ill-effects of various pesticides are:

1. *Destruction of natural enemies (parasites and predators) of insects, leading to massive "rebound" pest populations.* Most agricultural pests are held to generally low population levels by their natural enemies, though there might be occasional destructive outbreaks of pests. This is part of the dynamic "balance of nature," but this problem is aggravated by the practice of monoculture—the cultivation of large blocks of a single species of crop plant. There is frequently a "lag" period during which pest populations increase explosively before predator or parasite populations catch up. Further complicating the situation is the fact that many pest species have been accidentally imported from other parts of the world, while their enemies have been left behind. Thus, a reasonable position on the use of pesticides is that some use of pesticides is probably unavoidable if current

and future world populations are to be fed. Yet the first application of pesticide to a particular crop should be avoided unless there is a clear and present threat of destruction of a major portion of the crop. Then the pesticide to be applied should be chosen on the basis of a minimum of destruction of beneficial insects and other environmental damage. It should be borne in mind that the decision to make the first application of pesticide to a crop will usually commit the grower to further applications during the season.

2. *Outright killing of birds, fishes, and other wild animals.* Sometimes the cause and effect relationship here is quite obvious, as when pesticide contamination of a river results in millions of dead fish washing ashore. In other cases, the cause of death may be obscured. For example, the pesticide may be concentrated through the food chain, so that the bird or other animal killed may be quite remote from the point of application of the pesticide, either in distance or in time.

3. *Interference with the reproductive processes of birds, fishes, and other wildlife.* It has been clearly established that certain pesticides interfere with shell formation in bird eggs or with the sex hormones of both birds and mammals. Such reproductive interference by persistent pesticides in the environment has apparently already doomed several species of birds to near extinction. Even if all use of such pesticides stopped

Another side-effect of pesticide use is the threat to the natural life processes of some species. Along the West Coast of the United States, the number of brown pelicans is rapidly declining because of DDT-induced weakening of the shells of newly hatched eggs. *Photo by Joseph Jehl, Jr.*

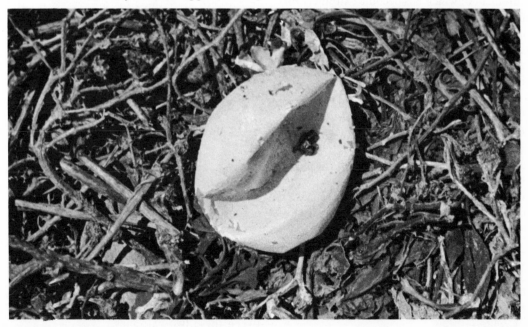

*19*

immediately, it is likely that they would persist in the environment longer than some of the threatened bird species could survive.

4. *Inhibition of photosynthesis in plants.* The exact mechanism of this is not known.

5. *Concentration of pesticides in fishes to unsafe levels for human consumption.* This occurs through the many steps of the food chain, with about a tenfold concentration with each step. We may eventually have to curtail consumption of the larger fish species, turning instead to the smaller species which, being the product of a shorter food chain, should have lower pesticide levels. A parallel situation resulted in the high levels of mercury in swordfish which led, in 1971, to the virtual elimination of this fish as a part of the American diet.

6. *Presence in cow's milk of levels beyond legal tolerance for human consumption.* Production of pesticide-free milk requires pesticide-free hay and other feeds, the procurement of which has become extremely difficult. Large areas of many states are now unsuitable for the growth of hay for milk cows due to the high levels of pesticide used in those areas—the drift of pesticides onto hay crops being inevitable.

7. *Birth defects in animals (and man?) attributed to commonly used herbicides (weed killers).* The herbicide 2,4,5–T has enjoyed widespread use as a brush killer. Typical applications have included clearing of brush from rangeland and defoliation in jungle warfare. While this herbicide was, for years, considered safe, birth defects similar to thalidomide damage were noticed in animals in areas treated with 2,4,5–T. These results were confirmed in laboratory studies with mice and other animals. Whether such defects are also caused in man is not known, but the possibility has led to the curtailment of use of 2,4,5–T.

8. *Acute and chronic impairment of the health of workers who apply and otherwise handle pesticides.* Each pesticide presents its own particular set of hazards to its handlers, ranging from the risk of swift death if only a few drops are spilled on the skin to such obscure possible hazards as genetic mutations which may affect future generations.

9. *Illness and death of farmworkers laboring in treated crop areas.* Following the application of any pesticide, there is a period of time during which workers should stay out of the treated area. This period varies greatly, depending on the chemical used and such environmental conditions as temperature, wind, and rainfall. Too often, growers have sent crews into recently treated fields for thinning, weeding, and similar operations, resulting in illness and occasionally death for the workers.

10. *Development of pesticide resistance in over 200 species of insects.* Continuing to show the great adaptability that has enabled them to survive for millions of years, most pest species have developed resistance to any pesticide to which they have been exposed over a period of several years. For example, the common housefly, once easily controlled with DDT, can now withstand a dose over 1000 times as great as that which once proved fatal in every case.

Inevitably there are other serious problems yet undiscovered and unforeseen that will arise from the use of pesticides.

*Alternate Methods of Pest Control.* It is obvious that continued haphazard and reckless use of pesticides will result in worldwide environmental destruction and the extinction of countless species of organisms, perhaps even man. Yet, the abrupt abandonment of all pesticides would result in widespread starvation and insect-borne disease. The answer to pest control must lie somewhere between these two extremes.

An imperative first step is to shift immediately from the persistent chlorinated-hydrocarbon pesticides to the more rapidly decomposing organic phosphates and carbamates. Even the less persistent pesticides should be used with caution, however, since their generally higher acute toxicity may result in immediate ecological changes caused by massive wildlife death. In addition, the effects of long-term human exposure to these chemicals are not really known. The table on common pesticides gives the acute toxicity count and other information on various pesticides (pp. 22 and 23).

Chemical pest control should be integrated into the many other effective methods of control and used only as a "last resort" when all other methods fail. Some of the alternatives to chemical control include relying on predators and parasites, insect-disease-producing organisms (bacteria, fungi, and viruses which cause insect diseases only); releasing sterilized insects (especially effective in species that mate only once); developing pest-resistant crop varieties; and using cultural control practices, such as rotating crops and timing plantings and harvests to escape insect attacks.

Consumers and government agencies have contributed to the pesticide problem by demanding that insect damage to fruits and vegetables be kept to unreasonably low levels. Some relaxation of the standards for insect damage or contamination could allow a great reduction in pesticide usage.

### Pollutants in Food

One of the favorite topics among people concerned with maintaining overall health standards is the matter of substances added to food. On one side are people who claim that all types of dangerous chemicals are being added to food without due regard to the consequences. On the other, food-industry spokesmen are quick to point out that purposely added substances are used with justification and safety. These chemicals retard spoilage, enhance flavor, improve color, improve consistency, retard drying, or help to retain crispness. Some are added as nutritional supplements, such as thiamine to bread, iodine to salt, fluoride to water, and vitamins A and D to milk.

Some substances, including insecticides, hormones, antibiotics, and disinfectants, enter food accidentally and unintentionally. Some of these enter from the wrappers or containers which touch the food.

Certain federal agencies are going to great lengths to protect the consumer against injurious substances. Before we point out these areas of concern, however, we should define several terms. A *food additive* is a substance, other than a basic foodstuff, which is intentionally present in food as a result of any aspect of production, processing, storage, or packaging. This definition does not include chance contaminants. *Toxicity* is the capacity of a substance to produce injury. *Safety* is the practical certainty that injury will not result from use of a substance in a proposed quantity and manner. *Hazard* is the probability that injury will result from use of a substance in a proposed quantity and manner. An *adulterant* is a foreign or inferior substance added to a food product in place of a more valuable substance. The adulterant might be actually harmful when consumed, or merely deceptive, such as the inclusion of horsemeat or cereal in hamburger. A *residue* is a quantity of a pesticide or other contaminant remaining unintentionally on a food product as a result of treatments made during its growing or processing. A *tolerance* is a quantity of residue, presumed to be safe for consumption, legally permitted to be present in food.

# SOME COMMON PESTICIDES

| PESTICIDE (OTHER NAMES) | RELATIVE ACUTE TOXICITY[a] | COMMENTS |
|---|---|---|
| **CHLORINATED HYDROCARBON GROUP** *(Characterized, in general, by long-term persistence in the environment.)* | | |
| DDT | Toxic[b] $LD_{50}$ = 250 mg/kg | Has been world's most used insecticide |
| DDD (TDE, Rhothane®) | Slightly toxic $LD_{50}$ = 3400 mg/kg | A breakdown product of DDT |
| Dicofol (Kelthane®) | Moderately toxic $LD_{50}$ = 575 mg/kg | Used to kill mites |
| Methoxychlor | Essentially nontoxic $LD_{50}$ = 6000 mg/kg | |
| Benzene Hexachloride (BHC, Lindane) | Toxic $LD_{50}$ = 125 mg/kg | Very stable |
| Chlordane | Toxic $LD_{50}$ = 225 mg/kg | Very stable Absorbed through skin |
| Heptachlor | Toxic $LD_{50}$ = 90 mg/kg | |
| Aldrin | Toxic $LD_{50}$ = 55 mg/kg | |
| Dieldrin | Toxic $LD_{50}$ = 60 mg/kg | Absorbed through skin Has been very damaging to wildlife |
| Endrin | Highly toxic $LD_{50}$ = 5-45 mg/kg | Absorbed through skin Very poisonous to birds Very stable |
| Endosulfan (Thiodan®) | Toxic $LD_{50}$ = 110 mg/kg | Absorbed through skin |
| Toxaphene | Toxic $LD_{50}$ = 69 mg/kg | Less persistent than others in group |
| **ORGANIC PHOSPHATE GROUP** *(Generally less persistent than chlorinated hydrocarbons, but often of greater acute toxicity. Same mode of action as nerve gases of warfare.)* | | |
| Azodrin® | Toxic $LD_{50}$ = 21 mg/kg | Reportedly very harmful to beneficial insects |
| Bidrin® | Toxic $LD_{50}$ = 22 mg/kg | |
| Ciodrin® | Toxic $LD_{50}$ = 125 mg/kg | Rapid decomposition in environment |
| Diazinon (Spectracide®) | Toxic $LD_{50}$ = 150 mg/kg | Widely promoted for home use |
| Dichlorovos (DDVP, Vapona®) | Toxic $LD_{50}$ = 56-80 mg/kg | Widely promoted for home use |

## SOME COMMON PESTICIDES (Continued)

| PESTICIDE (OTHER NAMES) | RELATIVE ACUTE TOXICITY[a] | COMMENTS |
|---|---|---|
| Malathion | Moderately toxic $LD_{50}$ = 900-5800 mg/kg | Relatively safe for home use |
| Parathion | Extremely toxic $LD_{50}$ = 3-15 mg/kg | Readily absorbed through skin. Too toxic for home use Cause of many deaths |
| Phorate (Thimet®) | Extremely toxic $LD_{50}$ = 2-4 mg/kg | A systemic insecticide, translocated through vascular system of plant Not for home use |
| Mevinphos (Phosdrin®) | Extremely toxic $LD_{50}$ = 6-7 mg/kg | Readily absorbed through skin. Many professional applicators refuse to work with this chemical |
| CARBAMATE GROUP *(Not persistent in the environment)* | | |
| Baygon® | Toxic $LD_{50}$ = 95 mg/kg | Has been widely used by exterminators |
| Sevin® (carbaryl) | Moderately toxic $LD_{50}$ = 500 mg/kg | Relatively safe for home use. Extremely toxic to honeybees and beneficial wild bees |
| Bux® | Toxic $LD_{50}$ = 170 mg/kg | |
| BOTANICAL GROUP *(Extracted from plants)* | | |
| Nicotine (Black Leaf 40®) | Highly toxic $LD_{50}$ = 10 mg/kg | Absorbed through skin Long a standard for home garden use |
| Pyrethrum | Slightly toxic $LD_{50}$ = 2000 mg/kg | Among least toxic to man Safely used around foods and as ''fog'' for quick kill without residue |
| Rotenone | Toxic $LD_{50}$ = 300 mg/kg | Extremely toxic to fish |

[a]Acute toxicity refers to the amount required to cause immediate death, but does not take into account any possible long-term effects such as accumulation in tissues of body, carcinogenesis (cancer production), mutagenesis (stimulus of mutations), or any other long-term effect.

[b]$LD_{50}$ is the *median lethal dose,* the amount required to kill 50 percent of the test animals. Figures given are for oral doses for rats. Human toxicity is generally comparable.

SOURCE: Sun, Yun-Pei, *Pesticide Reference Standards,* Bulletin of the Entomological Society of America, Vol. 14, No. 3 (September 1968), 238–248.

*Pesticide Residues in Foods.* Modern food-production practices include the use of hundreds of pesticide chemicals—insecticides, miticides, herbicides, nematocides, fungicides, and so on. There is now mounting concern about the possible immediate and long-term adverse effects of the consumption of food containing residual traces of various pesticides.

All pesticides must be registered with the federal Environmental Protection Agency (E.P.A.) before application to crops is allowed. Such registration is granted only after extensive safety testing, which includes feeding the pesticide in measured quantities to test animals over long periods of time, as well as analyzing treated crops for the amount of pesticide residue. Registrations are quite specific in the quantity of pesticide that may be applied and in the conditions of the application, such as the interval between application and harvest. Pesticide registrations have been granted on the basis of a "zero tolerance" (no trace of residue permitted) or on the basis of a specific tolerance (generally a few parts per million permitted). In the case of specific tolerance the government insists on a residue safety margin of a hundredfold; in other words, only one one-hundredth of the presumed safety level of residue is allowed in consumer foods.

Fearing the possibility of yet unknown effects of long-term consumption of even small amounts of pesticides, some authorities now question the wisdom of allowing any tolerance. They often cite possible genetic damage, cancer, and metabolic disorders as effects that might show up after many years of exposure.

A more immediate danger lies in the occasional cases of improper use of pesticides. Excessively heavy or frequent application, improper formulation, or application too close to harvest times are examples of practices that may result in residues above the legal tolerance. Although many such cases are detected by E.P.A. inspectors—with the subsequent destruction of the contaminated foods—it must be assumed that much food carrying illegal residues is reaching the consumer.

Some though not all pesticide residues can be removed from foods in the home by thorough washing, peeling, removing outer leaves, and similar processes. Foods showing visible residues or having unusual smells should not be purchased.

*Intentional Food Additives.* Shifting our attention now to chemicals purposely added to foods, we find that some of the prepared "convenience" food products contain up to a dozen or more chemical additives. As with pesticides, new food additives must undergo intensive testing before their use is approved. Food additives are approved by the Food and Drug Administration (F.D.A.) of the Department of Health, Education, and Welfare. However, many additives that were introduced prior to 1958 did not receive the safety testing now required, yet they have been permitted to remain in use. The withdrawal of cyclamates from general use in 1969 illustrates that some of the older additives may not be as safe as had been presumed.

Increasing numbers of authorities are questioning the wisdom of our consumption of substantial quantities of food additives. While it is unlikely that the amount contained in one food product presents any great threat to health, the individual or family relying on convenience foods could potentially consume quantities and combinations of additives that might disturb the metabolism or result in genetic damage, cancer, or other

## URBAN AND RURAL POPULATIONS, UNITED STATES, 1790–1970

| BY MILLIONS OF PEOPLE | 1790 | 1910 | 1920 | 1930 | 1940 | 1950 | 1960 | 1970 |
|---|---|---|---|---|---|---|---|---|
| Urban | 0.2 | 42 | 54 | 69 | 74 | 96 | 125 | 149 |
| Rural | 3.8 | 50 | 52 | 54 | 57 | 54 | 54 | 56 |
| Total | 4.0 | 92 | 106 | 123 | 131 | 150 | 179 | 205 |
| By percentage of total | | | | | | | | |
| Urban | 5 | 45.7 | 51.2 | 56.2 | 56.5 | 64.0 | 69.9 | 73.5 |
| Rural | 95 | 54.3 | 48.8 | 43.8 | 43.5 | 36.0 | 30.1 | 26.5 |

NOTE: Urban population is defined as those persons residing in cities of over 2500 persons.

SOURCE: U.S. Bureau of the Census, *Statistical Abstracts of the United States: 1970* (91st ed.), Washington, D.C., 1970.

serious disorders. It seems only sensible to minimize the intake of additives by selecting simple, basic food ingredients rather than premixed, additive-laden prepared foods.

## THE URBAN ENVIRONMENT

The United States is an urban nation. When the first national census was taken, in 1790, only 5 percent of the people lived in cities of over 2500 population, whereas 95 percent lived in the country or in very small villages. By 1970, 73.5 percent of the people lived in urban areas and the trend toward urbanization continued strongly. Thus, both numerically and by percentage, more and more Americans are living in cities. (See the table on urban and rural populations.)

Surprisingly, the Western states are the most urbanized, with 82.9 percent of their population concentrated into the cities. California is the nation's most urbanized state, with 90.9 percent of its population living in urban areas.

While there is no clear-cut line between "urban" and "suburban" areas, the suburbs are, in general, the ring of younger and smaller cities surrounding the older central city areas. Census figures show that in recent years the greatest population growth has been in such suburban areas. For example, between 1960 and 1970, the entire United States population grew by 11 percent. However, this growth was concentrated in the suburbs, where population grew by about 25 percent. During this same period, the central cities grew by only 1 percent.

Another problem in population distribution is that the coasts seem to have a magnetic attraction for people. For many years the nation has experienced a migration of population out of the central states and into the coastal areas. By 1970, 53 percent of all Americans were living in counties lying at least partly within 50 miles of a seacoast. This trend continues today with no end in sight. We are becoming a nation of people jammed into strip cities extending the length of each coast, with relatively few people living in the vast spaces between.

## INTENSITY OF SOME COMMON SOUNDS

| SOUND | INTENSITY IN DECIBELS[a] |
|---|---|
| Human whisper | 30 |
| Normal conversation | 60 |
| City traffic | 80 |
| Garbage disposal unit | 80 |
| Vacuum cleaner | 85 |
| Garbage truck | 85 |
| Food blender | 93 |
| Subway train | 95 |
| Jackhammer | 95 |
| Power lawnmower | 96 |
| Printing press | 97 |
| Farm tractor | 98 |
| Punch press | 105 |
| Boiler shop | 105 |
| Textile looms | 106 |
| Motorcycle | 110 |
| Riveting gun | 110 |
| Rock band (amplified) | 114 |
| Drop hammer | 130 |
| Jet airplane | 135 to 150 |

[a] A *decibel* is the smallest difference in intensity of sound that the human ear can detect. The scale is logarithmic; a difference of ten decibels represents a tenfold increase in energy.

SOURCE: Compiled from *Medical World News*, Vol. 10, No. 24 (June 13, 1969), 42–47, and other sources.

From almost every health-related standpoint, there are disadvantages in this intense urbanization. Environmental quality problems become overwhelming, including air pollution, sewage disposal, acquisition of safe water, noise abatement, space for outdoor recreation, substandard housing, lack of privacy, and a host of other problems. Emotional stress is great, leading to a multitude of physical and emotional problems. Yet, the social, cultural, and economic advantages of city life continue to hold a powerful attraction for the majority of Americans today.

### Noise Pollution

One of the more recently "discovered" pollutants in the modern environment is noise. For the city dweller, noise may be the most significant environmental pollutant. He is constantly buffeted by the noise of aircraft, trains, motorcycles, buses, sirens, machinery at home and at work, his neighbor's stereo, and his neighbor's toilet flushing. (See table on the intensity of some common sounds.) One study showed that the average noise level in residential areas rose as much as 9 decibels between 1954 and 1967. (The decibel scale is logarithmic—an increase of 10 decibels indicates a tenfold increase in energy.)

Some of the effects of noise have been known or suspected for years. Fatigue, emotional stress, and permanent loss of hearing acuity are well-documented effects of excessive noise. Other studies have shown that noise, either prolonged or sudden, produces involuntary responses by the circulatory, digestive, and nervous systems. Noise can cause adrenalin to be shot into the blood, as during stress and anxiety periods; it can cause the heart to beat rapidly, the blood vessels to constrict, the pupils to dilate, and the stomach, esophagus, and intestines to be seized by spasms. A three-year study of university students showed that noise of only 70 decibels consistently caused constriction of the coronary arteries supplying oxygen to the heart muscle. Permanent hearing loss occurs with prolonged exposure to sounds of over 90 decibels. High-decibel sounds destroy the hair cells of the inner ear.

Probably the most damaging effect of noise on the quality of human life is its disruption of our psychic balance. Loud, harsh, or persistent noise robs us of our peace of mind, puts our nerves "on edge" so that our personal relationships are strained and often explosive, interferes with our concentration, and impairs the efficient functioning of our minds. Noise must be regarded as far more than just an annoyance: it is a serious threat to the quality of our lives.

In our concern with other forms of environmental decay, we have largely overlooked the importance of noise control, and noise levels continue to creep upward. Like any other form of pollution control, noise control will require legislated limits on noise levels, strict enforcement of those limits, and a personal concern for the rights of others to live in a decent environment.

### Substandard Housing

About 34 million Americans are now living in some 11 million dwelling units that are either grossly overcrowded or have serious structural or plumbing deficiencies. Such dwellings occur most often in large cities or rural areas, less commonly in suburban areas.

The infant mortality (death in first year of life) in such housing is from three to five times the national average. Accidental injuries, burns, and poisonings occur five to eight times more frequently than the national average. In addition, more than 14,000 rat bites are officially recorded each year in such surroundings—certainly a much larger number is never reported.

Lead poisoning of children is a particular problem in substandard housing. In older, uncared-for homes, woodwork, walls, and furniture are often covered with multiple coats of old lead-based paint. Babies and young children often chew on furniture and woodwork, ingesting large amounts of lead. In addition, old paint may flake off walls and ceilings, falling into food and entering the body in the form of dustlike particles.

Lead poisoning can cause serious brain damage, mental retardation, and even death. Even in mild cases, a child's learning ability may be impaired.

Lead poisoning usually does not result in dramatic, sudden changes in a child's health. Instead, the child gradually becomes lethargic, loses appetite, and is less attentive to the world around him. Later, he may vomit, complain of vague stomach or arm or leg pains, and become irritable. Eventually, symptoms of brain damage, such as convulsions, appear. By then, the brain has suffered permanent damage.

If a specific check is not made for lead poisoning in the early stages, the symptoms are so vague that they will likely be overlooked. If the poisoning is detected in its early stages, however, the child can often be treated successfully. Of course, lead poisoning will recur unless the home environment is changed to remove this hazard.

Of the 12,000 to 16,000 cases reported every year in the United States, about 200 children die of lead poisoning. Thousands more are left with mental retardation and other impairments. The loss to the individual and to society from impaired learning ability due to lead poisoning is really incalculable.

Other results of substandard housing are more difficult to translate into figures. The psychological and sociological implications of poor housing are overwhelming. For example, privacy may be nonexistent. Quiet reflection, important to emotional stability, or successful schoolwork may be impossible in crowded living conditions. Marital relationships, sexual and otherwise, may be severely strained by lack of privacy, contributing to the decay of the family unit. Insufficient sanitary facilities (as results when several families are sharing one bathroom) make personal cleanliness and grooming difficult or impossible, putting residents of substandard housing at a social disadvantage.

To date, efforts toward upgrading housing on a national basis have had only limited success. In many cases, substandard housing has been removed in urban renewal projects, only to be replaced with units beyond the financial means of those who previously lived there. In addition, we are now facing the paradoxical situation of renewal projects postponed because sufficient housing on a temporary basis for the displaced residents is not even available.

While there are no simple answers to the national housing crisis, an immense need does exist for upgraded housing units. It seems likely that this need will have to be met through the combined efforts of government and private enterprise. Obviously, the basic problem is poverty; any long-term gains in housing quality must be the result of improved family economic units.

### Stress

As will be discussed in the chapter on Emotional Problems, prolonged stress can have severe damaging effects on both the physical and emotional health of a person. Just a few among the many urban stressors are the problems of high-density housing, with its attendant noise, lack of privacy, and lack of play areas; substandard housing, with its rats and inadequate sanitation; deficient and crowded urban transportation; strikes, blackouts, and other service problems; ethnic tensions; and the ever-present fear of crime.

Many of the physical effects of stress can be objectively measured, such as increases in pulse rate and blood pressure, dilation of the pupils of the eyes, sweating, respiratory rate, and so forth. Studies have shown that the typical commuter, driving home at peak rush hours, experiences more of the deleterious effects of stress than have some of the astronauts during reentry into the earth's atmosphere.

### The Future of the City

Poor housing, noise, stress, and congestion are only part of the total urban environmental problem. Even those city dwellers fortunate enough to be able to afford relatively pleasant living conditions and facilities still face many serious environmental concerns. People who live in cities bear the greatest burden of land, air, and water pollution. They are subject to the stresses of noise, crowding, high crime rates, estrangement from the natural environment, and the multitude of inconveniences and frustrations that characterize the urban development. The urban poor, of course, bear the greatest burden.

While cities have always been associated with an abundance of problems and deleterious effects on the human spirit, the quality of city life in the United States has seriously deteriorated in recent years. During this period, several important trends have emerged. First, there has been the previously mentioned shift from rural to urban areas. Second, the growth pattern of the cities has, in general, been haphazard, with little or no master planning. The almost formless lateral spread of many cities has been determined largely by the predominant form of transportation—the automobile. Development has simply spread along the paths of major traffic arteries. Sociological and ecological factors have been largely ignored.

Almost all population growth in metropolitan areas has been concentrated at their suburban edges. Suburbs of metropolitan areas now often meet back-to-back. We are currently witnessing the development of several "strip cities," one extending from San Francisco to San Diego, one from Chicago to Pittsburgh, and one from Boston to Washington, D.C.

Most of the middle-income population of the central cities gradually moves to suburbs in search of space, privacy, newer housing, and a pleasant life-style. In the central city, housing deteriorates into slums, the crime rate rises, and major businesses follow the money into the suburbs.

Another trend is that the black populations become concentrated into the deteriorated central portions of the cities. In less than 30 years, as the need for farm labor decreased, the black population shifted from a primarily rural to a primarily urban setting. Today,

over three-quarters of the nation's black population is concentrated in cities, and their movement away from rural areas still continues. For most migrating blacks, the move is advantageous, leading to higher income, better housing, better health, and better schools. But for many it is merely a change from rural exploitation to an even worse exploitation system in the cities. On arriving in the cities of the North and West, the new migrants have faced the discriminatory practices of those areas, a lack of adequate housing, and the impact of automation on job opportunities for uneducated, unskilled workers. The jobs that helped previous generations of foreign immigrants and rural American migrants adjust to urban life are becoming increasingly scarce. For urban blacks today, the unemployment rate is high. For those fortunate enough to have jobs, the pay is often low, rents are inordinately high for the quality of the dwellings, and commodities and services are priced well above similar goods or services in the suburbs.

Within ghetto areas, an estimated 60 to 70 percent of the families have an income below that required for a minimum decent standard of living (no luxuries, just the bare essentials). The result is badly overcrowded housing, inadequate diet, poor medical care, and few books and magazines. Thus, the paths to upward mobility are largely blocked by poor health and limited educational opportunities. Poverty frequently perpetuates itself generation after generation.

A study of city government in the United States reveals, for better or worse, an amazing degree of stability. The same "powers that be" may control a city for decades or even for generations. Within this stability lie both strengths and weaknesses. If the system of local government could be easily changed, it would probably be intolerably unstable. Many elements are involved in maintaining the status quo, including powerful vested interests, the established bureaucracy, special interest groups with favored tax positions, political differences among different sections of the city, and the general lack of strong community bonds.

Barring any major upheavals, such as nuclear warfare or total revolution, there are no indications of any drastic shift from current urban trends. Changes may be expected to come very slowly. This is true of both the physical design and growth of cities as well as of the social structure.

The concept of the "planned city" is gaining popularity. Considerable evidence suggests that there is a maximum desirable size for any type of system, above which efficiency is decreased. This principle seems to apply to living organisms, machines, factories, schools, and to cities. Rather than encouraging further expansion of existing cities, communities might be planned in terms of maximum population, educational and public service facilities, businesses, wide-open areas, and quality housing.

There is a current trend among college students to prefer urban life because of its social, educational, and cultural advantages. The pressure from young people to improve the quality of urban life might well encourage city planners to consider new ways of making cities "livable."

# 2

# Population Dynamics

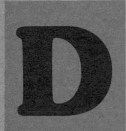

**D**uring past centuries, the increase in the number of human beings had been governed by three regulators—disease, war, and starvation. Consequently, each major upward step in population followed some major discovery or development which acted to control one of these regulators—the advent of agriculture, the initiation of urban life and trade, the harnessing of nonhuman power, or the progress of modern medicine. As a more sophisticated and economically responsible group of societies developed, the ability to maintain a higher population level became a reality.

## THE MECHANISM OF POPULATION INCREASE

### The Past

Only fragmentary data are available to indicate the past growth rate of the population of the world. A regular census of population was not conducted before 1800, although registers were maintained for small groups prior to that time. Therefore, the commonly accepted population figures of the world before 1800 are only informed guesses. Nevertheless, it is possible to piece together a consistent series of estimates for the past two centuries. This information, supplemented by rough guesses of the number of persons alive at selected earlier periods, provides the background for a graphic estimate of the world population from 1 to 2000 A.D. This graph reveals a spectacular spurt during recent decades (see p. 33).

World population is estimated to have reached its first billion mark sometime between 1810 and 1850 A.D. The second billion mark was reached in 1925, the third in 1960, and the fourth is expected by 1975. It took most of man's history to reach one billion, about 100 years to reach two billion, 35 years to reach three billion, and an estimated 15 years to reach four billion.

According to two early reports on world demography (Carr-Saunders and Willcox), the population of Europe increased more than fourfold between 1650 and 1900, whereas the population of Asia increased only about two and one-half times. Moreover, the population in the area of European settlement, including Europe and the Americas, increased about five times. As a result of these differential rates of growth in Asia and Europe, the proportion of the world's population living in Asia declined from around 60 percent in 1650 to about 53 percent in 1900. But since 1900, the proportion of the world's population living in Asia has been increasing and, according to the Population Reference Bureau figures, by 1972 it climbed to over 56 percent. The proportion living in Europe and North America has been declining, and by 1972 it constituted only about 18 percent of the world's total.

The discoveries of sulfa drugs, antibiotics, insecticides, and other means of combating disease-carrying organisms radically altered the situation of population dynamics. It became possible to lower mortality rates irrespective of economic development. This was man's first major victory over death. Within a few years, this victory was to be responsible for the rapid population explosion that now

jeopardizes the economic growth of all developing nations.

In the developed countries of the Western world, the reduction in the death rate came slowly. Its effect on population growth was influenced by factors which reduced the birth rate; namely, a rising standard of living and industrialization. This meant that children were no longer an economic asset because many menial tasks were assumed by machines. The death rates per year in advanced countries have been reduced from the traditional thirty-five to forty per thousand to less than ten per thousand. The average life span (life expectancy at birth) has almost doubled in the western world since the mid-nineteenth century. It now stands at over seventy years in Europe and North America. This part of the world had time to adjust to lowered death rates while also accepting factors that lowered birth rates as well. In contrast, lowered death rates in developing countries occurred so fast that they have not had time to undergo a simultaneous rise in living standard and industrialization. Thus their populations have mushroomed. The table at the left shows how longer life spans have evolved in many regions of the world.

During the early years of the United States, the high rate of population growth was a source of great pride. With seemingly limitless resources and room for westward expansion, the fertility rate reached levels seldom exceeded anywhere on earth. During the colonial period the average family included about eight children. Even with the high death rate, the population more than doubled every generation. At that time, a large family was considered a definite asset. The more children a family produced, the more help it had to clear and cultivate land.

In addition to this high fertility rate, the United States for many years practiced an open-door policy of immigration. Prior to the 1921 Immigration Act, about 35 million im-

### LIFE EXPECTANCY AT BIRTH

| YEARS | LIFE EXPECTANCY AT BIRTH IN YEARS[a] |
|---|---|
| 1840 | 41.0 |
| 1900 | 50.5 |
| 1930 | 61.7 |
| 1940 | 64.6 |
| 1955 to 1972 | 71.0 + |

[a]The average of six European countries and one state in the United States. The countries are Denmark, England and Wales, France, the Netherlands, Norway, and Sweden; the state in the United States is Massachusetts.

SOURCE: *Population Bulletin of the United Nations*, No. 6, United Nations Publication Sales No. 62, XVII.2, Table IV.1.

migrants entered the country, accounting for about one-third of the population growth up to that time. Since 1921, immigration has accounted for less than 10 percent of the population growth.

But long before 1921, the women of the United States slowly began to limit the size of their families. Actually, neither the government nor the women had yet become concerned about the threat of overpopulation. The government restricted immigration because of the diminishing need for unskilled labor. The women restricted their family size because their interests were beginning to extend beyond the farm, kitchen, and nursery toward the city, school, and labor force. By the middle 1920s the average family size had dropped to 2.5 children.

During the 1930s the birth rate dropped still further to a low of just over two children per family. Although the low birth rate characterized those years, the trend toward it actually had started in about 1880. Actually, then (as now) poor economic conditions were only a slight deterrent to large family size. Traditionally, the poorest families have the most children. At what point the birth rate might have leveled off without the Depression is purely a matter of speculation. But even with this low birth rate the population of the country continued to grow due to a diminishing death rate.

After World War II, a temporary surge in the birth rate was expected in order to make up for births "postponed" during the war years. But the birth rate, rather than rising and returning to "normal," continued to rise year after year until, in 1957, it reached a peak which resulted in an average family size of almost 3.8 children. Station wagons and four-bedroom houses suddenly became very popular. After 1957, the birth rate started dropping, at first slowly, then sharply during the 1960s. Possible future trends will be discussed later in this chapter. During the 1950s

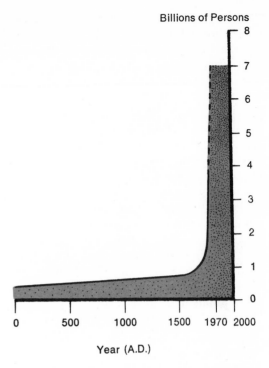

Estimated world population, 0 to 2000 A.D. Based on estimates of the Population Reference Bureau and other sources.

and 1960s the death rate has stayed virtually constant.

### The Present

The world population continues to grow at an accelerating rate. According to the Population Reference Bureau, the world population in 1972 was increasing by over 1.46 million per week. By 1972 the world population had surpassed 3.7 billion and was expected to reach 4 billion by 1975, fully five years ahead of the 1965 predictions. Current growth rates, if continued, will result in a world population of 6.5 billion by the year 2000, now less than 30 years away.

In general, the fastest growing countries are those with the lowest standard of living, the "have-not" nations—politely called the developing nations. The growth rate of many of these countries averages almost 3 percent per year, in contrast with an average of under 1 percent in the wealthier countries such as Europe and North America. Of the babies being born each day now, over 83 percent are in Asia, Africa, and South America. If a 3-percent annual population growth rate does not sound very high, let us point out that such a rate doubles a population in just twenty-three years.

During the past decade, six out of every ten persons added to the world's population were born in Asia; another two out of ten were born in Latin America and Africa. Undoubtedly, this increase will change the world's balance of power, and influence world affairs in coming years.

Equally important is the population growth potential of a country. This is reflected in the percentage of a population now under 15 years of age. In Africa, Asia, and Latin America 40 percent or more of the population is under 15 years of age. This compares with 25 to 29 percent for the United States, the U.S.S.R., and Europe. The greater proportion of people in their prereproductive years in the developing nations represents an explosive growth potential. As these young people grow up and move into their reproductive years, the size of the childbearing fraction of the population will increase automatically. Even though significant progress is made immediately in reducing the number of births per female in these countries, it will be at least 30 years before such birth control could significantly slow population growth due to the large number of females of childbearing age.

The reduction of the death rate in the developing countries of the world was introduced with startling speed. Ancient diseases were brought under control or totally

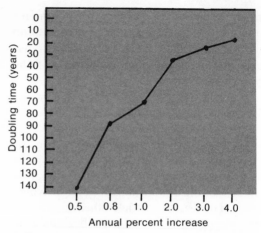

Time needed for a population to double.

abolished in the space of a few decades, or even a few years. But the initiation of effective birth-control measures on a national basis generally lags by many years (about a generation) after the accomplishment of "death control." In the interim, the birth rate remains very high because the majority of the children being born are, for the first time in the history of the nation, maturing and having children of their own. Consequently, the developing countries are now in a stage of explosive population growth. There are many factors contributing to the birth-control lag. One belief held by many developing countries is that their emergence as world powers depends on producing and maintaining very large populations. In addition, there are powerful religious sanctions against birth control in many countries, and there is the lingering belief that many children must be born to insure the survival of a few to maturity. There are strong social or cultural influences favoring large families. There are still countries in which the status of women is so low as to preclude their having any authority over the number of children they produce. There are people so poor that the cost of many birth-control methods seems

## WORLD BIRTH AND DEATH RATES, 1970

| | BIRTH RATE[a] | DEATH RATE[b] | CURRENT ANNUAL GROWTH RATE[c] | DOUBLING TIME | POPULATION UNDER 15 YEARS |
|---|---|---|---|---|---|
| World | 33. | 13. | 2.0% | 35 | 37.% |
| United States | 17.3 | 9.3 | 1.0% | 70 | 29.% |
| Europe | 16. | 10. | 0.7% | 99 | 25.% |
| USSR | 17.4 | 8.2 | 0.9% | 77 | 28.% |
| Asia | 37. | 14. | 2.3% | 30 | 40.% |
| Africa | 47. | 21. | 2.6% | 23 | 44.% |
| Latin America | 38. | 10. | 2.8% | 25 | 42.% |

[a]Births per thousand population.
[b]Deaths per thousand population.
[c]Net rate, including immigration and emigration.

SOURCE: *1972 World Population Data Sheet,* Population Reference Bureau, Washington, D.C., 1972.

prohibitive. There are countries whose availability of health services is so sparse that many women lack access to effective birth-control methods. There are countries where the education level is so low that the majority of the people are either unaware of the need for birth control, unaware of the availability of effective methods, or lack the knowledge or motivation to use them effectively.

The rate of human reproduction in any part of the globe directly affects the health and welfare of the rest of the human race. The birth rates in Africa, Asia, and Latin America are presently around forty births per thousand population, whereas their death rates are about ten to twenty-two per thousand. (See table on world birth and death rates.) The most rapid increase of population in the world today is reported to be in Costa Rica, where a birth rate of forty-five per thousand and a death rate of seven per thousand is causing an increase of almost 4 per in the world today is reported to be in Kuwait, where a birth rate of forty-three per thousand and a death rate of seven per thousand is causing an increase of almost 8.2 percent per year, which means they will double in 9 years. Similar rapid increases are taking place all over Latin America, where the population is expected to double within the next 25 years if the present rate of increase continues.

Such population increases intensify the existing imbalance between the distribution of the world's population and the distribution of wealth, resources, and the use of non-human energy. Probably for the first time in human history, there is universal aspiration for rapid improvement in the standard of living and a growing impatience with conditions that appear to stand in the way of its attainment. Millions of persons in Asia, Africa, and Latin America now are aware of the standard of living enjoyed by Europeans and North Americans. They are demanding the opportunity to attain the same standard and resisting the idea that they must be permanently content with less. But continuation of the present high rate of human multiplication in these areas will act as a brake on the already painfully slow improvement in the level of living. Just to maintain their current standard of living, let alone improve it, Latin America with a doubling time of 25 years will need to double *all* services (schools, roads, offices, hospitals, stores) within this time. This is patently impossible. This factor will increase political unrest and possibly bring about changes in governments.

The capital and technological skills that Africa, Asia, and Latin America require in order to produce enough food and to raise per-capita income simultaneously exceed their existing national resources and abilities. An immediate supply of the necessary capital is available, but only from wealthier nations that do not want to support the economic development of less advanced nations on the level they desire. Even if such support were extended, it is not as yet clear how long the wealthier nations would be able to support the uncontrolled propagation of the populations receiving assistance. General application of such a foreign-aid program will postpone for only a few decades the inevitable reckoning with the results of unregulated human multiplication.

The complexities of the United States growth rate are worth our attention here. The birth rate in the more affluent countries reflects the influences of social and economic differentiation not found in the developing forces not found in the developing nations. In those countries, the population is generally skewed either toward the very high or the very low borders of the economic scale. In the more affluent nations, the existence of a large middle class introduces other factors. The middle class consumes more of the world's resources. Its members buy more, travel more, dispose of more materials than lower classes. Increased use of these limited

resources offsets the "safe" lower birth rate of middle class families.

In addition to the total rate of population growth, it is significant to compare the relative birth rates of various segments of the population. Some of the groups we should examine for possible differences are those of differing racial composition, financial level, and educational background.

*Birth Rate and Race.* Let us first consider birth rate in relation to color, ignoring possible differences in education or income between the groups. According to figures published in 1972 by the U.S. Census Bureau, 82.5 percent of the population of the United States is white, about 11.1 percent is black, and 1.4 percent is composed of other nonwhites, including primarily North American Indians and Orientals.

In the table comparing the fertility rates of white and nonwhite women in different years, the fertility rate is the number of children born per 1000 women within a given group. From the table it can be seen that in the last two decades, nonwhite women had more children than white women. These figures, of course, do not indicate whether the greater fertility rate is due to greater inherent fertility, desire for a larger family, or less effective use of contraceptive measures.

## BIRTH RATES IN THE UNITED STATES BY RACE

| RACE | 1950 | 1955 | 1960 | 1965 | 1970 |
|---|---|---|---|---|---|
| Nonwhite | 33.3 | 34.7 | 32.1 | 27.6 | 25.0 |
| White | 23.0 | 23.8 | 22.7 | 18.3 | 16.5 |
| TOTAL | 24.1 | 25.0 | 23.7 | 19.4 | 17.6 |

NOTE: Number given is the number of children born per 1000 population.

SOURCE: U.S. Bureau of the Census, *Statistical Abstracts of the United States: 1972* (93rd ed.), Washington, D.C., 1972.

## FAMILY SIZE AND INCOME

| | AGE 25–34 | | AGE 35–44 | |
| FAMILY INCOME | WHITE | NONWHITE | WHITE | NONWHITE |
|---|---|---|---|---|
| Under $3000 | 2.74 | 3.69 | 3.23 | 4.57 |
| $3000 to $4999 | 2.66 | 3.19 | 3.89 | 4.47 |
| $5000 to $7499 | 2.38 | 2.98 | 3.50 | 4.10 |
| $7500 to $9999 | 2.20 | 2.77 | 3.30 | 3.60 |
| $10,000 to $14,999 | 2.15 | 2.41 | 3.06 | 3.45 |
| $15,000 to $25,000 | 1.78 | 1.92 | 2.97 | 2.92 |

NOTE: Numbers given are for the average number of children ever born per woman of two age groups, by family income and race. As of June 1972.

SOURCE: U.S. Bureau of the Census, *Current Population Reports: Population Characteristics*, Report P-20 (248), Table 20, Washington, D.C., April 1973.

*Birth Rate and Income.* In the United States, low income is often accompanied by large family size ("the rich get richer and the poor get children"). This is shown in the table on family size and income. In 1969, the last year for which such figures are available, those families with the lowest income had the most children. As incomes increased, family size decreased until an income of over $15,000 was reached. At this level there was an upturn in family size. The apparent significance of these figures is that the middle-income groups desired smaller families and made more effective use of contraceptive measures than did the lower income groups. Possible reasons may include greater motivation to control family size; better education, enabling more efficient use of contraceptives; household conditions more favorable to contraceptive use; and income sufficient to engage medical assistance in the selection and prescription of contraceptives. Another possible reason is the high infant-mortality rate of the poor (three to five times the national average). The resulting feeling of uncertainty whether each child will survive may act to motivate a higher birth rate. Until living conditions are improved, the poor will probably continue to conceive more children.

*Birth Rate and Education.* Another table relates the number of children born to the educational level of the woman. The relationship here is similar to that between income and number of children. The higher the level of education, the fewer children produced. Unlike the income comparison, no upturn in number of offspring exists at the upper end of the scale. The racial breakdown is also similar to that found in the income comparison. The poorly educated nonwhite woman has more children than the similarly educated white woman; conversely, the well-educated nonwhite woman has fewer children than the similarly educated white woman. Among women who finish high school, the number of children produced by the two racial groups is about equal.

These sets of data have been the subject of serious analysis by political scientists, sociologists, demographers, and historians. Information of this type can be used to produce an organized view of American society and its priorities.

## FAMILY SIZE AND EDUCATION

| WOMAN'S EDUCATIONAL LEVEL | WHITE | NONWHITE | ALL RACES |
|---|---|---|---|
| Not high school graduate | 2.65 | 3.53 | 2.76 |
| High school graduate | 1.99 | 2.29 | 2.01 |
| College, one year or more | 1.52 | 1.67 | 1.53 |

NOTE: Numbers given are for the average number of children ever born per woman, 14–39 years of age. As of June 1972.

SOURCE: U.S. Bureau of the Census, *Current Population Reports: Population Characteristics*, Report P-20 (248), Table 9, Washington, D.C., April 1973.

In the writings of Rufus E. Miles, Jr., we find good examples. He is Chairman of the Board of the Population Reference Bureau and has specified seven major influences which promote large families in the United States; he calls these the "pronatalist" influences:

1. Large numbers of adult Americans, both male and female, feel that procreation is the best way for them to find self-fulfillment.

2. For many parents—primarily mothers—large families are a psychological defense against lack of interesting employment, lack of a sense of belonging to a satisfying social group, or lack of other forms of self-realization.

3. Smaller numbers of people—mainly those in or near poverty areas—lack the knowledge or medical services available to higher-income people which would facilitate the control of their family size.

4. Large numbers of parents desire a child of a particular sex and will keep trying until they produce such a child, regardless of how many children they have in the process.

5. Many people are influenced by the "growthmania" of the American way of life.

They believe that any system which is growing is healthy and good, while any which is not growing is stagnant and bad.

6. Governmental policies have reinforced the pronatalist influences of society and have partially offset the economic disadvantages of children through such provisions as high taxes on single people, tax deductions for children, provision of public housing and public assistance only for families with children, and other measures which provide similar encouragement to childbearing.

7. Too little educational information has come from leadership sources or from the mass media to counteract the effects of the six pronatalist influences listed above. Most of the information presented always seems to imply that population problems are in "other" countries, or that the problem is most serious among the poor.

The rate of population growth for the United States declined during the 1960s. As the table on population growth shows, in 1960 the population increased only by 1.8 percent; by 1972 the annual rate of increase has dropped to less than 1 percent. The trend in declining birth rates continued in 1972 though the population will probably continue to increase for some years due to the large number of girls just now reaching reproductive age. If the downward trend continues however, there appears to be a good chance of eventually achieving population stability in this country.

### The Future

Is the present spurt of worldwide population growth a temporary phenomenon, or will it continue until the former biological regulators—war, disease, and famine—once again take control?

Future populations of individual nations, of regions, or of the entire world cannot be predicted with any degree of accuracy for more than a few decades at a time. Just as Thomas Malthus could not foresee the tremendous changes that have taken place in Europe since the eighteenth century, we really cannot foresee the future extent and consequences of population growth.* There are too many unpredictable influences on population. In addition, it is usually difficult to predict what the exact effect of a particular event or condition will be. Starvation, political turmoil, natural disasters, industrialization and agricultural improvements have all caused both higher *and* lower population growth rates at different times.

---

*Robert Thomas Malthus (1766–1834), an English economist and theologian, was among the first to foresee overpopulation as a major world problem. His basic thesis, very unpopular at the time, was that human populations increase by a geometric progression (2, 4, 8, 16, 32, 64, 128, etc.) while food supplies can increase only by an arithmetic progression (1, 2, 3, 4, 5, 6, etc.). Malthus was, surprisingly, an outspoken foe of contraceptive techniques, urging, rather, late marriage and "moral restraint" as a means of controlling population. It should be remembered however, that in the eighteenth and early nineteenth centuries, there were few other reliable methods of controlling the birth rate.

The basic tendency in population prediction unfortunately has been to steadily underestimate future population levels. It is difficult to choose those specific factors which can reliably be extrapolated into the future. For example, the average annual rate of population growth in the United States from 1790 to 1964 (174 years) was 2.2 percent. Simply projecting this rate for another 174 years (until the year 2138) would give this country a population of 8.8 billion, several times the current population of the entire world. Undoubtedly, long before this level is achieved, drastic measures would be taken to curtail reproduction. Actually, the level at which the population of the United States will stabilize might be as low as 300 to 400 million people, yet this too is far larger than our present population.

Our most immediate concern is with the "boom babies" born between 1950 and 1960. In 1960 there were 11 million women in the 20 to 30 year age group. In 1980 there will be 20 million women in this prime reproductive group. This statistic is not just a guess or a rough speculation—these females have already been born and are now growing up. The only question remaining is the rate at which they will reproduce. Will the current trend toward smaller families continue, or will a larger family again become "fashionable"? If the latter takes place, the baby boom of the 1950s will compare to the boom of the 1980s like a cap gun compares to a cannon.

The future may witness a dramatic increase in man's ability to control his environment. Man has been able to modify or control many natural phenomena, but he has not yet discovered how to evade the consequences of biological laws. No species has ever been able to multiply without limit. Fundamentally, there are only two methods of population control—high mortality or low fertility. Man can choose which of these checks will be

| YEAR | FERTILITY RATE[a] | BIRTH RATE[b] | DEATH RATE[c] | TOTAL U.S. POPULATION ON JULY 1 (MILLIONS) | PERCENT ANNUAL POPULATION GROWTH[d] |
|---|---|---|---|---|---|
| 1960 | 119.1 | 23.8 | 9.5 | 179.3 | 1.7 |
| 1961 | 118.4 | 23.5 | 9.3 | 183.1 | 1.7 |
| 1962 | 113.2 | 22.6 | 9.4 | 185.9 | 1.5 |
| 1963 | 109.4 | 21.9 | 9.6 | 188.7 | 1.4 |
| 1964 | 105.8 | 21.2 | 9.4 | 191.4 | 1.4 |
| 1965 | 97.3 | 19.6 | 9.4 | 193.6 | 1.3 |
| 1966 | 91.8 | 18.5 | 9.5 | 195.7 | 1.1 |
| 1967 | 88.1 | 17.9 | 9.4 | 198.8 | 1.1 |
| 1968 | 86.1 | 17.6 | 9.7 | 201.2 | 1.0 |
| 1969 | 86.2 | 17.8 | 9.5 | 203.1 | 1.0 |
| 1970 | 88.0 | 18.3 | 9.4 | 205.2 | 1.0 |
| 1971 | 82.6 | 17.3 | 9.3 | 206.2 | 0.9 |
| 1972[e] | 77.2 | 15.5 | 9.6 | 208.2 | 0.8 |

[a]Fertility rate is the number of births per 1000 women ages 15 through 44.
[b]Birth rate is the number of births per 1000 total population.
[c]Death rate is the number of deaths per 1000 total population.
[d]Includes immigration and emigration.
[e]Figures for the year 1972 are provisional.

SOURCE: U.S. Public Health Service and Bureau of Census Reports.

applied—but one of them *must* be. Whether or not we use scientific knowledge to guide the future of man on this planet, some control will be instituted—possibly only by the blind forces of nature.

## THE BOUNDARIES OF POPULATION GROWTH

Unfortunately, discussion of the population problem often centers on two issues—space and food—as though finding enough standing room and enough food per person to allow survival would resolve the problem. Such oversimplification misses the vastness of the problem for many reasons:

1. Most of the world's people are already living under such poor conditions that it is not sufficient for food production merely to keep pace with population growth. A great increase in food production would be necessary just to feed the *current* population properly

2. Many of the methods that have been proposed to increase food production (such as insecticides, fertilizers, and land reclamation) are, even at their current level of application, proving harmful to the total environment.

3. World production of many commodities (not only food) must be increased sharply to meet the reasonable needs and demands of people seeking an adequate existence.

4. The production of waste products (pollutants) increases with the population. The ability of the environment to "absorb" pollu-

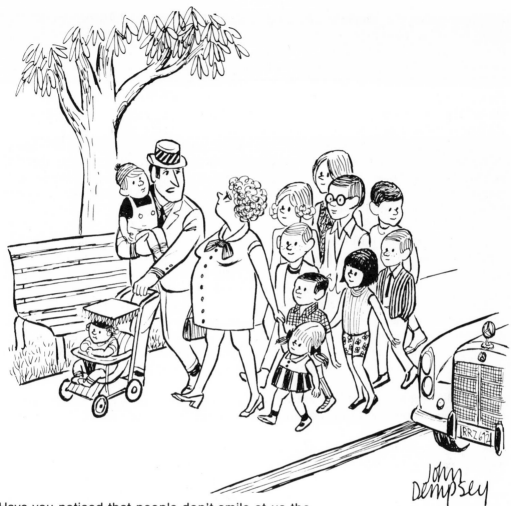

**Have you noticed that people don't smile at us the way they used to?**

tants is limited. Even the disposal of human wastes becomes a serious problem at high population densities.

5. Frustration of the growing desires among all people for decent living conditions, education, and economic opportunity is creating tremendous political and social tensions throughout the world.

6. The world is not one big, unified reservoir of space, skills, resources, knowledge, and capital from which nations can procure their respective needs for unlimited time.

7. There is a wide gap between what is technologically or theoretically possible and what can be applied with safety and at reasonable cost.

The population problem is based on the procurement and distribution of resources. The alarming differentials in consumption of resources between different nations and regions of the world cause additional problems. Furthermore, a society devoted to supporting maximum numbers of people at a bare subsistence level is incompatible with any humane standards of civilization. To what extent are we willing to sacrifice quality of life in order to attain quantity of life? And if the quality of life is sacrificed, how long will we be able to maintain the quantity? Our environment could be so severely damaged in the process that it might eventually be able to support only a small number of people at a very low level of existence.

Some people argue that we really do not have to worry about population control—that "nature" will take care of the problem. Unfortunately, however, nature's population control methods are often inimical to the quality of life. Those who would rely on starvation, drought, natural disasters, suicide, and the other serious consequences of population excess evidence a callous disregard for humanitarian values. The question of quality must be a major concern in our approach to world population problems.

In the following pages, we are going to consider the various factors that are either potential or actual brakes on population growth. It is time to take a careful look at these factors and determine which can be useful or detrimental to the quality of human life.

### The Fixed Factors

*Space.* In relating space needs to population, it is essential that our thinking go beyond the question of how many people could survive on the land surface of the earth. Most people are concerned about the quality of life, rather than the attainment of a minimal level of survival.

Space is needed for decent living conditions, without the constant sight and sound of neighbors. Space is needed for recreation and for the opportunity to enjoy solitude from the ever-present crowds. Space is needed for food production; natural watershed area is essential for replenishment of water supplies. Undeveloped wilderness area is required for the maintenance of such natural cycles as the oxygen cycle and for the total ecological balance of the earth.

With regard to space for living or agriculture, some experts point to the deserts of the world as room for expansion. But most people do not want to live in a hot, dry desert climate. If people really wanted to live on the deserts, these areas would have been settled some time ago.

The use of the deserts for agricultural purposes on any large scale is still only a theoretical possibility. The cost, both in terms of dollars for irrigation and transport and in terms of environmental damage from widespread irrigation, is staggering. For the deserts are not vacuums in the ecological system of this planet; they are an important element in the earth's natural balance, and cannot be tampered with.

*Resources.* We are living in a world where a rapidly increasing number of people must share a fixed, or in some cases decreasing, supply of natural resources. The world population problem is the total of all the population problems of the major countries of the world. Through modern transportation and communication, the world has become so "small" that a population problem in any one country may have serious effects in other countries.

The earth's capacity to provide raw materials is limited. Many minerals and most of the presently used energy sources are nonrenewable. In some places the scarcity of forests limits the use of wood and wood products. More and more cities are finding it necessary to curtail their water service or to make use of new, and more remote, sources of fresh water.

If the entire world were to develop industrially on a level comparable to that of the United States and Europe, our known reserves of coal, petroleum, and natural gas would not be sufficient for the proportionately increased energy requirements. It has been forecast that the high point in petroleum production will be reached in the relatively near future—sometime before the year 2000. The pressure to produce petroleum in increasing amounts is pushing the oil companies toward more and more ambitious and possibly ecologically catastrophic systems, such as the Alaska pipeline and the huge oil tankers now being built. The fossil fuels (natural gas, petroleum, and coal) are expected to provide the world's energy needs for no more than several hundred years.

Our traditional sources of energy are water (which provides about 10 percent of our electrical power), coal, gas, and oil. In fulfilling an ever-increasing demand for power by burning the fossil fuels, we are depleting stores that cannot be replaced. These are nonrenewable natural resources and, in time (an alarmingly short time if the demand keeps growing as it has in the past quarter of a century), these fuels will be gone. However, there are two energy sources that may be substitutes for fossil fuels, one is radiation from the sun (solar energy) and the other is nuclear energy—that derived from the fission (splitting of heavy atoms) and the fusion (union of light atoms).

Considering the inherent dangers of atomic energy, it would seem that capturing solar energy directly is preferable to utilizing nuclear energy. However, the practical utilization of solar energy at present is restricted to rather small solar batteries. It is possible that this source of energy will be further developed, but at the moment atomic energy is the far more practical alternative.

The adoption of fission power will be slow and its rate of development will depend ultimately on the exhaustion of fossil fuel reserves. Fusion power, while potentially having many advantages over fission power, including an inexhaustible fuel supply of negligible cost, has not yet been established as feasible and its costs cannot be readily assessed.

The two major problems with the adoption of atomic power as a major energy source are the problems of waste-heat disposal and the possibility of nuclear accident. Actually, the latter should not be a significant worry; nuclear reactors as planned for power plants are probably quite safe. Yet, the possibility of a "leak" and the resulting public pressure against the building of nuclear power stations near populated areas is slowing the adoption of this method of power production.

The waste disposal problem is probably more significant. The water circulating through the nuclear power plant picks up the excess heat given off by the operating nuclear reactor. Unless cooling bins are installed, the heated water then flows directly into a living community of fish, birds, and aquatic plant life. The effects of continual "washing" by heated water have not been completely evaluated, but most ecologists predict that the effects can be serious indeed.

It might seem strange that heat is considered a pollutant; after all, it is a form of energy and a potentially useful one. A recent study at Oak Ridge National Laboratory in Tennessee has presented encouraging evidence that this same "thermal pollution" can be cycled directly in the heating system of a city the size of Philadelphia and thus reduce the possibility of ecological damage. The most important point, however, is that careful study is required before nuclear power plants can be safely incorporated into the environment.

Since the most easily obtained minerals

and sources of energy have already been used, the continuing mining of less accessible deposits will cost this country considerably in the future. Yet, even this low-yield extraction has its limits. Each of the acts just mentioned represents an unnecessary borrowing on the future, or solving the problems of today while creating potential problems for our grandchildren.

Borrowing on the future is taking place with the resources of the United States, as well as with those elsewhere in the world. Although North Americans compose only about 6 percent of the world's population, they consume half of the world's production of major minerals; they consume twice as much commercial energy per person as the British and four times as much as the people of India. It is estimated that each year the average American utilizes an amount of natural resources equal to that used by 25 to 30 Indians. In relation to these facts, the increase of this country's population appears frightening. In light of the aspirations of many parts of the world for better living standards, it is questionable whether 6 percent of the population is justified in continuing this extraordinary level of consumption.

*The Absorption of Pollution.* As previously discussed, the environment has a limited ability to absorb and assimilate pollutants. But the quantities of many population-related pollutants *now* being dumped into the environment exceed this ability. Disposal of one of the most directly population-related pollutants, human sewage, has become a particularly critical problem. Even after treatment, sewage still contains large quantities of inorganic nitrates and phosphates that overstimulate the growth of algae, leading to "dead" rivers and lakes, such as Lake Erie. But much sewage in the United States, and most sewage on a world basis,

does not receive any treatment. It is dumped into the most convenient lake, river, or ocean as raw sewage—teeming with living disease organisms and laden with nitrates and phosphates. Consequently, since 1960 there has been a great world increase in the incidence of sewage-borne diseases, particularly cholera and other dysenteric (diarrheal) diseases.

The gap between sewage production and sewage treatment is growing, not closing, as world populations increase. It is easy to offer the solution of increased sewage treatment facilities, but the reality of the situation is that such facilities are economically impossible for much of the world at this time. How can the developing countries hope for adequate sewage treatment when this goal cannot be attained by even the wealthy United States?

In addition, the quantity of almost every other pollutant also relates to population levels. The more people, the more need for transportation, food, power, housing, and so forth, all of which contribute to environmental decline. Thus, it is obvious that population control is the first requirement for the maintenance of a livable environment on this planet.

### The Flexible Factors

*Food Production.* Most people do not have enough food to eat. As the table on food consumption shows, more than half of the people in the world today live on 2100 calories per person per day, although the Food and Agricultural Organization (FAO) of the United Nations recommends a daily minimum of 3200 calories per man, and 2300 calories per woman. By 2000 the average daily intake is estimated to be 1340; 1350 per day is starvation level. The amount of calories in food is only one consideration. Equally important is how well the diet is balanced with various kinds of foods. The

## LEVELS OF DAILY PER CAPITA CONSUMPTION OF FOOD BY REGIONS AND GROUPS OF COUNTRIES

| REGIONS | CALORIES | TOTAL PROTEIN (GRAMS) | ANIMAL PROTEIN (GRAMS) |
|---|---|---|---|
| Far East | 1910 | 54 | 6 |
| Near East | 2190 | 70 | 14 |
| Africa | 2100 | 61 | 15 |
| Latin America | 2380 | 67 | 29 |
| Europe | 2870 | 91 | 31 |
| Northern America | 3120 | 90 | 60 |
| World | 2260 | 66 | 18 |

[a]The postwar levels of consumption were used.

SOURCE: Stuart Mudd, ed., The Population Crisis and the Use of World Resources, Bloomington, Ind., Indiana University Press, 1964.

low-calorie diets of the world consist primarily of plant foods and cannot be considered balanced. Though the majority of Americans enjoy adequate diets, millions of people in this country suffer from diets deficient in quantity, quality, or both.

Most of the world's population increase is occurring in poorly developed areas that are already short of food—Asia, Africa, and Latin America. The basis for most food production is land. But an increasing population itself requires even more land for housing, industries, businesses, roads, schools, and all the other services necessary for a satisfactory standard of living. In too many places, the choicest agricultural land is being taken out of production to provide for increasing populations. As a result, farming operations must move onto less suitable land where the production of adequate crops requires greatly increased expenditures for land leveling, irrigation, and fertilization. Although this adjustment can usually be made in the United States with relative ease, the more limited economies of most of the world's countries cannot bear an increased cost for food.

The most important techniques for increased food production have included extensive use of insecticides and mineral fertilizers. Only through their use is the world being fed as well as it is, though that is not really very well. But insecticides cannot be used in limitless amounts without inflicting severe damage on man's environment and perhaps on man himself. Evidence now indicates that excessive nitrates from fertilizer applications are present in food and water supplies at levels which may be harmful to humans, especially infants, and are contributing to the pollution of rivers and lakes.

Thus, it seems that the cost of greatly increased food production will be much higher than predicted and that this cost will be measured not only in economic terms but also in damage to the environment. Optimistic viewpoints should be further dampened by the fact that during the past 60 years, food production has actually increased much more slowly than has the population. Theoretically a much greater population than that

that the world's population is getting hungrier by the day.

How much food could be produced throughout the world? The table below shows the production of organic matter per year by the vegetation of the earth; thus it indicates the earth's potential food-producing capacity based on current standards of cultivation.

Cultivated vegetation is shown to be less efficient than forests in producing organic matter, yielding a smaller overall output. Yet despite its impracticality, this type of vegetation will replace all others for the production of food. Also, total land vegetation leads sea vegetation in efficiency and in net tonnage. This comparison implies that reaching into the sea is not the ultimate answer to food production problems.

Since the most easily cultivated land—both in terms of cost and energy—is already in use, higher yields, as well as conservation of existing lands, offer the best means of in-

made to feed the present hungry people of the world will mean little if the world's population continues to grow unabated. The best hope combines increased food production and a reduction of birth and death rates to replacement levels.

*Population and Health.* Public health agencies have been highly successful in their battle against long-established infectious diseases. Through measures such as antimalarial programs, it has been possible (in Ceylon, for example) to open huge areas for habitation and cultivation that were formerly uninhabitable. Public concern over health problems has resulted in improved sanitation, purer and more adequate water supplies, and prevention and control of communicable diseases through immunization, insecticides, antibiotics, and increased attention to nutritional disorders. These improvements have contributed toward a lowered death rate and an increased life expectancy.

It is mistakenly assumed by some that the

## ANNUAL PRODUCTION OF ORGANIC MATTER

| TYPE OF VEGETATION | AREA IN MILLIONS OF SQUARE KILOMETERS | NET PRODUCTION PER YEAR | |
|---|---|---|---|
| | | GRAMS OF CARBON PER SQUARE METER | MILLIONS OF TONS OF CARBON |
| Cultivated | 13.31 | 204 | 2,728 |
| Forest | 44.41 | 874 | 48,100 |
| Grassland | 36.90 | 103 | 3,286 |
| Other (desert, swamp, etc.) | 53.90 | 178 | 2,706 |
| Total | | | |
| Land | 148.5 | 373 (mean) | 56,820 |
| Sea | 371.0 | 90 (mean) | 33,400 |

SOURCE: Based on data in "The Human Population" by Edward S. Deevey, Jr., *Scientific American*, Vol. 203, No. 3 (September 1960), 203.

present world population problem is due solely to the great efficiency of health programs. It is true that as countries develop economically, better living conditions and improved nutrition usually result. These in turn lead to a drop in death rates. After a lag of several generations, however, the birth rate also tends to decline. In the past, owing to infant mortality, parents conceived more children than they expected to raise to maturity. For example, parents may have conceived six children in order to raise three to maturity. As medical services improve and as they are made available to larger numbers of people, infant mortality drops. But it takes time for parents to realize that they can be assured of the survival of most of their children. If this lag could be reduced from several generations to a single generation, the total population growth in economically developing countries could decrease.

Health programs, therefore, may prove to be one of the best prospects for solving the population problem, especially if a corresponding emphasis on family planning is also provided. Ideally, parents would feel secure enough about the health of their children to decide upon, and practice, birth control measures. As a result of the logical relationship that can and does exist between health programs and population control, national family planning programs are commonly assigned to health services. These have pioneered in Japan, India, Korea, Taiwan, Pakistan, Egypt, Turkey, Czechoslovakia, and Poland.

As we have implied, the success of family-control programs lies in sufficiently motivating the entire population. Historically, when food or living conditions became too bad, people voluntarily controlled population through methods they would normally consider objectionable or immoral. During the potato famines in Ireland a century ago, the excessive population was decreased by late marriages, emigration, and inheritance legislation favoring eldest sons. Japan currently legalizes abortion as a principal method of population control—with the number of abortions exceeding the number of live births. In mainland China there are indications that the population is returning to the old custom of female infanticide. These examples of population controls lead some authorities to doubt that the "standing room only" prophecies will ever become a reality. In preference to such practices as infanticide, people must be motivated to accept the use of contraceptives in family planning.

### The Underlying Problems

Many people look to science for the answer to world population problems, believing that when the "ideal" means of fertility control is developed, population control will automatically follow. Unfortunately, there is very little evidence to support this belief. The methods of fertility control now available (sterilization, contraception, and abortion) are more than adequate for the purpose of stabilizing world population. The problem is that even with ready access to family-planning methods, many couples will plan to have three, four, or even more children. Thus, controlling population is primarily an economic, cultural, and political problem, not a scientific one.

The United Nations Declaration on Population states, "The opportunity to decide the number and spacing of children is a basic human right." The intent of the statement was to encourage the availability of birth control information and facilities, but it can be, and has been, interpreted as an approval of large families and high birth rates.

In the past, the official policy of the United States government has been limited to family

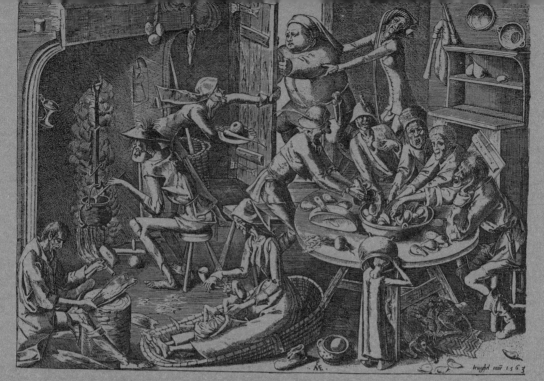

La Cuisine Maigre describes itself — it has little food in it. "Everything, everyone is lean, scrawny, half starved in this poor kitchen."

La Cuisine Grasse is occupied by "Mynheer Fatman and his friends . . . A suckling pig is being basted, while an overfed cat laps the drippings . . ."

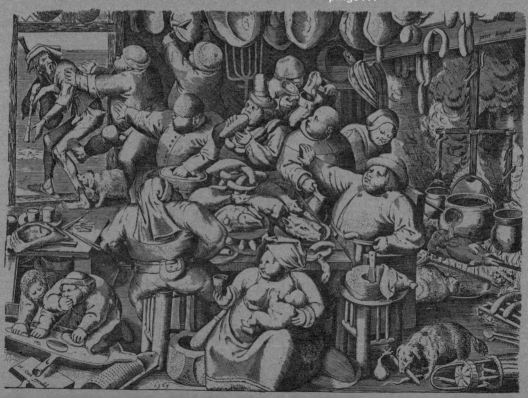

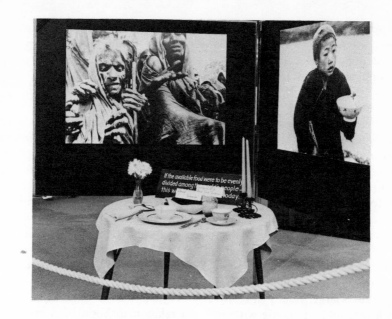

Exhibits such as this one are helping to inform Americans of the food scarcity problem we face *right now.* This attractive table setting actually demonstrates a frightening fact — if the present food resources of the world were equally divided among all the people of the earth, each person's share would amount to a small glass of soybean milk, a cup of rice, and a dish of seaweed. *Photo by Malcolm McWhorter.*

planning assistance for those who would like to restrict family size. It was not until 1971, when the Commission on Population and the American Future issued its interim report, that the need for an "explicit U.S. population policy" was indicated. The report brought home the question of excessive population growth, and how it contrasts with the long-range goal of achieving a good standard of living for all Americans.

To date, most birth control programs have been oriented toward low-income families. But studies show that poor families account for less than one-third of all births in the United States. Although "unwanted" births pose a major problem in all income groups, the real problem, in relation to population control, is not the unwanted but the *wanted*

child. There is a definite distinction between "family planning" and "population planning." Family planning by millions of couples may have no effect at all in terms of world-wide population control.

*Personal Responsibilities.* Any hope for controlling the population explosion must lie in motivating individual couples to limit their familes to two children (actually, an average of 2.1 children would achieve stability, since some persons never marry or else die in childhood).

Millions of couples today who could afford (financially and emotionally) more children are voluntarily limiting their family size out of concern for the population crisis. Many couples who want to raise more than two children are adopting additional children.

Couples who are not motivated by a concern for world population can perhaps be reached through an appeal to their more selfish interests. For example, the cost of raising a child to the age of eighteen should be widely publicized. It now costs the family of average income over $25,000 to raise each child through high school graduation, not to mention the cost of college. In making the decision whether to have another child, it is very difficult for a couple to foresee the cost of the food, clothing, shoes, medical and dental care, school expenses, and so forth, that would be required to raise that child. For the great majority of couples, the choice is simply between raising a small family in relative comfort or a larger family in relative hardship, with the children "doing without" such advantages as vacation trips, orthodontia, and adequate medical care.

*Social and Governmental Factors.* The status of women in society is, according to Rufus E. Miles, Jr., Chairman of the Board of Population Reference Bureau, one of the key determinants of the birth rate. He feels that the more satisfying the employment opportunities for women, the less likely it is that they will want large families. Women who lack the satisfactions that come from decent employment—a sense of belonging to a group, a sense of self-esteem from being able to express a talent or make a contribution to society and be paid fairly for it—must find self-fulfillment in some other way. If, in addition to lacking satisfactory employment, women lack membership in any social group with which they have rapport, they are strongly motivated to create a social group of their own by producing babies.

If Miles' assumption is true, and there is considerable proof that it is, then greatly enlarged employment opportunities for women may be one of the most important factors in reducing average family size. There is much evidence that many if not most women of childbearing age prefer employment at decent jobs to being fulltime homemakers. If our society genuinely desires to lower its birth rate, it must find more numerous, more satisfying, and better-paying opportunities for women, particularly those of childbearing age. An important step in freeing women for meaningful employment is the creation, either by government or by private enterprise, of expanded neighborhood child-care centers. In many areas, such centers are either nonexistent, prohibitively expensive, or of such poor quality that concerned mothers are reluctant to leave their children there.

As previously mentioned, the real problem in relation to population control is not the unwanted child, but the wanted one. Yet unwanted children do add significantly to the birth rate, as well as to a multitude of social and psychological problems. According to several surveys, it's believed that at least one American child in five is unwanted. Certainly, most out-of-wedlock babies (about 1 out of 12 births in the United States) can be considered unwanted, as can the majority of infants born to mothers under 17 years old. Preventing the birth of unwanted children would reduce the birth rate to below the magic 2.1—the level of zero population growth.

The obvious solution is to make contraceptives and abortion cheaper and easily available. It is imperative that every woman have access to family planning assistance, regardless of her age, marital status, or financial condition. It has been estimated that there are about 5 million women in the United States who need publicly supported family planning services.

Although current forms of fertility control could decrease population growth if properly utilized, new methods are also needed. None of the currently available methods is entirely satisfactory, either in relation to its safety, effectiveness, or ease of use. Fertility-control research must be given high priority in the allotment of federal funds.

Finally, there must be a reversal of the numerous social and government pressures and incentives favoring marriage and child-bearing. Unmarried women have been made to feel that they are social failures, when in reality a person of either sex can live a personally satisfying, socially useful life without marriage. Tax laws have generally penalized single people, while heavily favoring those with large families. Welfare programs, public housing projects, and many other govern-ment policies clearly display a bias in favor of the social norm, which holds that everybody should marry and have children. Not only are such policies damaging from the population standpoint, they are sociologically and psychologically destructive as well.

It is our emphatic belief that man, as an intelligent being, can and must maintain his population at such a level that every individual is able to achieve his full biological potential for a long and worthwhile life. It is obvious that if our population continues to increase at its present rate, each individual's "slice of the pie" of life is going to get smaller and smaller until life becomes a burden to be borne rather than a joy to live.

## FOR FURTHER READING

Anderson, Walt (ed.), *Politics and Environment*. Pacific Palisades: Goodyear, 1970. *A collection of some of the most important papers on the ecological crisis.*

Chamberlain, Neil W., *Beyond Malthus*. New York: Basic Books, 1970. *The business and economic views of world population growth and its impact on economics and trade.*

Dasmann, Raymond, *The U.S. Environment: A Time to Decide*. Washington, D.C.: Population Reference Bureau, 1968. *A factual basis for action to improve the environment.*

Ehrlich, Paul R., and Anne H. Ehrlich, *Population—Resources—Environment*. San Francisco: W. H. Freeman, 1970. *A probing examination of our environmental crisis together with suggested political and personal solutions.*

Fraser, Dean, *The People Problem: What You Should Know About Growing Population and Vanishing Resources*. Bloomington, Indiana: Indiana University Press, 1971. *Explains the biological and mathematical laws regulating population growth and what can be done.*

Odum, Eugene P., *Fundamentals of Ecology*. 3rd rev. ed. Philadelphia: Saunders, 1972. *A thorough, updated treatment of basic ecological concepts.*

Paddock, William and Paul, *Famine Nineteen Seventy-Five: America's Decision, Who Will Survive*. Boston: Little, Brown, 1968. *An excellent book tracing the projected effects of unchecked population growth in the United States.*

Sears, Paul B., *This is Our World*. Norman, Olahoma: University of Oklahoma Press, 1971. *First published in 1937, now a classic exploring how society's values and standards will determine what is done concerning the environmental problems of today.*

Wagner, Richard H., *Environment and Man*. New York: W. W. Norton, 1971. *A systematic review of today's environmental problems with suggestions on what man can do to survive.*

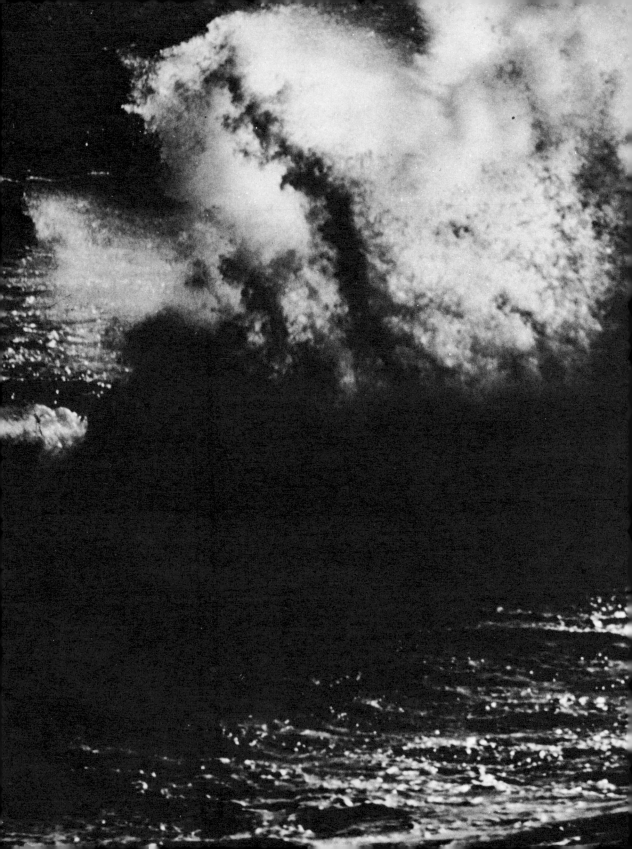

**2**

# Emotional Health

# 3  The Structure of Personality

Personality • The Self and Identity • Basic Human Needs • Characteristics of Good Emotional Health • Developing Emotional Maturity • Developing a Value System • Dealing with Emotional Stress

# 4  Emotional Problems

Effects of Emotional Problems in the United States • Emotional Dysorganization • Treatment of Emotional Disorders • Professional Workers for the Emotionally Disturbed • Treatment Facilities for Emotional Illness

# 3
# The Structure of Personality

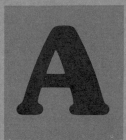basic characteristic of all living things is their attempt to adjust to their environment. In man, this adjustment is much more complicated than in the simpler animals, because we are capable of reasoning. We try to establish and maintain an equilibrium; and since the environment is constantly changing, our attempts at equilibrium demand constant attention.

The demands of our environment are further complicated by our inner needs, so that our life becomes a matter of constantly adapting to changes in the environment, while we still try to satisfy the basic inner needs. Very often we find that environmental situations make the satisfaction of inner needs difficult or even impossible. All of us are frustrated to some extent in our attempts to satisfy our needs. The ways in which we react to this frustration are indications of our emotional health, and vary with each personality.

## PERSONALITY

Personality is made up of a number of behavior patterns, traits, attitudes, and all other interactions a person has with his environment. Everything that has ever happened to him has produced some effect on his personality. An infant is born with a certain genetic makeup, and the personality he eventually develops depends on his original endowment and how the environment acts upon it. His personality will also include the ways in which he looks at his environment and how he learns to deal with the conflicts between his basic inner needs and the obstacles presented by the outer world (the environment).

Thus, we find four forces that influence the personality: genetic makeup, environment, interpretation of the environment, and the learned ways of coping (the coping behavior). The first two forces are largely beyond our power of control. We have no control over those things we inherit, like basic intellectual capacity, body build, skin color, and so forth. We have limited ability to influence our environment. It is in the third and fourth categories—our interpretation of the environment and our methods of coping—that we can improve our personality makeup.

Many attempts have been made to describe the makeup of personality. For example, pioneer psychoanalyst Sigmund Freud conceived of personality as being divided into three "processes": the *id,* which is unconscious; the *ego,* which is mostly conscious; and the *superego,* which has both conscious and unconscious elements. According to this scheme, the mind is like an iceberg, with the conscious mind visible and the great bulk of the unconscious mind below the surface.

Although psychoanalysis no longer enjoys the level of professional popularity it once held, the psychoanalytic concepts of id, ego, and superego may still serve to describe the structures of personality.

### The Id

The id, which is unconscious, is the most primitive of the three portions of the personality. It contains all the basic instinctive drives. These instincts, which are present at birth, represent the unconscious urges to survive and enjoy life. Throughout life, the id remains as the storage place for the primitive instincts.

Since the id works for the individual's biological survival, it is aggressive and selfish, and operates purely for pleasure and gratification. The id makes no distinction between good and evil, or between what is realistic and possible and what is not. Thus, aggression is seen by many authorities as a fundamental, inherent human characteristic, capable of being expressed in both harmful and beneficial ways. Competition, in business, politics, and sports, for example, is seen as an acceptable expression of basic human aggression. Harmful outlets of aggression include physical violence directed toward other persons or even self-directed, like suicide. It should be stressed that not all psychologists accept these concepts, especially the

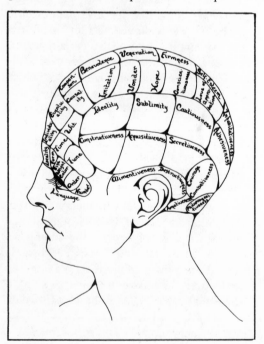

Man's age-old curiosity about the functioning of the human mind has inspired the invention of many notions and systems which seem strange to us today. Phrenology analyzes behavior and personality by reading of the lumps on the skull. It is based on the theory that certain areas of the brain, controlling specific characteristics and forms of behavior, grow larger or smaller, reflecting their relative importance in the individual's psychological makeup.

relationship of aggression to violence and suicide.

### The Ego

The ego represents the conscious mind, and acts as a moderator between the id and the outer world. It is in contact with the environment (reality) and with the id and the superego (judgments of goodness and worthiness). The ego must integrate all factors and determine appropriate behavior for the situation. The ego must decide which urges can be allowed satisfaction and which urges must be suppressed.

The ego is not present at birth; it develops gradually in response to experience and the pressures of society. The most important ego development occurs during the first years of life, but in the emotionally healthy person, the ego continues to grow throughout life. New experiences constantly modify, strengthen, and enlarge the ego. The older person, with his more highly developed ego, is usually able to control and postpone instinct gratification. The infant, on the other hand, has only a weakly developed ego—he is largely driven by id forces. Maturity can thus be measured by the degree to which the ego is able to control the id.

Even in the healthy, mature individual, the ego has a difficult task, but in the emotionally disturbed person, the ego is limited in strength and has increased difficulty in controlling the id and the superego.

### The Superego

The superego represents the judgment mechanisms regarding right and wrong, good and evil. It advises and threatens the ego. The very young child has little concept of what is right and wrong, but as codes and values of society are impressed upon him he gradually develops his superego. The main basis of the child's superego is his concept of his parents as he sees them in his own mind. He therefore uses his parents as a guide for his own behavior. His superego is based on his own impression of his parents, rather than how they may really be.

The attitudes that a child perceives in his parents, and his interpretation of what he perceives, become his basis for judging the morality of situations. Since social values do change, these attitudes may be a source of trouble years after he has become an adult. He may still be carrying childhood values that may have become outdated. Or he may have picked up overly strict or very lax ideals from his parents.

The word "conscience" is sometimes used to describe the superego, but actually the conscience is only part of the superego. It is this portion of the well-developed superego that makes cheating or stealing difficult or impossible, because the person knows that these actions are wrong and that he would feel guilty if he did them.

Another important element of the superego is the "ego-ideal," which is a model of acceptability and worthiness, also gained from his parents. It is important to realize that any violation of the judgment of the superego produces guilt, and that guilt is an extremely uncomfortable feeling. As a result, an individual will go to great lengths, both consciously and unconsciously, to avoid guilt and to avoid behavior that would produce guilt. Or he may use certain ego-defense mechanisms to escape guilt, such as blaming his behavior on someone else or denying behavior that doesn't seem consistent with his ego-ideal.

Punishment is a way of dealing with guilt, so a person who feels guilt may unconsciously seek punishment in various disguised ways. A criminal sometimes purposely leaves clues so that he may be caught and punished. The accident-prone individual may suffer from unconscious guilt, so he unconsciously allows "accidents" to happen to him to serve as punishment and release him from his guilt.

It is possible for a person with a weakly developed superego to live according to the principle of personal pleasure alone, without regard for the rights and privileges of others, yet suffer little or no guilt. On the other hand, it is possible for the superego to be so rigid and severe that it prevents almost all pleasure, regardless of the situation. The most healthy superego is one that fits within the demands of society and yet allows adequate individual pleasure.

## THE SELF AND IDENTITY

The *self* is an individual's awareness or perception of his own personality. It is a composite based on the individual's own feelings about himself and how he imagines that other people feel about him. Much of what we "know" about ourselves is based on our experiences with other people. Our chief sources of information about ourselves are the reactions of others to us. Of course, we evaluate these reactions subjectively and it is possible for a person to see himself somewhat differently than others see him.

Many influences contribute to a person's self-image. The kinds of experiences that he has are very important in determining what his self-perception will be like. He finds that his appearance and personality elicit responses of acceptance or rejection, kindness or hostility, attention or indifference. He hears (or overhears) himself described by other people in terms of various personality traits, and when these traits are consistently applied to him, he usually accepts them as descriptions of himself. Praise and attention help him to form a picture of himself as a desirable person. Rejection, indifference,

criticism, or hostility can lead to a poor self-image, with resulting inferiority feelings.

The treatment that a person receives from others may or may not reflect accurately his own traits and abilities. For example, we tend to react most positively to those whose traits are most like our own. Thus, a person may meet with indifference or rejection merely on the basis of his racial, religious, or cultural background. As a result, an effective and pleasant person may come to perceive of himself as inadequate, inferior, or undesirable in reflection of the prejudices or misconceptions of others. Conversely, the child of admiring and doting parents who excessively praise even his poor performance may grow up with a somewhat inflated self-image.

Knowing a person's self-image helps us to understand his behavior, especially when he sees himself much differently from the way others see him. Behavior is largely determined by how a person perceives a situation with reference to himself.

When a person's self-image is too different from his true or objective personality, serious adjustment problems may arise. He must constantly either explain or ignore circumstances that are inconsistent with his view of himself. Heavy use is made of the ego-defense mechanisms, discussed later in this chapter. Consider, for example, the just-average student who has somehow come to think of himself as an intellectual giant, but is faced with the conflicting evidence of his poor grades. He may rationalize his failure, probably blaming his instructors, or repress the perception of his low grades so that his self-image is not damaged.

But the problem shared by the great majority of us is that we tend to underestimate our capabilities. We fall into the trap of feeling that our lives are completely structured for us by circumstances beyond our control and that we are impotent to make

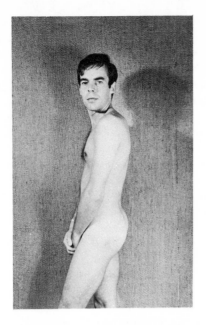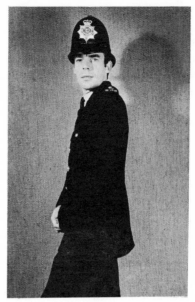

Often the apparel proclaims and explains the man. Little can be said of a man unadorned, other than that he has a unique face and body. Fully clothed, his person and personality often become clear. His bearing and expression take on a particular significance. *Photo by Frank Halbicht.*

any significant change in their course. In reality, each one of us has an amazing ability to accomplish things, if we just accept and believe in this ability. This is the concept of *self-determination.*

Self-determination depends on two basic beliefs. First, it is necessary to believe that human beings in general are self-determining and have considerable control over the courses of their lives. Second is a belief or confidence in your own personal ability to accomplish what you want. This belief in self is based on faith and experience. When a person learns that he is successful in most of the things he attempts, he develops faith in himself. Even his failures do not bother him excessively, because he has confidence

in his ability to recover from failure. Through his experiences in living he has learned what he can and cannot do and he has a basis for self-determination.

When a person does not believe in himself, he acts in ways that are limiting or even self-destructive. When a person "knows" he is going to fail, his failure is assured. This concept is valid in every realm of life. It is true for the student in his courses; for the athlete in competition; for anyone in his relations with people, especially in sexual relationships; and for the patient balanced between life and death with a critical illness.

An integral part of our concept of self is our sense of *identity*. This is our appraisal of who we are, what we mean to ourselves and others, and where we fit into the general scheme of things, especially in our relations with other people. The process of establishing identity is a source of much internal conflict for many people. Most of us suffer our greatest identity conflicts during our high school and college years when we are separating our identity from that of our parents and finding our own place in the world. But changes in identity (and identity crises resulting from conflicts in identity) can occur at any age throughout life. Since the development of personality continues from birth to death, it follows naturally that one's identity must also change. In the past, most people made only minor changes in their identity once they "found" their identity as adults. But the rate of change in all aspects of life has accelerated tremendously (and continues to accelerate) so that an identity which is satisfactory for a young adult today is very unlikely to remain satisfactory for the rest of his life. In fact, even ten years from now, it would probably seem woefully inappropriate to his life situation at that time. The person who goes through life with one career field and one spouse will probably be the exception, where once he was the majority.

Many people never do really discover their own identity. They may go through life hiding in a career, a marriage, organizations, or a succession of "causes." Or they identify themselves in terms of what they have, rather than what they are. Either of these approaches is just a way of dodging the difficult task of defining one's true identity. But for a truly fulfilling life, one must find his own identity, as an individual. The rewards are well worth the cost.

## BASIC HUMAN NEEDS

One of the first requirements for good emotional health is to know ourselves. Why do we feel the way we do? Why do we do the things we do? The answers to these questions will come largely from our understanding of our basic needs, the extent to which these needs are fulfilled in us, and how we react to the frustration of these needs.

We might expect all authorities on the subject to be in complete agreement on something as basic as the needs of man. But actually we find disagreement on this subject. Perhaps the needs of all of us are not exactly the same, and each authority interprets and generalizes his own needs as being true for everyone.

A. H. Maslow, in his classic book *Motivation and Personality,* made an interesting presentation of his interpretation of human needs. He arranged these needs in sequence from the most basic needs to the higher needs. Maslow believes that the higher needs develop only when the basic needs are fulfilled. For example, since food is a very basic need, a person who is starving may have little interest in fulfilling higher needs such as pursuing knowledge or reaching his full artistic potential.

In the following discussion we shall examine some of the basic human needs presented by Maslow.

### The Physiological Needs

The most basic of human needs are the physical drives of man. Among them are hunger, thirst, sleep, sexual drive, and many others. When a person's physiological needs are unsatisfied, he pushes all other needs into the background. Not only is his immediate interest in the higher needs lost, but also his whole plan for the future is modified. For example, an extremely hungry man thinks of Utopia merely as a place where there is plenty of food. He thinks that if only he were guaranteed enough to eat for the rest of his life, he would never want anything more.

Similarly, a young person feeling youthful sexual tensions may direct his behavior toward obtaining sexual satisfaction and have little regard for the present or future fulfillment of his higher emotional needs. Such behavior is frequently demonstrated by both boys and girls. This is why so many marriages are based on sexual attraction alone, without consideration for the higher emotional needs of the marriage partners.

Observations of behavior in a concentration camp suggest that among the physiological needs, those immediately related to survival dominate. Acts related to survival so dominated the individuals' thoughts and actions that no overt sexual activity was evident, and even dreams were reported to be free of sexual content typical of a more normal environment.*

But what happens when the physiological needs are satisfied? Immediately, other and higher needs emerge and begin to dominate the person. As long as a need is satisfied, it has little effect on behavior. Behavior is governed much more by unsatisfied needs.

### The Safety (Security) Needs

Maslow rates the safety needs as second only to the physiological needs. After the physiological needs are fairly well satisfied, the safety needs emerge, and they make everything else appear less important. The safety needs are most easily seen in the fright reactions of infants and children, because adults in our society have been taught to hide or inhibit these reactions at any cost. Thus, even when some adults feel their security threatened, they are not likely to react in a visible manner, but rather with masked anxiety and such physical changes as increased heartbeat.

Actually, knowledge and experience in the

*Victor Frankel, *Man's Search for Meaning*, New York: Washington Square Press, 1963.

adult should eliminate many of the fright reactions shown by the child. One of the most important functions of education is to neutralize apparent dangers through knowledge. Much unnecessary fear results from ignorance. For example, a sonic boom may be quite upsetting to someone who does not understand it. But one who understands sonic booms, although he still may not enjoy them, is not panic-stricken by them.

Parents raising a child must provide him with a feeling of security in the home. The relationship between parents is especially important to a child. Their quarreling, physical abuse, separation, or divorce may be particularly frightening to him. When the parents' anger is directed toward a child, as in speaking harshly to him, handling him roughly, or administering physical punishment, the child often reacts with such total terror that it is clear that his distress involves more than just the physical pain of the punishment. He fears that his parents' love will be taken from him.

Another indication of the child's need for security is his preference for a certain amount of routine and ritual in the daily schedule of the family. He likes a more predictable, orderly world. A young child seems to thrive under a system that has some structure and presents a framework of certain ground rules of conduct. He prefers and needs permissiveness *within limits,* rather than total permissiveness. Basic consistency is more important, however, than the degree of rigidity or permissiveness. A child raised under a consistent system is happier and develops better emotionally than one who is not because he feels more secure. He knows what his parents expect of him and how they will react to his behavior.

The adult in our society usually feels fairly secure as long as he believes his physical and emotional health are good and his source of income is reasonably stable. Many adults express their safety needs in such ways as looking for a job offering more security, saving money for emergencies, and maintaining various kinds of insurance.

Another result of the adult's need for security is the commonly seen preference for familiar rather than unfamiliar things—for the known rather than the unknown. This preference often increases with age, and it is one of the sources of the differences between generations, sometimes called the "generation gap." The older generation has often been dismayed by the new and unfamiliar actions, attitudes, clothing, and so forth, of the younger generation. A person who makes a conscious effort to overcome

a rigid preference for familiar things should be able to face new ideas and challenges without fear.

### The Needs for Love and Belonging

Maslow rates the needs for love and belonging (companionship) after the physiological and safety needs. The person whose physiological and safety needs are fulfilled "somewhat consistently" feels motivated to satisfy his needs for love and belonging. He feels a strong need for friends or a mate. He has a need for companionship with people in general, for a feeling of belongingness and acceptance by his group, and a need to love and be loved.

A feeling of group belonging and accept-

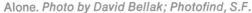

*Alone. Photo by David Bellak; Photofind, S.F.*

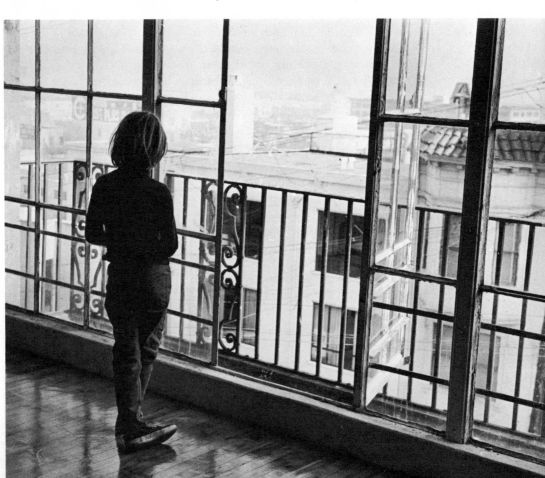

ance has particular value to a person because social life generally centers around group activity. One of the greatest causes of unhappiness is the lack of this feeling of group acceptance. Along with the immediate social satisfaction derived from group belonging are other possible benefits to the individual, such as giving him the security needed to become more independent of his family, exposing him to values different from those of his parents, and providing him with experience in reacting as an equal with his peers. School, church, play, and even work provide many opportunities for group involvement.

Our society has a rather inhibited and cautious attitude toward love and affection, and especially their possible expression in sexuality. This attitude has made it difficult for many people to establish close interpersonal relationships, including those in which sex would play no role. Love and sex are not synonymous. There may be strong love relationships in which sex is not involved, just as there may be sexual relationships in which love is not a factor. The most characteristic feature of love is a genuine concern for the welfare of the loved one.

It is of the utmost importance that parents be responsive to a child's love needs. The child who feels unloved and rejected by his parents will have a poor self-image and may be the source of much trouble at home and at school, and he may grow into a juvenile delinquent or an adult lawbreaker. Parental rejection may leave life-long emotional scars in a child (if he cannot find an adult love relationship elsewhere). The child who has been rejected may later be reluctant to establish close personal relationships for fear of further rejection, and may never be able to give and receive love, thus going through life as a "loner." The person who has "loved and lost" may also withdraw due to fear of further rejection. But to a reasonably secure

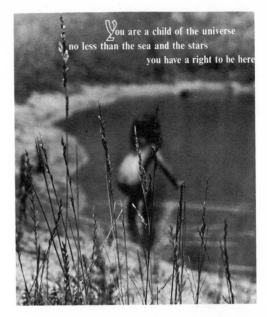

You are a child of the universe no less than the sea and the stars you have a right to be here

© 1971 by Celestial Arts.

person, the fulfilling of love needs is worth the risk involved.

### The Esteem Needs

Every normal person has a need for self-esteem, which means a feeling of personal value or worth, of success, achievement, self-respect, and confidence in the face of the world. In addition, most people have a need for respect or esteem from other people, as seen in their striving for status, dominance, attention, and appreciation.

We shall first consider the need for *self-esteem*. Satisfaction of this need leads to feelings of self-confidence, value, strength, adequacy, and usefulness. Inability to satisfy the self-esteem need produces feelings of dependence, inferiority, weakness, helplessness, and despair.

The most obvious way to build self-respect is to do something of value well—to excel. The specific area in which to excel should be determined by one's interests and ability.

Anyone who makes the effort can find some constructive activity in which to excel. It is especially fortunate if a person receives a feeling of satisfaction from his work, since he devotes a great amount of time to it. But a sport or hobby can be equally rewarding in building self-respect, as can social and love experiences.

It can be seen that the feelings gained through satisfaction of the need for self-esteem are likely to give rise to accomplishments that further build self-respect. A person who suffers from a lack of self-respect and who feels helpless finds it difficult to accomplish anything that will help build his self-respect. Something must be done to break his cycle of insignificance and begin the building of his self-esteem.

The second of the esteem needs concerns the desire for respect from *other* people, in the form of reputation or prestige. It seems that as a person's self-respect is strengthened, his need for the esteem of others is diminished. The person who feels confident of his own worth is less dependent on the praise of others. It is certainly better for him to base his self-respect on *his* actual achievement rather than on the opinions of others, which often are either higher or lower than the truth warrants.

The constant seeking of praise may suggest insecurity on the part of the seeker, but it is important in dealing with people to recognize that everyone has a need for some recognition from others. Sincere praise is one of the foundations of good interpersonal relationships. It is important to give praise when praise is due. Too often we tell people when we are annoyed with them, but forget to tell them when we are pleased.

### The Need for Self-Actualization

The need for self-actualization is merely the need to do what one is capable of doing, to achieve self-fulfillment. If he is to be at peace with himself, an artist must paint, a poet must write, and a musician must make music. Maslow says, "What a man can be, he must be." This statement means that in order to feel fulfilled a person must not only do the kind of thing he is able to do, but also do it as well as he is capable of doing. Most of us (Maslow says 99 percent) are not operating at this level, we are hung-up or stuck at a lower level of motivation.

### The Need to Know and Understand

Among the higher needs of man are his impulses to satisfy curiosity, to know, to explain, and to understand. Curiosity is a natural rather than a learned characteristic of man. The young child is naturally curious. He may lose this curiosity, however, through overly strict discipline at home or too much regimentation at school. The home and school must be careful not to destroy this

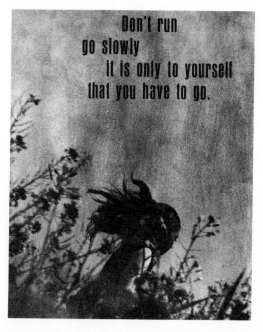

Don't run
go slowly
it is only to yourself
that you have to go.

valuable characteristic. When curiosity has already been suppressed, every effort should be made to restore it, for curiosity leads to creativity and invention.

Although many people can live fairly satisfying lives without much intellectual stimulation, these would not be highly fulfilling lives. The person whose thoughts are confined to the mundane may become bored, feel constantly tired, and have little zest for life. In contrast, the satisfaction of the need to know and understand often gives a person a bright, happy feeling of fulfillment in his emotional life.

### The Aesthetic Needs

Beauty is a subjective quality that defies any scientific measurement. But it is a basic need for many adults and probably for all normal children. Like curiosity, an appreciation of beauty may or may not be retained into adulthood.

Most women and girls in our culture very readily show their appreciation of beauty. But many men and boys are embarrassed by their love of beauty, because they are afraid it may be an effeminate trait or be seen as such by their friends. Therefore, they may actually hide or suppress their enjoyment of beauty. But the male should realize that his love of beauty is perfectly natural and that he can enjoy beauty without risking his masculinity. He should be able to feel and express enjoyment of the beauty of a flower, a tree, a skillfully designed building, a well-designed car, or an attractive girl.

## CHARACTERISTICS OF GOOD EMOTIONAL HEALTH

It would be very difficult to set up an exact standard by which an individual's level of emotional health could be judged. There certainly is no line that neatly divides the emotionally healthy from the emotionally ill. There are many different degrees of emotional health. The following characteristics are all signs of good emotional health. But the lack of one or more of them in a person does not indicate emotional illness. Actually, no one has all the traits of good emotional health at all times. At the very least, an emotionally healthy, fully functioning, or self-actualizing, person "feels good," he enjoys himself and his personal existence.

### Ability to Deal Constructively with Reality

The healthy person accepts reality, whether it is pleasant or not. He does not generally attempt to escape from reality by mental fantasies or by excessive use of drugs or alcohol. Nor does he take the opposite path, becoming preoccupied with his own problems and spending much time worrying or brooding.

Dealing constructively with reality means that a person must learn to acknowledge and accept his own capabilities and limitations. Then when a problem arises, he can do something about it (if the solution is within his ability) or else realistically accept the problem as beyond his ability to solve. In situations in which someone else has a greater ability to solve the problem, the mature person does not hesitate to ask for help. When it is apparent that he is dealing with a problem that is impossible to solve even with help, he then adjusts to the situation.

The healthy person sets realistic goals for himself. He tries to make the fullest use of his natural abilities, but he also realizes his natural limitations and does not frustrate himself trying to do something that is obviously beyond his present ability. A person usually is happiest when he is working at or near his full ability. He usually is not very happy when he is working far below his ability or when he is trying to work far above it.

Another indication of emotional health is the acceptance of responsibilities. An unhealthy person may actually work harder at evasion than he would if he accepted his responsibilities and did whatever was necessary to fulfill them. The more healthy person not only accepts responsibility, but also enjoys and needs a certain amount of it.

### Ability to Adapt to Change

There is a natural tendency to resist change and even to fear the future. This results from the basic need for safety and security, as discussed previously. But the healthy person is more confident of his ability to adapt to change. He realizes that the world constantly changes, and he expects to change with it. He plans ahead and does not live in fear of the future.

Many aspects of maturity improve with increasing age, but one characteristic that often is gained at a young age and then lessened is the ability to adapt readily to change. Most young people welcome new experiences and new ideas. They should try to keep this open-minded approach to life as time passes. In past generations this adaptive ability was less important than it is now, because then conditions changed much more slowly than they do today.

### Ability to Make Long-Range Choices

An important characteristic of self-actualization is the ability to give up some immediate pleasure for the sake of long-term values. The more mature person has certain goals for the future and realizes that he must make some sacrifices in order to reach those goals. The less mature person, in contrast, wants his pleasures "here and now" without concern for the future. The more mature person also cares about pleasure, but he plans his life to give himself the greatest amount of pleas-ure over the long term—and his plans sometimes require passing up an immediate pleasure.

This principle applies to many areas of our lives. We may pass up rich desserts in order to gain a more attractive figure. We may save money now in order to pay college expenses later. We may skip a favorite television show in order to study for an examination. We may avoid casual sexual relationships for the sake of long-term values. There are many other similar situations in our lives.

### Reasonable Degree of Autonomy

A person in good emotional health can function autonomously, think for himself, and make the most of his own decisions. He can plan his life and follow through with his plans. The inability to make decisions is very common in the immature, insecure person. He may spend much time in confusion, not knowing what to do. He is afraid to face the consequences of whatever decisions he makes, so he makes as few as possible. Growth involves mistakes as well as successes.

Yet, a certain amount of dependence is also desirable. A person should not try to divorce himself completely from the society in which he lives and of which he is a part. For example, it is normal to enjoy being loved by another person (a form of dependence on that person). In our complex society we are dependent on other people in many ways. Healthy people enjoy this interdependency.

### Freedom from Stresses of Tensions and Anxieties

The emotionally healthy person is more able to properly control his emotions. He is not overpowered by fears, anger, hatred, jealousy, guilt, or worries. He can take life's disappointments in his stride, minimizing the

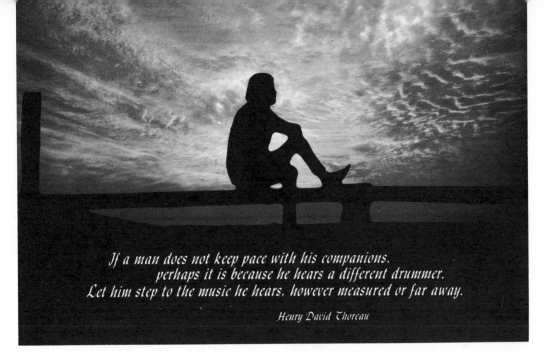

*If a man does not keep pace with his companions,*
*perhaps it is because he hears a different drummer.*
*Let him step to the music he hears, however measured or far away.*

Henry David Thoreau

unpleasant aspects. He has a more tolerant attitude toward himself as well as others. He is inclined to look at the brighter side of life, rather than to concentrate on his troubles. He can laugh at himself. This attitude tends to minimize problems and may make them more effectively solvable.

Good emotional control has two requirements: proper degree and desirable methods of control. These requirements are discussed later in this chapter.

### Concern for Other People

The healthy personality combines self-respect with a concern for the rights and happiness of other people. Such a person truly finds as much satisfaction in giving as in receiving. He respects the differences he finds among other people, accepting them as they are. He does not bully or use them unreasonably in reaching his own goals. He is careful in his words and actions to avoid offending others. He avoids saying things to build his own ego at the expense of others.

### Satisfactory Relationships with Other People

The person who enjoys better emotional health is able to relate to other people in a more consistent manner with mutual satisfaction and happiness. He likes and trusts most people and expects that people will like and trust him. His relationships with others are satisfying and lasting. He has enough self-confidence to be able to feel a part of a group. He feels accepted by a group and, conversely, makes others feel accepted.

The person who seems to have trouble dealing with people should examine his own attitudes and actions. He may mistakenly think that he is always right and that everyone else is wrong, or that he is being rejected by others when he has actually been hostile or inconsiderate himself.

### The Ability to Love

The mature person does not have a large number of childish needs that must be expressed. He is able to express affection for other people. Even a rather immature person can receive love, but it takes a mature person to give love unselfishly. Although we refer to this type of love as "unselfish," it is actually very emotionally rewarding; it is one of the most fulfilling actions of man.

It must be stressed that the love to which we are referring is not just sexual love, but includes a love for children (not just our own, but all children) and for all people, regardless of their racial, religious, or cultural backgrounds. It is a love for humanity. Only the person with a well-developed sense of inner security can freely express such acceptance of others. Before a person can love others, he must learn to accept himself, and really love and respect himself.

### The Ability to Work Productively

It is widely agreed among authorities today that one of the prime indicators of good emotional health is the ability to work effectively and productively. The inability to be productive may be considered a symptom of emotional illness. Many examples can be found. In school, it is often found that the student who has trouble completing his work suffers from emotional conflicts. The chronically unemployed adult often suffers from emotional problems that inhibit him from actively looking for a job, work against him during job interviews, or lower his productivity to the point where he repeatedly loses jobs.

The housewife may similarly reflect her emotional problems in her inability to keep up with her housework or in the fact that routine household chores consume so much of her energy that she is able to do little else.

## DEVELOPING EMOTIONAL MATURITY

We have now seen some of the characteristics of the emotionally mature person. But how does a person who lacks these characteristics develop them? For most of us, the passage of time and the gaining of various experiences bring on a degree of maturity. For example, we expect different levels of maturity in 3-, 10-, 16-, and 30-year-old people. But for various reasons some people do not act at the level of maturity we expect of them, and there are times when everyone seems less mature than usual.

There are two basic forms of immaturity. One is called *fixation*, in which a person remains emotionally at an earlier level of development. A fixated person is one who has never grown up in certain attitudes, ideas, or behaviors. The other type is called *regression*, a return to an earlier level of maturity. Many people show signs of regression temporarily while they are under stress. Some examples of their behavior during difficult periods might include pouting or throwing temper tantrums. During regression people display behavior patterns that are more characteristic of children than of adults. If a person's behavior seems to fit the description of either fixation or regression, we may wonder why and what can be done about it.

First, let us consider why a person might be immature. It may be that he has never developed the traits of responsibility, courage, or the ability to view problems objectively. Sometimes an individual behaves as though he wants someone to protect him. He may be the child of parents who have encouraged him to remain childlike by rewarding his immature behavior in devious ways. Such parents themselves fear and dislike adult life and are trying to protect their child from it by keeping him immature.

Maturity is an ongoing process, rather than a condition finally reached. Maturity involves your relationship with others and with yourself as well. Maturity involves both actions and attitudes. The following points may be of value in developing maturity.

1. Draw others out in conversation. In doing this, you are exposed to many new ideas and attitudes.

2. Accept the differences in others. Really accept these differences, do not just tolerate them, which is patronizing. Learn to appreciate, and enjoy them!

3. Learn not to feel that you must establish a rightness or wrongness about everything. Most things (including beliefs and attitudes) are simply different, not necessarily better or worse than others. This does not mean that you should have no standards of your own. It is very important that you do have a set of values, but you should not believe that all values other than your own are wrong.

4. You can probably really learn about yourself only through exposure to others. It is not enough to merely expose your intellectual ideas—you must expose your feelings as well. Such exposure of true feelings encourages others to reveal their feelings. People can hope to understand each other only when their true feelings are revealed. Emotions are normal and human.

## DEVELOPING A VALUE SYSTEM

Values are those things—acts, ideas, beliefs, traits—to which we attach worth. A value system is how we organize our values in such a way that they influence how we live our lives. A value system is actually a philosophy of life. Regardless of whether a person has ever given the matter any conscious thought or not, he has at least some basic values that govern his life. These values are expressed in the way he spends his time and money, and in all his other actions.

A person's philosophy of life is often more truthfully expressed by what he does than by what he says. We often meet people who express very lofty ideals, but whose actions betray their true values.

Value systems range from the purely selfish to the overly idealistic. The person whose value system lies at either one of these extremes is likely to be unhappy and frustrated much of the time. The most emotionally rewarding philosophy lies somewhere between these extremes.

A person's value system is influenced by many factors, some of which are beyond his control. All the following factors have a degree of influence on a person's values:

1. Places he has lived
   (a) Nations
   (b) Regions
   (c) City, suburban, or rural areas
2. Era in which he was born
3. Values of parents, as influenced by their
   (a) Ethnic group
   (b) Religion
   (c) Economic level
   (d) Age
   (e) Occupation
   (f) Education
4. Values of his age group and friends
5. School experiences
6. Religious training
7. *Everything* that has happened to him in life

If a person has never done so, it would be helpful for him to spend time in an honest appraisal of his current value system. Does it seem adequate for the future he has planned for himself—such as marriage, a career, and the raising of children? Is it even adequate for his current situation?

One characteristic of a truly successful value system is that it is never rigid. It is constantly being modified and changed as a person undergoes new experiences and gains in maturity, and as the world he lives in continues to change. Change and flexibility are values too!

There is no cut-and-dried approach to developing a satisfying value system. Much depends on personal factors such as the religion (if any) that a person accepts and the many experiences that are exclusively his own. But a few general suggestions may be helpful.

1. *Draw on the experiences of others.* Spend some time reading the works of the great philosophers of the past as well as those of the present. Talk to more experienced people whose lives you admire and study their value systems and how they express their values in their daily actions.

2. *Accept only that which is meaningful.* Evaluate what you read in respect to your own experiences. From all the conflicting ideas presented, you should accept only the ideas that seem personally meaningful and significant to you. It is not that some value systems are basically right and others wrong, but that ideas often conflict because a philosophy or value system is highly personal and individual. What is right for one person may be very wrong for another. You should not automatically accept the philosophy of another, regardless of how famous he may be. If your philosophy is not really your own, it is inadequate.

3. *Respect the rights of others.* A value system can work successfully only if it takes into consideration the reality that the freedom of the individual is limited by the rights and freedoms of others. A value system is unrealistic and will be unsuccessful as a guide through life if it demands rights and freedoms for one individual, while denying these same rights to others. For example, the person who demands the right to freely express his own ideas must extend this same right to all others. This concept would seem to eliminate violence as a part of one's philosophy. Anyone who is willing to inflict violence upon another person should be equally willing to receive violence, and this seems rather unlikely.

Several value systems today are totally self-centered. The pleasure and comfort of the individual is the only consideration. But such philosophies are self-defeating. It has been shown repeatedly that most people are happiest and their emotional health is best when their concern extends beyond their own material comfort to include the welfare of mankind in general. This type of value system indirectly leads to the greatest individual happiness, so it actually accomplishes that which the more selfish philosophies fail to produce. The person who is totally occupied with the satisfaction of his own desires is destined for much frustration, because he must share this planet with millions of other people having similar desires and competing for the same goals. The person who is satisfied with his fair share and who can feel satisfaction in the happiness of others will receive the greatest pleasure from life.

4. *Re-evaluate your values periodically.* From time to time your philosophy should be re-evaluated in the light of the kind of life it is producing for you. Are you truly satisfied with the way things are going? Perhaps your values are inadequate or could be on a higher plane. As you gain in wisdom and experience, it is normal to alter your value system accordingly. Values that are perfectly normal and acceptable for a 15-

year-old could well seem immature and inappropriate for a 30-year-old person.

## DEALING WITH EMOTIONAL STRESS

The word "stress" appears in almost every discussion of emotional health, yet the word is used in many different ways. To avoid any misunderstanding, we will use the word in the following ways in this book.

1. *Stress,* in its most general sense, and as defined by the noted Canadian physiologist Hans Selye, is a group of nonspecifically induced changes within a living system (such as a person) resulting from the imposition on the system of any harmful external force.

2. A *stressor* is any force that produces stress. It may be emotional conflict, fear, fatigue, physical injury, disease germs, poison, radiation, or any other harmful force.

3. *Emotional stress* is a condition involving tension, frustration, or conflict. Anxiety may or may not be present.

### The General Adaptation Syndrome

Prolonged stress can have severe damaging effects on both the physical and emotional health of a person. The sympathetic division of the autonomic nervous system reacts to emotional stress by preparing the body for emergency action. Among the many effects of sympathetic stimulation are increased speed and strength of heartbeat; diversion of the blood supply away from the digestive organs and to the body muscles; dilation of the pupil of the eye; changes in hormone levels (especially in the adrenal hormones); increase in blood sugar level; and inhibition of the digestive glands. Such effects, although useful while actually responding to emergencies, become harmful when continued over long periods of time.

Many aspects of contemporary life produce the kinds of emotional stress that stimulate the sympathetic nervous system. Typical of these stress-producing factors are marital and home tensions, indecision over career goals, grades, the draft, and the deteriorating urban environment with its housing and transportation problems, noise, threat of crime, and in general the effect of *novelty, diversity,* and *acceleration* on all aspects of our environment. Toffler, in his book *Future Shock* (1970), describes these three *forces* as the significant factors which test the adaptational capacity of every member of a technological society.

If a person suffers from prolonged emotional stress, such as chronic conflict, anxiety, frustration, or hostility that smolders on month after month, then the resulting autonomic (sympathetic) stimulation can also continue without letup. A multitude of physical problems can result from such prolonged stress, including high blood pressure, asthma, peptic ulcers, skin disorders, impotence, and menstrual irregularities. Such disorders are termed *psychosomatic* (*psyche* meaning mind and *soma* meaning body), because they may be caused by psychological stresses. Of course, any of these disorders may also have purely physical causes, or be the result of a combination of both physical and psychological factors. Emotional stress, however, is the precipitating cause of many cases of these disorders.

Hans Selye explained the physical manifestations of stress, applying the term "*general adaptation syndrome* (GAS)." A syndrome is a group of symptoms. He emphasized that this same reaction is elicited by any type of stressor to which we are subjected, be it emotional stress, a physical injury, infection with disease organisms, fatigue, or exposure to extremes of heat or cold.

The general adaptation syndrome includes three successive stages. The first is the *alarm reaction,* consisting of the immediate mobilization of the body's defense mechanisms,

71

consisting of those just mentioned and similar responses. If the stress continues for some time, however, the person enters the second stage, called *resistance to stress.* This is the stage of maximum ability to withstand the stressor. It may continue for days, weeks, or even months, depending on the vitality of the person and the amount of rest he is able to obtain during this period of maximum effort. Such endurance, however, puts a considerable strain on the body's resources and often results in the psychosomatic disorders. If the stress continues long enough, the third stage, *exhaustion,* may be reached, in which the person becomes progressively devitalized, and his ability to resist the stress diminishes. He has exhausted his internal resources for dealing with continued stress. Every function of the body is weakened. If this stage continues long enough, death results.

A key concept in the general adaptation syndrome is that, since all types of stressors produce the same reaction, exposure to any one type of stressor reduces our ability to defend ourselves against all other types of stressors. For example, prolonged emotional stress interferes with our ability to fight off infectious diseases; thus, we may become physically ill more readily while under a state of emotional stress. Or, conversely, physical illness lowers our ability to resist emotional stresses. Thus, the health of the body and of the mind are inseparably interrelated and interdependent. Because of this interdependence the full range of practices identified for the maintenance of "good health" serve as preventatives against physical and emotional stress. Conversely, their repeated neglect increases the potential for physical and emotional stress and illness.

### Defense Mechanisms

Stress situations are a part of every life and everyone develops methods for coping with them. The purpose of these coping methods is to avoid a conscious feeling of stress. These stress-preventing devices have been called "ego-defense mechanisms" or just "defense mechanisms."

There is no disagreement that defense mechanisms do exist. But there has been disagreement on how many of these defenses there are and to which defense mechanism a particular behavior pattern should be attributed. The problem has come about through man's efforts to neatly classify every type of behavior as the result of a particular mechanism. Actually, no such concrete classification is possible, since the same behavior can often result from any of several causes. Defense mechanisms are thought to be called into play whenever a situation, or impulse, or feeling comes up that is in conflict with the person's self-concept.

These defense mechanisms should not be thought of as abnormal. Everyone makes use of them. They are recognized by most authorities today as necessary and valuable in dealing with the stress situations that we all face throughout life. It is doubtful that anyone could successfully go through life without making use of them. However, excessive reliance upon them, or inability to acknowledge or accept them, can be a sign of low ego strength. This becomes difficult when we realize that most defense mechanisms are unconsciously motivated—that is, we don't know why we do them.

In examining a few of the more widely accepted defense mechanisms, we will make no attempt to classify these mechanisms as good or bad. In most cases, the value of a particular mechanism depends on the extent to which it is used. Used in moderation and in the proper situation, a mechanism might be of great value. Yet the same mechanism, used in excess or in inappropriate situations, might be definitely harmful.

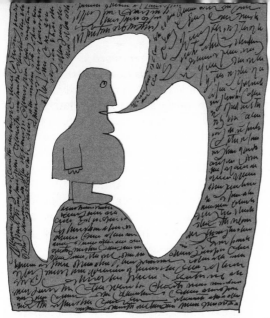
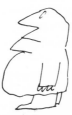

*Avoidance.* One of the simplest and most common methods of defense against anxiety is to avoid situations that produce it. We all use this defense to some extent. The person who fears airplanes travels by car or train. The person who is bothered by speaking in front of groups tries to avoid situations in which he must make public speeches. The boy who still feels uneasy in a personal relationship with girls avoids this anxiety by not asking them for dates.

Certainly, none of these examples of avoidance could be considered abnormal or even unusual. But avoidance can become so intense that it does indicate a serious emotional conflict. Such would be the case if a person became so fearful that he refused to leave his house for any reason, or if he lacked the self-confidence to perform any kind of job at all. Thus it can be seen that the same defense mechanism can be normal and harmless or seriously disabling, depending on the degree to which it is used.

*Denial of Reality.* In using this mechanism, a person protects his ego from a stressful situation by refusing to perceive it. Denial of reality is usually an unconscious process, or at least partly so. The individual usually is not consciously aware that he is denying anything.

Denial appears in several forms. One is merely to refuse to see or hear certain things that might lead to stress reactions, such as a child "tuning out" his mother's call for him to come home. Children and elderly persons often use this mechanism. Another form is to deny the existence of a reality. A motorcyclist, for example, may avoid anxiety by vigorously denying that motorcycles are dangerous.

Still another variation is the denial of inward feelings. A boy might deny his feelings of desire for a beautiful girl if he knows he has no chance of winning her. He might even find something about her to criticize or ridicule. We also tend to react in the same way to material things that we believe are entirely out of our reach. We usually avoid anxiety by restricting our serious desire to that which is attainable, or nearly so.

Like avoidance, denial can be either a helpful or harmful defense, depending on the situation in which it is used and the extent to which it is used. For example, we must admit that the world is, to some extent, a dangerous place. Every day, each one of us faces the possibility of being cut down by fatal disease, war, murder, automobile accident, fire, flood, tornado, lightning, or building collapse, to name but a few of life's hazards. But the probability of anything happening to a given person on a given day is extremely remote. If we continually considered all the dangers we face, we would be in a constant state of anxiety. Through denial, we can ignore the remote dangers and live a normal life.

But denial can be harmful if it results in failure to take precautions against more immediate dangers. For example, some people fail to get immunizations or physical examinations because they deny the possibility of illness; others fail to use automobile seat belts because they deny the possibility of an accident. When any clear and present danger is denied, that is obviously a misuse of the mechanism of denial.

*Repression.* Repression is the process of forgetting (or more accurately, restricting to the unconscious mind) an event, feeling, or memory that would produce anxiety. The repressed material, though blocked from entering the conscious mind, continues to have an influence. It constantly seeks expression in some indirect way. It may cause tension in certain situations, or it may influence preferences, decisions, attitudes, or beliefs. It may require the use of other defense mechanisms in order to keep the material repressed and to prevent anxiety from rising to the conscious mind.

Material that is repressed is pushed back into the unconscious mind much more rapidly than material that is ordinarily forgotten. It may happen almost immediately in response to the urgent need to defend the ego against the awareness of anxiety. This occurrence is especially true of frightening experiences in childhood, such as a bad fall or an attack by an animal. Adults similarly tend to repress such occurrences as accidents, attacks, socially unacceptable feelings or actions, and other frightening events. Interestingly, repression underlies most of the other defense mechanisms.

In the area of psychology called "psychoanalysis," repressed conflicts are seen as the cause of much vague anxiety. Psychoanalysts make elaborate efforts to bring these conflicts from the unconscious mind into the conscious mind so that they can be rationally discussed and the anxiety of the patient relieved. This approach has been used much less frequently in recent years, although it still has followers and is of value in certain situations.

*Projection.* Projection is the way in which a person bolsters his own self-image by unconsciously attributing his own feelings or characteristics to other people. This is generally done with some characteristic that we unconsciously consider to be undesirable. For example, a person who lies, cheats, or steals usually believes that everyone lies, cheats, or steals. Thus, he can feel that his own behavior is really not too bad because "everybody does it." Very often the thing that a person accuses others of doing is exactly the things that he himself is doing (or would like to be doing).

*Rationalization.* In rationalization, closely related to projection, an individual explains his behavior in such a way as to assign a socially acceptable motive to it and disguise the unacceptable motive his behavior actually expresses. Rationalization is among the most commonly used of the defense mechanisms and we probably all use it to some extent. A student who fails an exam or course often blames the instructor, the curriculum, in fact anything but his own lack of aptitude or inadequate effort. A person who gets fired from his job or gets a traffic ticket similarly finds someone or something else to blame. A person using rationalization really believes what he is saying. He uses this mechanism to protect his own opinion of himself, not just the opinion that others have of him.

*Regression.* Regression occurs when, in times of acute stress, a person unconsciously tries to return to an earlier stage of his life in order to escape his current anxiety. As a person gains in age and maturity, he finds that his responsibilities are equally increased. He becomes particularly responsible for the consequences of his own behavior and therefore must maintain a greater degree of control over his emotions and impulses. This naturally tends to produce some stress.

Most people can look back at the earlier stages of their lives as being less stressful than their current stage of development. This situation may be actually true, or it may be that the less pleasant aspects of the earlier ages have been forgotten or repressed. But when stress occurs, a person may behave in ways that were characteristic of the earlier period, usually involving less responsibility and greater dependency.

Many examples of regression can be cited. The wife or husband who deserts a marriage and "goes home to mama" is demonstrating regression. The satisfaction received from sucking on a cigarette has been attributed to regression. A most extreme example of regression is the emotionally ill person who curls up, mute and withdrawn, into the fetal position (knees tucked under the chin).

*Fixation.* Fixation is closely related to regres-sion. In fixation, however, a person does not regress from an advanced point of development; he simply never reaches it. He remains emotionally immature, either in all phases of his personality or only in certain phases of it. Such a person may never gain emotional maturity, or he may gain it at a later than average age.

*Sublimation.* The word "sublimation" was used originally to indicate the process of satisfying frustrated sexual desires in non-sexual substitute activities. The term is now used more loosely by many authorities to include any substitution of lower need satisfaction by the satisfaction of a higher need.

Through sublimation, thoughts and actions that we consider to be undesirable can be repressed by developing forms of behavior that are more socially acceptable. Instead of expressing aggressive impulses toward others in the form of destructive acts or behavior that is not socially acceptable, we can express these impulses with socially acceptable forms of competition, as in sports, politics, and business.

Sublimation thus means converting basic emotional drives, sexual and otherwise, into acceptable and useful activities. In Freudian terms, it is the taming of the id by the ego under the direction of the superego. Sublimation is considered by many authorities to be among the most constructive of the defense mechanisms. Though difficult to achieve, it can be both personally and socially beneficial, and can bring a social approval that strengthens the ego by satisfying one of the higher needs.

Sublimation can operate both unconsciously and as the result of conscious thought and effort. Unconsciously, it often keeps us from even being aware of undesirable motives. Most people would be very surprised to learn of the hostile and lustful impulses

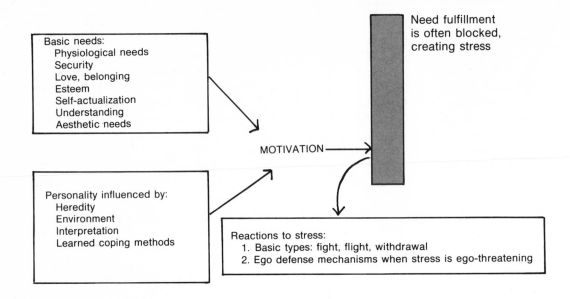

The personality adjustment process. Basic needs and personality create motivation, but the fulfillment of needs and motivations is often blocked, creating stress. Reactions to stress may then influence personality, possibly altering motivations.

that they have been able to repress through the mechanism of sublimation. Through conscious effort, a person can sublimate conscious undesirable impulses and work toward more desirable personal and social goals.

### Everyday Coping Devices

The defense mechanisms as well as many similar mechanisms are necessary for the avoidance of anxiety. Yet, at the same time, the use of these mechanisms often creates a stress in itself.

The ability to tolerate this tension varies considerably among different individuals. Some can stand much more tension than others, but each has his limit. When the tension reaches this limit, it must be relieved in some personally satisfying way or the defense mechanisms will fail. Such a failure is commonly but incorrectly called a "nervous breakdown."

In order to obtain relief from tension, people use many types of behavior called "everyday coping devices" (Menninger, 1963). The purpose of these devices is to drain off the tension that may result from the use of the ego-defense mechanisms. According to Menninger, an important distinction between the defense mechanisms and the coping devices is that the defense mechanisms function on an unconscious level, while the coping devices are often consciously and purposely used to relieve tension. Some of these coping devices are as follows:

1. *Touch, rhythm, and sound.* These stimuli give pleasant sensations that relieve tension. For example, playing, singing or listening to music is often useful in reducing tension. Dancing to rhythmic music is especially good.

2. *Eating, smoking, and chewing gum.* There are several theories on how these oral

activities work to reduce tension. Obesity is often the result of tension.

3. *Alcohol and drugs.* These work by dulling or altering one's perception and are among the least desirable coping devices.

4. *Laughing, crying, and swearing.* Such open expressions of tension may be very useful in relieving that tension.

5. *Sleeping.* This may be another device for escaping reality or boredom.

6. *Talking out a problem.* Discussing one's problems with a trusted person can greatly relieve tension, even if the person does no more than listen. It reduces the sense of loneliness, even if the listener is a perfect stranger, as is often the case.

7. *Thinking through a situation.* Just a few minutes of clear, unemotional thinking can often place a problem in its proper perspective.

8. *Physical exercise.* It is now widely agreed that physical exercise is valuable in working off tension.

9. *Pointless activity.* This includes some of the less desirable tension-reducing devices, such as pacing the floor, hand wringing, nail biting, finger tapping, and scratching.

10. *Daydreaming.* Daydreaming is a retreat into fantasy, usually into a fantasy in which one's problems do not exist or have been solved. Occasional brief periods of daydreaming may be helpful in reducing tension, but it is easy to spend too much time in the retreat from reality.

11. *Familiar activities.* Doing something familiar so that it involves no threat or, perhaps, which is associated with comfort and satisfaction in the past (for example, working at a hobby, washing the car, working overtime).

# 4
# Emotional Problems

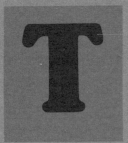he extent of emotional problems in the United States is high. There are no exact figures available, only estimates, and these vary considerably depending on the way in which emotional illness is defined. According to the concepts we will follow in this chapter, everyone can be considered emotionally disturbed at some time in his life. Of course, there are many degrees of emotional disturbance, but what we are concerned with is the number of people that have emotional problems serious enough to interfere with normal living patterns.

It is estimated that about one in every ten persons in the United States suffers from a serious emotional disturbance at some time in his life. This estimate means that about 10 percent of the people we know will at some time need professional help with their emotional problems; or that we, ourselves, have one in ten chances of being seriously disturbed at some time.

## EFFECTS OF EMOTIONAL PROBLEMS IN THE UNITED STATES

The high incidence of these problems places a heavy burden on the resources of our country. For example, every year over one million people are hospitalized in mental hospitals or psychiatric wards of general hospitals for treatment of emotional disorders. On any given day, more than half of all the hospital beds in the country are occupied by mental patients. The cost in terms of dollars and human suffering is staggering.

Since 1900 the rate of hospitalization for emotional problems has more than doubled. This increase is only partly the result of the greater stresses of modern life. Other important causes of this reported increase include a growing public awareness of the problems of emotional health, a higher percentage of the population living in large cities (where stress is greater), a growing population of elderly persons (who may suffer from senility, anxiety, or depression), and a great increase in the facilities available for treating emotional disorders.

Although the rate of hospitalization for emotional disturbance in the United States is one of the highest in the world, this does not necessarily mean that there is a higher incidence of emotional illness here than in other countries. This country has more facilities than any other country for treating emotional illness, and greater effort is made here to help the disturbed. In some countries, little or nothing is done to combat emotional illness.

Although the number of persons entering hospitals for emotional problems has increased, the number of patients requiring lengthy and full-time treatment has dropped considerably. For the great majority of patients now being treated, it has become more a matter of *when* they will be released rather than, as in former times, whether release would be possible. This more effective therapy is a result of new methods of treatment, which will be discussed later in this chapter.

## EMOTIONAL DYSORGANIZATION

The traditional approach to a discussion of emotional disturbance has been to describe various abnormal behavior patterns and give them definite labels and diagnoses. Unfortunately, these labels mainly describe the way in which the person is acting at the time, and they have little to do with the basic cause of the problem or the most effective approach to its treatment. They are only descriptions of signs and symptoms.

We have chosen to depart from tradition and instead present some of the ideas of Dr. Karl Menninger, one of the founders of the Menninger Clinic in Topeka, Kansas. This clinic is one of the most outstanding psychiatric hospitals in the United States, and Dr. Menninger is recognized as one of the country's leading psychiatrists. In his book *The Vital Balance,* Dr. Menninger proposes

doing away with much of the labeling of emotional problems and placing emotional problems into a range of severity that extends from relative emotional normalcy to a state of complete emotional collapse.

Dr. Menninger has coined the word *dysorganization* to describe the difficult or painful experiences a person must undergo in trying to maintain successful control over impulses. The prefix *dys-* means "painful" or "difficult." Dysorganization does not mean the same as disorganization, which is a common term meaning a lack of organization or a state of disarrangement. In dysorganization, the process of organization is difficult and painful, but there *is* organization.

According to Menninger's concept, the degree of emotional illness is in proportion to the amount of dysorganization present. There is, of course, a continuous range of degrees of organization. Menninger divides this range into five levels or steps of increasingly severe emotional disorder. Although these five levels are convenient for purposes of description, it should be stressed that they represent selected steps from a continuum and that there may be other levels of emotional dysorganization that lie between them.

### First Level of Dysorganization

The first level of dysorganization is what we commonly call "nervousness." This means that the person is having slightly more than the usual amount of difficulty in coping with his situation and feels an increased amount of tension as a result. He must deal with an increase in such impulses as fear, anger, and frustration. It takes more than the normal amount of effort for him to keep these internal tensions under control.

The nervous person often becomes unusually alert to events around him. He may hear small mysterious noises at night or notice the slightest change in the appearance of something. This alertness is one of the responses to stress that his body makes in preparation for emergency action. His entire perception is sharpened; his senses of sight, hearing, and smell become keener.

Since his body is alert, the nervous person may unconsciously refuse to relax at night, so sleep becomes difficult. He may awaken at the slightest noise. Other first-level symptoms include touchiness, tearfulness, irritability, nervous laughter, moodiness, or depression. Restless behavior is common, such as walking the floor, biting fingernails, chewing pencils, twirling hair, cracking knuckles, or drumming with the fingers.

At this level the person is often worried and spends an excessive amount of time thinking about some topic of concern. Or his mind may wander into a daydream so as to avoid reality, thus preventing effective thought or action.

Psychosomatic disorders are common among people at the first level. Itching skin, upset stomachs, headaches, and various vague pains can be examples of these disorders.

The symptoms of the first level are a response to stress. Anyone who is placed under enough stress will show some of the symptoms of nervousness or the first level of dysorganization. It is for this reason that Dr. Menninger states that everyone is emotionally dysorganized at times, for everyone reaches the first level at times. But when the unusual stress is gone, most people return to a level of optimum adjustment.

Other people are more limited in their ability to cope with stresses. These people chronically function at the first level, even when they are subject only to normal stresses. If these people are subjected to more than the usual amount of stress, or if they are no longer able to control behavior with the first-level devices, they must develop other self-maintenance devices. These new devices lead to the more serious second level of dysorganization.

### Second Level of Dysorganization

The symptoms of the second level are somewhat more serious than those of the first level. They may cause a definite detachment of a person from his environment. The second-level person is less realistic than the first-level person. His ego processes become more difficult, and his coping process becomes definitely unpleasant and emotionally painful. He is an unhappy individual who feels a sense of failure, uselessness, or depression. He sees other people either as indifferent or as definitely antagonistic, though they may actually be trying to help. His control over his words and actions is reduced. He says things he does not really want to say and does things he really would rather not do. His frustration tolerance is very low.

The second-level coping devices may be used temporarily by a usually normal person placed under great stress, or these devices may become a permanent part of the personality. He is still able to function in society, but his coping methods greatly reduce the pleasure he receives from life and also make him a difficult person with whom to associate. Although Menninger suggests that such terms be abandoned as obsolete, the common name for a person who lives at the second level is *neurotic*.

Let us now consider some of the common symptoms of the second level of dysorganization. These are all ways in which the person tries to keep unacceptable impulses (like hostility, guilt, or sexuality) under restraint. These may also be used normally, but not to this degree.

*Withdrawal.* A person may unconsciously withdraw from contact with the world temporarily. He may withdraw by fainting, developing amnesia (loss of memory), refusing to see or hear certain things, or developing *phobias*. Phobias are excessive and often crippling fears of objects or situations, such as high places, closed rooms, insects, cats, thunder, or darkness. Xeno, Hydra, claus

*Self-punishment.* Some people have such intense hostilities toward other people, groups, or situations that they take their hostilities out on themselves. This type of self-punishment is usually quiet and subtle. It often takes the form of an accidental injury or a psychosomatic disease.

*Compensating Acts. Rituals*—Not all ritual should be taken as indicating emotional conflict. For example, there is nothing particularly unhealthy about the ritual of getting up at the same time every morning, showering, shaving, combing hair, and dressing for school. These actions are a means to an end. A ritual indicates a problem when it becomes an end in itself, when the mere act of doing it becomes a kind of release. For example, a student might sharpen his pencil many times while taking a test, not because the pencil point was dull, but because sharpening the pencil relieved some of his anxiety about the test.

*Compensating Acts. Obsessional Thinking*—This is thinking that takes the place of action. Much time is spent in thinking the same thoughts. As such thinking becomes more intense, effective action and productivity decrease. Although this kind of thinking does indicate an emotional problem, it may be of value when a person merely thinks about dangerous aggressive action rather than actually taking such action. Too often, however, obsessional thinking takes the place of needed beneficial action.

*Compensating Acts. Compulsions*—These are irresistible desires or drives to perform acts that seem unreasonable and unnecessary to other people. Compulsive cleanliness is a common example. Many women are so concerned with the cleanliness of their houses that the normal use of the house becomes impossible. For example, a woman might not let her children walk on floors she had cleaned. Compulsive overeating is another example. Some compulsions can lead to serious trouble. Compulsive stealing (kleptomania) and setting fires (pyromania) may be motivated by an unconscious desire to be caught and punished.

Deviant sexual behavior is also a compulsion. Psychiatrists believe that sexual perversions, often aggressive in themselves, represent a cover-up or substitute for even deeper aggressions. Among the more common forms of sexual perversions are pedophilia, having sexual relationships with children; fetishism, gaining sexual satisfaction from objects (often articles of clothing); voyeurism, gaining gratification by watching the sexual activities of other people (the Peeping Tom); sadism, gaining satisfaction from cruelty to another person; and masochism, gaining satisfaction from suffering physical pain.

*Personality Deformities.* Probably the most common second-level symptoms, personality deformities are tendencies to adopt an emergency ego-defense device as a permanent part of one's personality. Many kinds of eccentricities, perversities, dependencies, and unpopular personality traits can be acquired as a chronic maladjustment to the stresses of normal life.

A person may become infantile (beautiful but helpless) or narcissistic (extremely egocentric); develop into a bully, a braggart, a worrier, or a liar; or become dependent on drugs or alcohol. The drug- or alcohol-dependent person is often emotionally immature and uses drugs or alcohol to escape from reality. If he had not turned to drugs or alcohol, he would probably have made use of one or more of the other second-level defense mechanisms.

*Hypochondria.* Another common characteristic of the second level is hypochondria —an exaggerated anxiety and concern about one's own health. The hypochondriac imagines that he is sick or else makes a big issue over very minor disorders. The psychosomatic disorders and hypochondria are processes the ego uses to protect itself from stressful situations. Illness can be an escape mechanism, a means of avoiding responsibilities. Many people go through life with a series of vague illnesses; these people are never really sick, but they are never well enough to assume normal responsibilities. If a doctor is able to cure one illness in such a person, the person replaces that illness with another one. Many more people use illness as a means of avoiding unpleasant situations. Consider the student who develops a sudden headache or upset stomach when an examination, a speech, or a term paper is due. These ailments are very real at the time to those experiencing them.

### Third Level of Dysorganization

This level is characterized by the display of aggressive impulses. The third-level person expresses open and direct aggression to the people and things around him. His id escapes the control of his ego, to utilize Freudian terms. Often the sick individual who commits an aggressive act is showing that all or nearly all of his restricting control has been lost.

In general, such an individual may be described as having the following traits.

1. His aggressive impulse is no longer concealed.
2. He shows disregard for laws and social customs and pays little attention to his conscience.
3. His judgment, consciousness, and perception may be reduced during the aggressive act.
4. He often feels or displays little or no remorse or guilt afterward.
5. After the aggressive act, his emotional tension is relieved.

As in the case of the first two levels of dysorganization, a person may drop to the third level for a short time while he is under great stress and then return to a healthier level of adjustment when the stress is gone, or he can remain at the third level, adopting repeated aggression as his way of life.

Even when a person reaches the third level only temporarily and briefly, the results may be spectacular. He may commit murder or assault, or he may become violent toward property, leaving a place in shambles. Suicide attempts sometimes occur at this level. The person who is constantly at the third level definitely needs treatment, as he presents a threat to society and to himself as well.

### Fourth Level of Dysorganization

The fourth level represents serious emotional disturbance. The severely disturbed person at this level has little or no ego control over his aggressive id impulses. His thought processes are greatly disrupted. Because he loses contact with reality, his interpretation of the outside world is badly distorted. His emotional reactions and behavior are inappropriate, exaggerated, and unpredictable. His behavior may be bizarre. His effective productivity, at home or on the job, is lost. Sometimes his actions are scarcely human.

This is the condition that in the past has been called lunacy or insanity. A more acceptable word for this fourth level today is *psychosis.* A psychotic person is one who suffers from a serious emotional disorder.

Some psychotic behavior patterns have been described as distinct kinds of emotional illness, but Menninger believes that we should consider these patterns merely as different symptoms of the same general disturbance. The fourth level of dysorganization often takes one of the following forms:

*Depression.* The depressed person may feel overwhelmingly sad, guilty, hopeless, or despondent. He may feel inadequate, incompetent, unworthy, or just no good. He often has a slowdown of physical body functions. Everyone feels depressed at times; only in its extreme forms is depression psychotic.

*Excess Excitement (Anxiety).* This person shows a great overflowing of poorly controlled energy. He talks rapidly, constantly, and incoherently. He may indulge in much bizarre activity, such as walking in a circle day after day or repeatedly stacking and restacking the same objects.

*Excess Concern with Self.* This person may be mute and totally withdrawn into himself. He may have delusions of his own importance, constantly telling people that he is God, Jesus, the President of the United States, or some other important figure.

*Persecution Complex (Paranoia).* This person may imagine that people are plotting to get him in some way and he may become very suspicious, resentful, and defensive.

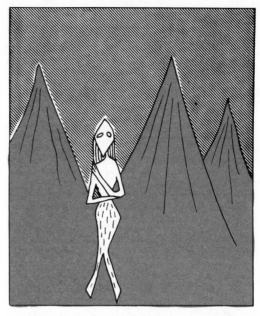

Artwork by the mentally ill, such as this painting by a schizophrenic, can be one of many indicators of what happens in the isolated mind of the emotionally disturbed. The altered perceptions reflected in a painting can be like a "broken twig in the forest" — important to the questioning therapist, but a clue which is difficult to interpret.

### Fifth Level of Dysorganization

The fifth level represents the greatest extreme to which the ego processes can be pushed. The ego completely disintegrates and rejects life itself; the will to live is gone. All that is left is a self-destructive determination to end life, or to settle for minimal existence.

The extremely ill person either commits suicide or becomes like a human vegetable, refusing to eat, drink, or make any contact with reality. Force-feeding may be necessary in order to prevent his starvation.

The earnest suicide attempts of the fifth-level person are quite different from the half-hearted suicide displays of people at the first three levels. In the exhibition suicide, the person is consciously or unconsciously hoping and planning for a last-minute rescue. This type includes the person who stands on a rooftop or at an open window while a crowd gathers and the fire department is called. It also includes the person who takes a few sleeping pills and immediately calls for help. These display efforts at suicide stem from various motivations. In general, however, these attempts should be interpreted as a desperate cry for help. The person who makes such an effort should have some professional psychiatric help, as it has been found that such persons often make repeated suicide attempts. The next time they might be serious and succeed.

### *Suicide*

Suicide is the tenth leading cause of death in the United States today. The "official" annual suicide rate is about 12 per 100,000 population and over 24,000 deaths are recorded as suicides each year. The actual suicide rate is probably closer to double the official rate as many suicides are disguised as accidents or natural deaths to avoid loss of insurance money or stigmatization of survivors.

No group or class of people is free of suicide. Every person is a potential suicide; and almost everyone at some time during his life gives some consideration to the possibility of suicide. However, the risk of suicide does relate to certain individual characteristics.

The most significant pattern in the incidence of suicide is the increase with advancing age. Suicide is rare among those under 14 years of age. The rate rises sharply in adolescence and sharply again among college students, for whom suicide is second only to accidents as a cause of death. Several factors are commonly associated with college suicides, the most frequent of which is academic failure. Failure brings not only the disappointment and disapproval of parents, but a shattering of personal self-confidence as well. The second leading cause of college suicide is the end of a love affair. When romance ends, there is more than just disappointment; there is the tumultuous feeling of being rejected and abandoned, the complete loss of self-esteem. College suicides often involve the reserved, introverted, or shy students who, lacking social contacts, tend to internalize their problems. Despite the alarming college suicide rate, many colleges offer little or no on-campus therapy for emotional problems.

The suicide rate rises again in middle age when the male realizes that his career goals have not been attained and are in fact now unattainable. The middle-aged woman may turn to suicide in reaction to menopause, if she feels "finished" as a woman, or upon the departure from home of her children, after which she may no longer feel useful and needed.

Finally, the suicide rate reaches its peak among the elderly, who today suffer from a host of emotionally crippling influences. Our society now emphasizes youth and young ideas. After a forced retirement at age 65, many people feel useless, lonely, bored, and frustrated. In addition, they may suffer great financial insecurity, physical pain from chronic ailments, or may have terminal illnesses. For persons over age 85, the suicide rate is 26 per 100,000.

For the United States in general, the suicide rate among men is greater than among women, though on the West Coast there are more successful female suicides than male. Nationally, women "attempt" suicide at least five times as frequently as men, though their attempts are often half-hearted and are really motivated by other desires. The bored housewife is the greatest suicide potential; she makes twice as many attempts as all other female classifications. For successful suicides, the percentage of male and female are 70 and 30, respectively. Among college students, males are twice as likely to commit suicide as females.

In recent years the suicide rate for women has risen sharply, while the rate for men has remained fairly static. This increase has been attributed to various causes. Possibly part of the increase is related to increasing opportunities and expectations for women. The opportunity to succeed in a career is also the opportunity to fail. It has been suggested that women are now committing suicide for reasons that were once more typical of males, such as despondency over unfulfilled career goals. On the other hand, a woman who spends her days at home in the traditional role of "wife and mother" may see herself as a failure as she perceives decreasing social approval of this role. There may be conflicts between her desires to succeed in the traditional role of homemaker and in a career as well. There is undoubtedly increasing marital dissatisfaction, as evidenced by the rapidly climbing divorce rate.

In general, suicide is less frequent among married persons, with the notable exception of those under 24 years of age in whom the rate is much higher than in single persons. In single people over 24 and in divorced people of any age, the rate is higher than among married people over 24. The rate among young widows (under 35) is quite high.

Racially, suicide is more than twice as prevalent among whites as blacks. Among young American Indians, however, the suicide rate is at an epidemic level.

There is a direct relationship between suicide and social status—the higher one stands on the social scale, the more susceptible he becomes to suicide. The rate is high among doctors, dentists, lawyers, business executives, and similar professionals. Among physicians in general, the rate is 33 per 100,000 (compared with 12 per 100,000 for the general public); among psychiatrists it is reported as between 60 and 70 per 100,000 in various surveys.

Suicide rates even relate to the time of year, soaring in the spring and during holiday periods, especially Christmas. Apparently, depression resulting from loneliness and business and social failures becomes unbearably painful during the supposedly "happy" times of the year.

*Theories on the Causes of Suicide.* Many psychological theories have been proposed to explain suicide, ranging from the Freudian to the behavioral. Most authorities agree that suicide may have a variety of motivations and that in a particular case there is rarely a single precipitating cause of suicide and that several causes are usually operative in an additive way. All of the following psychological factors are possible motives for suicide: severe depression in which life seems an unbearable burden; psychosis in which suicide is a response to hallucinations or delusions (this sometimes happens in LSD flashbacks); suicide for spite, in which the motive is to hurt the survivors (such as parents, a spouse, or a lover); poor impulse control, leading to suicide following some minor frustration; identification with celebrities or relatives that have committed suicide; and chronic or terminal illness.

Serious losses (or threats of loss) play a major role in the psychodynamics of suicide. These include loss of health, loved ones, money, earning power, job, pride, beauty, status, friends, children, and independence.

Social isolation is a common factor in those who resort to suicide. The more intimately one is involved with others, the less likely he is to consider suicide. Unfortunately, the severe depression that commonly precedes suicide is likely to lead to social alienation and isolation, further increasing the chance of suicide. Suicide may be considered the final outcome of a progressive failure of adaptation, with isolation and alienation from the usual network of human relationships that support us all and give meaning to our lives.

*Danger Signs of Impending Suicide.* It is not true that people who threaten to commit suicide never do so. Most people who attempt suicide actually give warnings, vocal or non-vocal, beforehand. Potential suicides can usually be recognized before they act. Knowledge of the danger signs can save a life. Any of the following indicates a definite risk of suicide (adapted from Solomon and Patch, 1971):

1. Previous attempts. Over half of those who successfully commit suicide have a history of a previous attempt.
2. Previous psychosis. A history of psychiatric disturbance indicates the possibility of a recurrence.
3. Suicide note.
4. Violent method. The more violent and painful the method chosen, the more serious the intent.
5. Presence of chronic disease.
6. Recent surgery or childbirth. The birth of a baby leads to a severe post-partum depression in some women.
7. Alcoholism or drug dependence. Drug or alcohol dependence indicates a person who needs to escape. The permanent escape of suicide is often appealing to such a person. Also, while actually under the influence of drugs or alcohol, the ability to resist the suicide impulse is weakened.
8. Hypochondriasis. Constant physical complaints often indicate underlying depression.
9. Advancing age.
10. Homosexuality. The suicide rate among homosexuals is high.
11. Social isolation. Indicates severe depression.
12. Chronic maladjustment.
13. Bankrupt resources. A person without money, job, or friends may see little to live for.
14. No obvious secondary gains. Many suicide threats are really attempts to manipulate others. For example, women often use the suicide threat to keep a dying marriage or love affair going. When there is no such motive and the threat is truly self-directed, the chance of suicide is much greater.
15. *Signs of grave risk:*
    a. The wish to die. Repeated statements by a person that he would be better off dead indicate very high suicide risk.
    b. Presence of psychosis. The psychotic person who is suspicious, fearful, or hears voices should be regarded as potentially suicidal.
    c. Depression is the most common cause of suicide. Any of the following symptoms indicates severe risk:
       (1) Guilt.
       (2) Feelings of worthlessness and despondency.
       (3) Intense wish for punishment.
       (4) Withdrawal and hopelessness.
       (5) Extreme agitation and anxiety.
       (6) Loss of the four appetites—food, sex, sleep, and activity.
       (7) Sudden well-being in a previously depressed person may reflect the feeling of relief at having made the decision to die.

*Prevention of Suicide.* Most suicidal people are not fully intent on dying. Though their wish to die may be extremely strong, there is almost always an underlying wish to live. But the suicidal person does not wish to live as he is living, for this he sees as being the same or even worse than death. Thus, the crucial element that makes suicide prevention possible is *ambivalence.* Even as suicidal impulses become almost overwhelming, the ebbing wish to live is a root of energy that can be tapped for suicide prevention.

The role of the layman in the suicide crisis is much the same as in any first-aid situation. It is to preserve life until professional help can be attained—it is not to play "doctor." In many cities there are 24-hour telephone services staffed by mental health professionals or volunteers specially trained in crisis intervention. If such a service is available, one's first efforts should be in aiding or encouraging the suicidal person to call for help. If a crisis intervention service is not available, or if the suicidal person will not cooperate in calling such a service, he must be kept from committing suicide until other professional help can be attained.

The first step in suicide intervention is to establish a relationship with the suicidal person and maintain contact with him. As an opening line, the National Save-A-Life League suggests asking, "Are you thinking of killing yourself?" Communication in crisis intervention must be open and direct. One must remain calm and convey attitudes of helpfulness, hopefulness, and genuine concern, building upon the suicidal person's ambivalence about dying, convincing him that he really does want to live. One must encourage him to relate all he can about his problems or troubles and show him that, with help, he can solve his problems too.

Everyone has some strengths. The severely depressed person often loses sight of his own strengths or his ability to use them. In talking to a suicidal person, one should keep emphasizing his strengths so as to decrease his feelings of helplessness and hopelessness.

As soon as the immediate crisis of threatened suicide seems to have abated, he should be encouraged to seek competent professional help. *Suicidal impulses recur,* and it is dangerous to assume that there will not be further suicide attempts. As many friends or relatives as possible should be involved in the emotional support of the person, because the chance of suicide is reduced through social interaction and increased through alienation.

### Recognizing the Severely Disturbed

With today's high incidence of emotional problems, there are few of us who do not occasionally encounter a severely disturbed person. Such a person may be a close relative, a neighbor, or a stranger encountered in a public place. In any case, it is important to be able to recognize the individual as disturbed and to know how to handle such a person. A person suffering from severe emotional disturbance will generally exhibit one or more observable symptoms.

*Changes in Behavior Pattern.* A normally quiet person may become suddenly very belligerent or overtalkative. Or conversely, the happy, outgoing person may become quiet and moody. Any sudden and radical change in a person's normal mood or behavior may indicate emotional conflict. What is important here is a change in the general pattern of behavior extending over a long period of time, not just a passing reaction to some stress or irritant.

*Loss of Touch with Reality.* The emotionally disturbed person usually (some authorities say always) suffers some degree of loss of contact with reality, ranging from slight to total. He may be unable to recall who he is, where he is, why he is there, the day or date, or similar information. Or he may withdraw totally from reality to the extent that he is completely unaware of his environment.

*Amnesia.* Temporary or permanent memory loss is a common symptom of mental disturbance. One of the mind's defense mechanisms is to repress those memories that are too painful for the conscious mind to bear. Loss of memory is also characteristic of the senile elderly person, often as a result of reduced blood supply to the brain due to arteriosclerosis.

*Delusions.* A delusion is a distorted belief or idea. Emotionally disturbed persons often harbor beliefs (called delusions of grandeur) that they are famous scientists or surgeons, prosperous executives, secret agents, or even God. Much harm may be done to themselves or to others when they act upon such delusions. Even more dangerous are delusions of persecution in which family members, neighbors, members of racial or religious groups, or just a vague "they" are believed to be plotting against the person. A person suffering from such delusions of persecution may be dangerous, as he may suddenly react to these beliefs by attacking those who he feels are "after" him.

*One-sided Conversations.* In the folk lore of emotional disorders one of the sure signs is "talking to yourself." Actually, just about everyone talks to himself from time to time. But a person carrying on an animated conversation to himself in a public place is very likely disturbed.

*Hallucinations.* Severely disturbed persons very commonly suffer hallucinations of one or more of the senses. They hear voices; they see, smell, taste, and feel imaginary things. Though such hallucinations may seem absurd to others, they are very real to those suffering from them, even to the point that they are acted upon, with serious or even fatal results. A frequent problem today is "flashback" halluncination following the use of hallucinogenic drugs, especially LSD and mescaline. Such flashbacks may occur many months after the last drug usage and may be severe enough to produce violent actions directed toward the hallucinating individual or others.

### Dealing with the Severely Disturbed

With increasing incidences of emotional disturbance, drug abuse, stressful situations, and increasing population density, the "psychiatric emergency" is becoming more commonplace. This may be defined as a situation in a public or private place in which an individual's behavior becomes dangerous to himself or others and for which prompt and decisive action must be taken. In dealing with a severely disturbed person, the immediate regard is for the safety of everyone concerned. In addition, the ability of the patient to recover and the speed of his recovery often depend on the handling he receives during the acute emergency phase of his illness.

The handling of the psychiatric emergency should be thought of as first aid and the basic rules of first aid applied. The prime rule is to recognize your own limitations as an untrained person. To attempt to play psychiatrist is to risk physical injury, lawsuit, and further deterioration of the condition of the disturbed person. Thus, the best course of action is to immediately call for assistance. A physician, even though not a psychiatrist, can often help calm the disturbed individual. Most policemen have both training and experience in handling disturbed persons, and are generally more readily available than physicians. While waiting for assistance, keep cool and calm and take only such action as is absolutely necessary to prevent someone from being hurt. Such action should involve a minimum of physical force or harsh words and should include efforts to reassure the disturbed person that you are his friend and are trying to protect and help him. If physical restraint becomes necessary, use only as much force as is absolutely necessary.

## TREATMENT OF EMOTIONAL DISORDERS

Fortunately, the methods and facilities for the treatment of emotional problems have been greatly improved during recent years. The person who becomes emotionally disturbed today, regardless of the level of dysorganization he reaches, stands an excellent chance of recovery if he receives the benefit of modern methods of treatment and if this treatment is begun promptly. Most patients today begin to show improvement very quickly. If they are hospitalized, they usually return home in only a few weeks, to continue treatment on an outpatient basis.

We shall consider some of the methods of treatment in use today, the different types of personnel working with the disturbed person, and the types of facilities that are now available for the treatment of emotional problems. Many different forms of treatment for emotional disorders have been used at one time or another in the past. Some have been abandoned as newer methods developed and others have been reduced in importance. Of those methods that remain today, some are administered in a hospital and others are used in outpatient clinics. These forms of treatment may be grouped into several main categories.

### Psychoanalysis

Psychoanalysis is a system of therapy dating back to Freud in which great importance is attached to the role of the subconscious mind causing emotional conflict. Psychoanalysis attempts to explore the unconscious mind through a long series of sessions in which the patient freely relates anything that happens to come to his mind. The therapist, called an analyst, interprets what the patient says, trying to help the patient recognize the subconscious feelings that have led to his problems.

Psychoanalysis has been of value to some patients with minor emotional conflicts, but is of little value for major mental disturbances. Also, this type of treatment for even a minor emotional problem may extend over several years at great expense to the patient. It is obvious that factors of effectiveness, time, and expense restrict the use of psychoanalysis to a rather limited clientele of only mildly disturbed patients.

### Other Individual Psychotherapies

Psychotherapy involves a dialogue between the patient and a specially qualified person. This therapy should result in the patient's having a better understanding of himself and of the ways to handle his affairs more effectively. The patient should learn to replace ineffective or undesirable coping devices with more appropriate methods. Psychotherapy is usually administered by a psychiatrist, psychoanalyst, or a clinical psychologist. (The distinctions among these types of therapists will be discussed later.) Psychotherapy is commonly given in outpatient clinics, offices, hospitals, and schools, and is of importance today for all levels of emotional problems, from the most minor to the most severe. Those with minor problems may need only a few sessions, but serious cases may need months or years of continued treatment.

### Reality Therapy

An interesting (though not universally accepted) concept of emotional conflict is presented by William Glasser, a psychiatrist, in his book *Reality Therapy* (Harper and Row, 1965). His belief is that everyone who is emotionally disturbed suffers from the same basic inadequacy—his inability to fulfill his basic human needs. The severity of the symptoms reflects the degree to which the individual is unable to fulfill his needs, and whatever the symptom, it disappears when the person's needs are successfully fulfilled.

Glasser sees another common characteristic among all his patients—they all deny the reality of the world around them. His concept of reality therapy is to lead patients toward reality through helping them find effective ways of fulfilling their needs.

According to Glasser, the two needs most often unfulfilled are the need to be loved and to love and the need for self-esteem. We all have these needs, but we vary in our ability to fulfill them. Central to the fulfillment of either need is involvement with other people—at the very least, one person, but hopefully many more than one. For good emotional health we must, at all times in our lives, have at least one person who cares about us and for whom we care ourselves. If we do not have this essential person, we will be unable to fulfill our basic needs. One characteristic is essential in the other person—he must be able to fulfill his own needs and thus be in touch with reality. In other words, he must be in good emotional health. Of course, it is common for two people to mutually fulfill their needs and thus maintain their emotional health through their involvement with each other. Glasser sees the role of the psychiatrist or psychologist as providing someone for temporary involvement until the patient learns to fulfill his need through involvement with others.

Another basic concept in reality therapy is *responsibility,* which Glasser defines as the ability to fulfill one's needs in a way that does not deprive others of the ability to fulfill their needs. This equation of emotional health with responsibility interjects a moral tone into reality therapy that is absent from conventional therapy. Conventional therapists generally consider deviant behavior to be a product of emotional illness, and the patient should not be held morally responsible because he is considered helpless to do anything about it. Glasser feels that in their effort to avoid the issue of morality, many conventional therapists accept behavior that does not lead to need fulfillment and that the irresponsibility of many patients is the

cause of their emotional disturbance, not its excusable result. Glasser claims particular success in the treatment of delinquent adolescents with his emphasis on responsibility.

Another departure from conventional therapy is that reality therapy does not probe into the patient's past life in a search for deep psychological roots for problems. The emphasis is, rather, on teaching the patient better ways to fulfill his needs within the confines of reality and responsibility. The past is discussed only enough to show the patient how and why his behavior has failed to fulfill his needs in a responsible manner.

It must be emphasized that reality therapy, like all other current theories on emotional disorder, is not universally accepted by all practicing therapists, but is favored by some therapists for some patients.

### Milieu Therapy

Severe emotional disorders generally require a period of hospitalization. The recovery process is greatly aided if the hospital is organized as a therapeutic community. Thus, milieu therapy refers to the conscious use of the social setting or environment in the treatment of psychiatric patients. It is concerned with physical environment, atmosphere within the psychiatric setting, attitudes, interaction among staff and patients, interaction among patients, and social organization. It adds use of the social system to individual therapy. In milieu therapy, the patient becomes an active participant instead of passively receiving treatment. His strengths are emphasized together with those areas in which he needs help; he is recognized as part of a community that has a culture of its own.

The doctors, nurses, and other members of the therapeutic team generally work in street clothes, rather than in uniforms, which tend to create communication barriers and detract from the therapeutic environment.

Since staff members act as role models for patients, it is accepted as part of milieu therapy that the appearance of the staff influences the patients. An attractive, vitally alive staff carries much nonverbal impact.

In milieu therapy, the environment is modified to facilitate more effective patterns of interaction. Social interaction is an important part of the treatment of the psychiatric patient. A well-organized milieu program includes provisions for patients and staff to make decisions on matters concerning themselves through the medium of community and small group meetings. Group therapy and patient-centered activities which are planned and carried out by patients are essential to a complete program. Work therapy or vocational rehabilitation is also an integral part of milieu therapy.

### Group Therapy

Group therapy, in its many forms, involves processes that occur in structured and protected groups and are calculated to cause rapid improvement in personality and behavior of individual members through controlled group interactions. Group psychotherapy was introduced into the United States in 1905 by Joseph Pratt, a Boston internist, to bolster the morale of his tuberculosis patients.

Group therapy is, to a large degree, based on the same theoretical principles as individual psychotherapy. However, it has additional dimensions and is often useful for problems not adequately met by individual therapy. Traditionally, group therapy has been conducted by psychiatrists, psychologists, and social workers. In response to the growing demand for it, many nurses, clergymen, educators, other professionals, and even laymen have become involved as leaders of group therapy sessions.

The criteria for success in group therapy are essentially the same as for individual therapy, such as relief from emotional distress, insight, enhanced personal dignity, and improved behavior and social relations. Individual therapy is sometimes preferable in achieving insight, but group therapy provides a better opportunity to "see ourselves as others see us."

The success of group therapy depends largely on the skill and degree of involvement of the therapist and the proper selection of patients. The therapist who considers group therapy to be an inferior form of psychotherapy tends to prescribe it for his least promising patients; if the results are then poor, his prejudice is reinforced.

While the lower cost of group therapy is one obvious advantage over individual therapy, it is not the only advantage, nor the most important one. Group therapy, for example, offers a remedy for the social isolation often resulting from the technological aspects of modern life. The group can multiply the effects of therapy by bringing many minds and viewpoints to bear upon each patient's individual problems. Group therapy offers the further advantage of providing each member with a "safe" human-relations laboratory. Within the protection of the group, each patient has the opportunity to test various ways of relating to others and to discover how others respond. The patient's dignity is enhanced when he is a giver as well as a receiver of help. Truly valuable insights and interpretations are often given by one patient to another. In an atmosphere of mutual help, the patient also becomes a therapist.

There are many human conditions for which group therapy is often more useful than individual therapy. Among these are shy and lonely people, whose very reluctance to enter group therapy is an indication that they could profit from it; patients who become

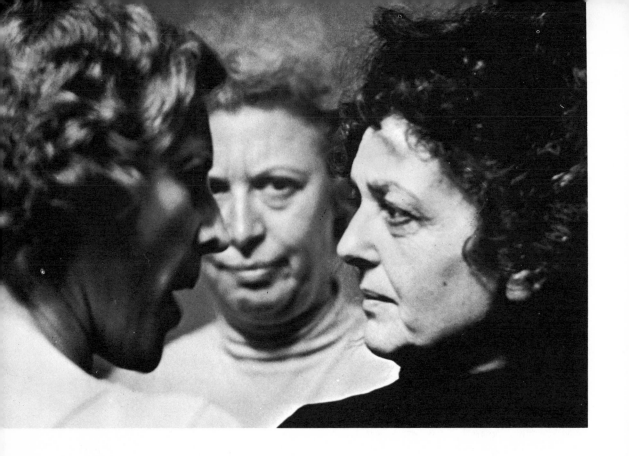

A group therapy session. The participants gain in self-awareness as they discuss their problems, question each other, and work with the therapist to better understand themselves. *Photo by Hella Hammid; Rapho-Guillumette.*

too dependent upon an individual therapist; patients trying to overcome phobias; patients who feel antagonism and fear toward parental and authority figures and thus withhold their true feelings from an individual therapist; patients who have had unsatisfactory relations with siblings or who have been without brothers or sisters; adolescents with confused sexual identification; patients with difficulty in getting along with others (those who demand much and give little, or have other ways of alienating people) are likely to show their characteristic behavior in the group and to be made aware of it by the others; patients with problems seen as shameful or unusual (such as homosexuals, bed-wetters, alcoholics, drug abusers, or obese persons) can be of great emotional support to one another; and married couples who, in couples groups, find that the problems they had considered unique to their marriage are often present in other marriages as well.

The many forms of group therapy can be broadly classified as evocative, directive, or didactic. Evocative methods of group therapy are those that encourage spontaneous expression of feelings by patients in an atmosphere of acceptance and of effort toward understanding those feelings. In group therapy the evocative leader promotes mutual interaction among patients in preference to exchanges between patient and therapist. The leader avoids authoritarianism. He does not demand that patients express the "right" attitude; he wants them to feel free to express their *real* attitudes. In evocative groups, the patients and leader generally sit in a circle. Thus, the therapist is not placed in any special position that would make him the focal point of the group's attention. Most group therapy today is of the evocative approach. Some specific forms include activity therapy, group psychoanalysis, T-groups (training groups), encounter groups, transactional analysis, sensitivity groups, and psychodrama.

Directive group therapy methods are those in which the leader asserts his authority, especially as an expert on proper attitudes and conduct. Advice and commands may be given. In directive groups the leader stands or sits in a special position, so that he is the focal point of the group's attention. Some examples of directive therapy include organized religion (the leader being the clergyman in his pulpit), Alcoholics Anonymous, and Synanon.

Didactic group methods aim at educating patients, often with factual knowledge about their problems and their treatment. The distinction between didactic and directive therapy is that the didactic approach seeks to educate, whereas the directive approach seeks to indoctrinate. Typical of didactic therapy

are classes and seminars for institutionalized patients with psychosis, sex deviations, and other problems that respond poorly to less structured approaches. Through understanding the nature, causes, and treatments of their conditions, the patients' fear and hostility toward treatment are diminished and they are motivated to cooperate with other forms of therapy.

### T-Groups, Encounter Groups, and Sensitivity Groups

T-groups are training groups that first came into use as a method of training psychiatrists and other mental health professionals, especially those interested in becoming group therapists. T-groups are not therapy groups—their participants are presumed to be well rather than ill. The T-group differs from the therapy group in that it is concerned with conscious or preconscious behavior rather than unconscious motivation. The participant learns human relations, communications, and leadership skills. He learns about the dynamics of his own behavior and that of others by being in the group under the guidance of a "trainer."

The objectives of training include self-insight, better understanding of other persons and awareness of one's impact upon them, better understanding of group processes and increased skill in achievement of group effectiveness, increased recognition of the characteristics of social systems, and greater awareness of the dynamics of change.

A T-group is typically composed of 12 to 15 persons who work together on an intensive schedule of perhaps 6 hours a day for 2 weeks or in marathon sessions that continue uninterrupted for 48 hours. If the group is to be successful in meeting its goals, the following conditions should be met: (1) each individual must share his thoughts and feelings; (2) a continuously operating feedback system must reflect the relevancy of each individual's behavior; (3) a group atmosphere of trust is necessary for persons to be able to reveal their thoughts and feelings; (4) each person needs enough knowledge of psychological theory to understand his own experience; and (5) each participant must have the opportunity to try new behavior patterns following the sessions. Unless these new learnings can be applied, they will soon be forgotten. Thus, the critical steps in the T-group process are presentation of feelings, feedback from others regarding those feelings, and experimentation with new behavior patterns.

The T-group method has been extended from mental health professionals to business executives, clergymen, medical students, and others whose work demands special ability in dealing with people. Recently, some T-groups have developed a new function as a social movement for overcoming "alienation" or emotional distance between people in general. Such groups are also called sensitivity groups or encounter groups and participation is not limited to special professional or occupational groups.

### Transactional Analysis

Transactional analysis focuses on the hidden meanings in interpersonal communications and is a useful tool in group therapy. It was popularized by Eric Berne in 1964 through his bestselling *Games People Play*. He called each unit of communication a transaction. When two or more people encounter each other, sooner or later one of them will speak or in some other way acknowledge the presence of the others. This first communication is called the transactional stimulus. Another person will then say or do something in response to this stimulus, and that is called the transactional response. Transactional analysis is concerned with diagnosing the real psychological motivations behind the transac-

tional stimulus and response. This approach is especially useful for groups of married couples, in whom it may reveal the playing of verbal and nonverbal games. Berne's "games" are repetitive, neurotic interactions with hidden meanings. Among the commonly played games described by Berne are "see what you made me do," "frigid woman," "if it weren't for you," and "look how hard I've tried."

### Behavior Therapy

Behavior therapy is the application to human beings of techniques derived from experiments with animal behavior. The behavior therapies differ in several important respects from traditional psychotherapy procedures. Perhaps the most important difference is that the behavior therapist addresses himself directly to the task of modifying objectionable behavior, rather than attempting to identify the "underlying unconscious disease process" that most psychotherapists (and all psychoanalysts) believe to be the cause of symptoms.

For this reason the behavior therapist does not deal with the unconscious, ego structures, or defense mechanisms, and does not employ insight as a prime treatment means. Behavior therapy is mainly used for patients with rather specific behavioral difficulties, rather than for those whose problems are more diverse.

The rationale of behavior therapy is that the undesirable behavior patterns were learned in the first place and, with proper training techniques, can be unlearned (behaviorists use the term "extinguished"). Extinction may involve either weakening the undesirable responses or learning new responses that are incompatible with the ones being extinguished.

There are several major types of behavior therapy. The *classical conditioning therapies* make use of unlearned, constitutional reflex behavior to modify or eliminate unwanted behavior. One of the major classical techniques is *counterconditioning,* in which new, more desirable responses are conditioned to the same stimuli that produce the undesirable responses. Varieties of counterconditioning include *aversion therapy,* in which the undesirable behavior response is accompanied by a nausea-producing drug, mild electric shock, or similar unpleasant experience; *reciprocal inhibition,* in which the patient is taught a response, such as relaxation, that is incompatible with the unwanted response to a given stimulus; and *desensitization,* in which the patient, under "safe" conditions, faces anxiety- or fear-arousing stimuli in gradually increasing degrees, so that other responses can be conditioned to them. This is particularly effective in treating phobias of many kinds.

Another type of behavior therapy is *operant conditioning,* in which the undesirable behavior is modified by the appropriate use of positive and negative reinforcers. (A reinforcer is a stimulus or event that changes the rate of a behavior when it follows that behavior.) In operant conditioning, positive reinforcers, such as food or desired objects or privileges, are used to reward desirable behavior; while negative reinforcers, such as pain, verbal reprimand, or the loss of desired objects or privileges, are used to "punish" undesirable behavior. By combining positive and negative reinforcement, a behavior therapist can do much to eliminate undesirable behavior and encourage suitable behavior patterns. This, of course, is basically how most parents raise their children.

Operant conditioning can be effective with relatively large groups of people in social situations. Entire wards in mental hospitals, for example, can be placed under a "token economy" in which coinlike tokens are given (and taken away) as reinforcement for certain behaviors. The hospital thereby becomes more like the world outside, and patients are led to interact with other people in useful ways. The tokens earned may be "spent" for such desired items as food, privacy, minor luxuries, or even leave from the hospital. The token economy can be an important part of milieu therapy, discussed earlier.

Behavior therapy has received a mixed reception among mental health professionals. Behavioral psychologists are highly in favor of it for almost every manner of mental disorder, while other psychologists and many psychiatrists remain unconvinced of its value. The true value of behavior therapy probably lies somewhere between these extremes of acceptance or rejection. As previously mentioned, it is best suited for the treatment of rather specific behavioral problems. It is of less value for most severe psychotic disorders and most general personality disorders.

The greatest success of behavior therapy has been in treating such problems as phobias, severe anxiety, obsessional thinking, sexual disorders of many kinds, overeating, gambling, and other compulsive behaviors. Drug dependence and alcoholism have also been treated, though with somewhat less success. Patients who have spent many years locked in the back wards of mental hospitals because they lack elementary social skills and competencies are often able to leave such wards following behavior modification procedures which teach them the rudiments of social skills. While they are not all able to leave the hospital, many actually do, and many more are able to spend their days in happier circumstances in less restrictive wards.

The advantages of behavior therapy, in cases for which it is suited, include: (1) It often works. (2) It may be administered by such nonprofessional therapists as psychiatric aides, parents, and school teachers, after only a few hours of training. (3) The procedures are clear-cut, unambiguous, and consistent; results may be achieved in a short period of time, often just a few weeks. (4) It is rare for a new behavioral problem to appear in the place of the old one.

### Drug Therapy (Chemotherapy)

The development of new drugs has had an important influence on the treatment of emotional illness in recent years; they have become a primary means of treating the seriously disturbed patient. The use of these drugs has reduced the time needed for improvement and recovery and has actually lowered the population of many mental hospitals.

The many drugs available fall into several basic groups. Among these are the tranquilizers, which are used to calm anxiety; the sedatives, which combat overactivity and insomnia as well as anxiety; the antidepressants, which help raise the mood of severely depressed patients; and antipsychotics, used to reduce or temporarily remove such symptoms as hallucinations.

Drugs are sometimes used as the primary treatment in cases of mild anxiety or mild depression. But in more serious cases, drugs are used in connection with psychotherapy. Often, the function of the drugs is to make the patient accessible for psychotherapy. Before these drugs were available, many patients were too agitated or too withdrawn to be reached by psychotherapy.

The old-time psychiatric hospital ward, with some patients wildly agitated and others mute and withdrawn, is fortunately becoming a thing of the past through the use of modern drugs. The drugs are not curing the patients, but they are making them calm and rational enough to participate in psychotherapy. After release from the hospital, many patients continue on drugs, and possibly psychotherapy, for varying periods of time.

Today, perhaps 90 percent of all cases of emotional disorder, including major and minor forms, are treated with psychotherapy, drugs, or a combination of the two. Although the use of other forms of treatment thus has become secondary, we will briefly describe two of them.

### Shock Therapy

Today shock therapy is used in only a few of the most severely disturbed patients. The most important of several kinds of shock therapy is called electroconvulsive therapy, in which violent muscular contractions, much like epileptic convulsions, are produced by carefully controlled electrical impulses. The purpose of shock therapy in severe cases is much the same as that of drugs—to make the patient accessible and receptive to psychotherapy. Insulin shock is also used to produce similar results.

### Lobotomy

Rarely necessary today, lobotomy is the surgical severing of the nerve tracts that connect the frontal lobes of the brain to the thalamus. The frontal lobes are centers for fear and anxiety. Today the same results produced by a lobotomy can almost always be achieved through drugs.

## PROFESSIONAL WORKERS FOR THE EMOTIONALLY DISTURBED

Many patients today are treated by a specially trained group of people, rather than by one individual. This group is sometimes called the psychiatric team. In addition to physicians and nurses, it may include psychologists, occupational therapists, social workers, and others who are concerned with specialized problems. Let us consider several members of this team.

*Psychiatrist.* A psychiatrist is a physician (M.D.) who has had additional specialized training in treating mental illness and has been licensed by the American Board of Psychiatry and Neurology. The psychiatrist may use any method of treatment he prefers, whether individual, group, drug, or shock therapy.

*Psychoanalyst.* A psychoanalyst is usually a physician who has had additional specialized training in psychoanalytic methodology and has fulfilled the requirements for membership in a psychoanalytic association. He uses some variation of Freudian theory.

*Clinical psychologist.* The clinical psychologist does not go through medical school, but instead does postgraduate study in psychology. He usually holds the degree of doctor of philosophy (Ph.D.) or master of arts (M.A.). He gives psychological tests, makes diagnoses, and engages in psychotherapy. He does not use drugs or shock therapy, since these may be employed only by a medically trained person. In mental institutions he often works in association with a psychiatrist.

*Psychiatric social worker.* The psychiatric social worker takes two years of postgraduate study and holds a master's degree in social work, with training in psychology. He makes contact with relatives, friends, employers, and others connected with the patient. He assists them in making any changes in the environment of the patient that seem necessary for the patient's recovery.

*Psychiatric registered nurse.* The psychiatric nurse is a registered nurse who has had special training and experience with the mentally ill. She may supervise a hospital ward and administer treatments under the supervision of a psychiatrist, as well as assisting in therapy.

*Mental health aide or assistant.* The aide or assistant, referred to as a *psychiatric technician* in several states, is charged with the actual physical care and custody of the hospitalized patient. The aide or technician is a paramedical staff person who has received on-the-job training. A few colleges now offer training programs for psychiatric technicians. Aides are important because of the great amount of time they spend with the patient and the personal influence they may have over him. A good relationship between the aide and the patient can greatly speed the recovery process.

## TREATMENT FACILITIES FOR EMOTIONAL ILLNESS

*Outpatient clinics.* Many patients with minor to moderately severe emotional illness can be treated today while they are still living at home. Psychotherapy sessions usually play an important part in such treatment. The psychiatrist or psychologist administering this care can be either in private practice, supported entirely by patient fees, or in a community clinic, supported by government or charity. Often these community clinics have a sliding scale of fees, determined by the ability of the patient to pay.

Outpatient clinics are also very important in providing care for the patient who has had short-term hospitalization during the acute stage of his illness and is completing his recovery at home. Such follow-up treatment can greatly reduce the chances of his needing to return to the hospital.

*Psychiatric sections of general hospitals.*

There is a growing trend for general hospitals to build or reserve certain sections specifically for the treatment of emotional disorders. These provide the patient with psychiatric treatment in a hospital setting without requiring him to travel far from home. They also help reduce the social stigma of emotional illness by treating it in the same context as any other disorder.

*State mental hospitals.* In the past, emotional problems often required prolonged hospitalization because no effective methods of treatment were available. Some patients received only custodial care, that is, they were given humane shelter, but no specific treatment. Since hospitalization was so prolonged, the responsibility for its cost was usually assumed by the state government. The main purpose of such hospitals was to confine the ill where they could not bother anyone.

Most states are now applying the newer approaches to the treatment of emotional problems, with results often comparable to those obtained in private hospitals. It has been shown that if a state is willing to spend the money to provide intensive care for newly admitted, acutely ill patients, money will be saved in the long run. Given this intensive care, many patients can leave the hospital in a short time. Without such care, the same patients may require hospitalization at state expense for years, and perhaps even for life. The states that recognize this principle have actually been able to reduce the population of their state mental hospitals during a period in which the population of the country has risen and the incidence of emotional problems has climbed.

*Private mental hospitals.* In recent years, increasing numbers of privately owned hospitals for the exclusive treatment of mental or emotional problems have opened. Some treat all kinds of mental problems, while others are restricted to such groups as adolescents, elderly persons, or alcoholics.

*Comprehensive community mental health centers.* Unfortunately, there is still an enormous gap between the best that could be done and what is actually being done for the emotionally disturbed. In many communities, facilities for treating emotional problems are nonexistent. Where available, such services are often priced beyond the reach of all but the most fortunate. Treatment for emotional problems is often specifically excluded from payment by health-insurance policies.

In order to stimulate the development of comprehensive community mental health centers, the federal government has made available financial aid to centers that meet certain standards of qualification. The following ten criteria describe the comprehensive community mental health center.

1. Inpatient services.
2. Outpatient services.
3. Partial hospitalization services such as day care, night care, and weekend care.
4. Emergency services available at all times.
5. Consultation and education services available to community agencies and professional personnel.
6. Diagnostic services.
7. Rehabilitative services, including vocational and educational programs.
8. Precare and aftercare services in the community, including foster-home placement, home visiting, and halfway houses.
9. Training.
10. Research and evaluation.

To date, the number of such comprehensive centers in the United States remains limited and they are especially scarce outside major metropolitan areas. But these criteria are an excellent yardstick by which a community can evaluate its own mental health facilities. While it is generally impossible for a small community to provide all these services, it is often feasible for several neighboring communities to collectively develop an excellent comprehensive mental health center. Adequate mental health facilities often can be established in a community through the efforts of concerned citizens, working in cooperation with interested professional personnel.

## FOR FURTHER READING

Berne, Eric, *Games People Play.* New York: Grove Press, 1964. *Describes the significance of specific patterns of interpersonal communication.*

Caprio, Frank, and Francis Leighton, *How to Avoid a Nervous Breakdown.* New York: Hawthorn, 1969. *Emphasizes the point that individuals must maintain a strong self-image in order to control the harmful effects of stress.*

Harris, Thomas, *I'm OK—You're OK: A Practical Guide to Transactional Analysis.* New York: Harper and Row, 1971. *Written for the layman, engagingly describes the insights and advantages of transactional analysis methods.*

James, Muriel, and Dorothy Jongeward, *Born to Win.* Menlo Park: Addison-Wesley, 1971. *Applies transactional analysis theory to everyday life.*

Janov, Arthur, *The Primal Scream.* New York: Dell Publishing, 1970. *An explanation of the author's Primal Therapy system, through which the patient's "primal" (early) experiences are relived, in order to avoid symptoms of neuroses.*

Maslow, Abraham, *Motivation and Personality,* 2nd ed. New York: Harper and Row, 1970. *Classic presentation of basic human emotional needs.*

Maslow, Abraham, *The Farther Reaches of Human Nature.* New York: The Viking Press, 1971. *Expands Maslow's prior observations on personality.*

Rogers, Carl, *Carl Rogers on Encounter Groups.* New York: Harper & Row, 1970. *A comprehensive and sensitive analysis of the encounter group—its implications for psychotherapy, its methods and procedures.*

Selye, Hans, *The Stress of Life.* New York: McGraw-Hill, 1956. *Explains Selye's widely accepted theory of the General Adaptation syndrome.*

Schutz, William, *Joy.* New York: Grove Press, 1967. *Description of Esalen Institute in Big Sur, California, and the methods of interpersonal encounter groups pioneered there.*

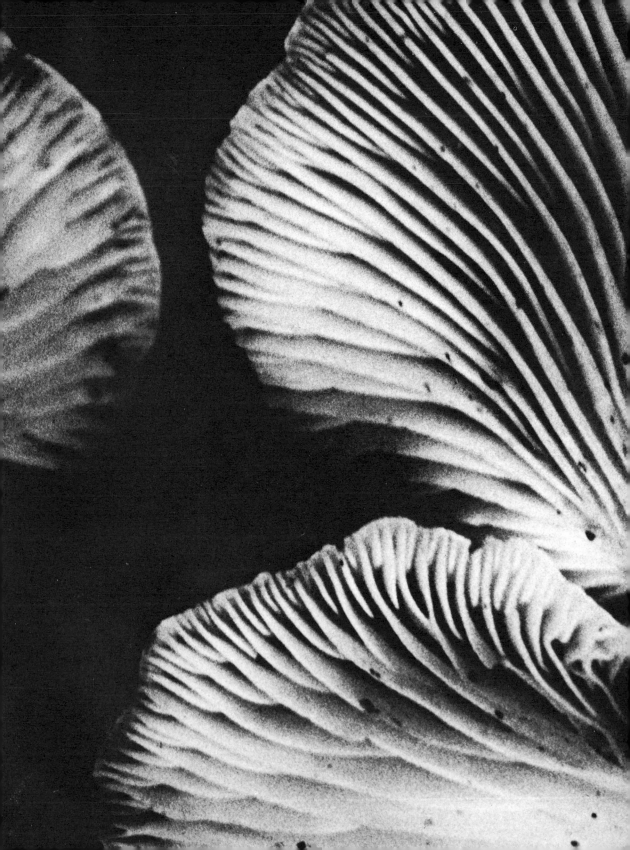

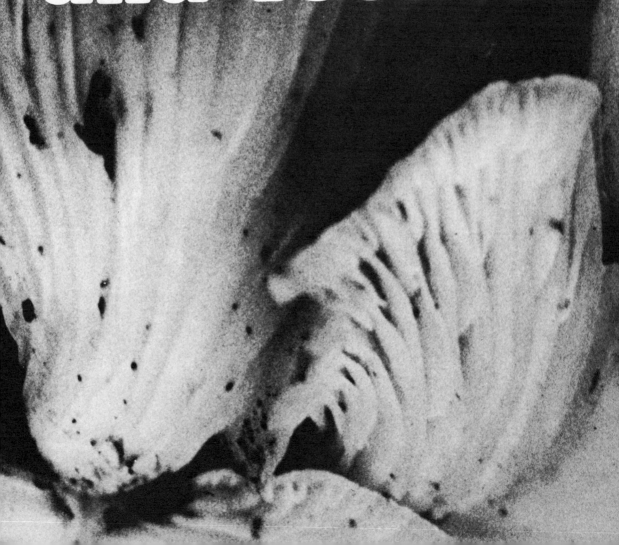

# 3 Drugs, Alcohol, and Tobacco

# 5

# Drugs — Their Use and Abuse

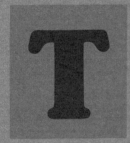

Today the word "drug" is a loaded term; in common usage, it now has two connotations—one positive, reflecting the crucial role of these natural and synthetic chemicals in medicine, and one negative, relating to self- and socially destructive patterns of misuse. A good definition of the term, which permits us to refer to both aspects, is, "A drug is any substance, other than food, which alters the body or its functions."

Many of society's problems with drugs come at the point where it has to deal with substances which have little or no medical value, or where nonmedical uses interfere with medical ones. Some drugs are so easily misused that there are laws prohibiting their being prescribed even by physicians. And some drugs, such as marijuana, have no current medical use and are not prescribed except for research purposes. In general, a drug is not considered safe for the public to use without prescription if its effects are dangerous enough to create a potential hazard for the person using them, or for the society in which he lives.

## DRUG USE—METHODS AND MEDICINE

The use of drugs dates back thousands of years. At first, they were used by early societies as part of religious healing ceremonies; in most of these societies, however, more reliance was placed on prayers, incantations, and charms than on the particular drugs used. Eventually, the powers of certain drugs became highly guarded secrets known only to the men who governed their use.

It was not until the latter half of the nineteenth century that scientists began to make accurate experiments to discover precisely what chemicals were contained in drugs and what effect individual drugs might have in alleviating pain or curing disease. Before that, prescribing drugs was a hit-or-miss affair; physicians and quacks often ascribed wonderful curative properties to "patent medicines" that were worthless or harmful.

In the past 30 years, new drugs have revolutionized the practice of medicine. Since the development of sulfa drugs and antibiotics in the 1930s, hundreds of new drugs have been introduced, many of them capable of reversing the course of serious disease and saving lives.

Because of the development of these "wonder" drugs and the ready acceptance of them by the medical profession, many people have built up unrealistic expectations about what drugs can do for them. The people of the United States are, in general, "drug users." In our zealous search for miraculous cures, we too often decide for ourselves what prescription drugs and what dosages we need instead of leaving this difficult and delicate decision where it belongs—in the hands of trained physicians. We feel that it is necessary for everyone to learn something about how drugs work. It is to be hoped that the more we know about drugs, the more cautious we will be regarding self-diagnosis, self-treatment, and the misuse of drugs.

Present knowledge of the chemical structure of drugs often enables scientists to predict what a drug will do and what the results of its actions will be. Drugs are administered to an individual for a specific purpose: to cure a disease or alleviate the pain or discomfort of an illness or injury. Any drug which is powerful enough to be effective has the potential to produce some adverse reactions which are not always predictable. These actions can be classified as either side effects or untoward effects. A side effect of a drug is any action or effect other than the one for which it is administered. Side effects are not necessarily harmful to the individual. Morphine is usually given to relieve pain, not for its ability to constrict the pupil of the eye. This constriction is a side effect. An untoward effect is a reaction regarded as harmful to an individual. The untoward effects of morphine—nausea, vomiting, constipation, and addiction—are obviously undesirable and harmful.

Doctors are very careful, and always conservative, about dosage size when prescribing drugs because of the possible untoward effects. A responsible physician is often reluctant to prescribe new drugs that have not been widely used and thoroughly tested, partly because of the risk of undesirable consequences.

Persons visiting a physician seeking relief from an illness sometimes respond with impatience and resentment when the doctor doesn't give them a prescription for drugs. But a doctor will not prescribe a medication until and unless he knows exactly what he is treating, and the process of making a diagnosis may take time. If a doctor too quickly prescribes drugs that temporarily relieve the symptoms of an illness, he may interfere with the diagnostic procedure and endanger the individual.

In addition, it is important to remember that most Americans are symptom-oriented. This might be a direct consequence of the standard methods of advertising medicines; television, radio, and magazine advertisements are designed to gear our attention toward symptoms, not underlying causes of illness or pain. Thus, many people seek immediate relief of symptoms and want their doctor's assistance. But if a doctor prescribes a drug that eliminates symptoms, most patients do not feel the same urgency to continue with diagnosis and treatment—the phases of medical attention which are really most important in terms of the individual's long-range health.

As the next figure shows, drugs can be introduced into the body in various ways. Some drugs, penicillin, for example, can be taken orally in the form of capsules or can be injected. Other drugs, such as insulin,

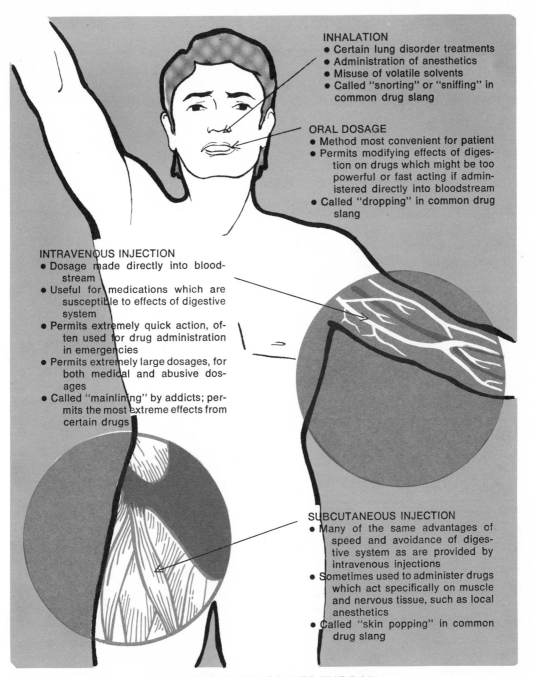

**INHALATION**
- Certain lung disorder treatments
- Administration of anesthetics
- Misuse of volatile solvents
- Called "snorting" or "sniffing" in common drug slang

**ORAL DOSAGE**
- Method most convenient for patient
- Permits modifying effects of digestion on drugs which might be too powerful or fast acting if administered directly into bloodstream
- Called "dropping" in common drug slang

**INTRAVENOUS INJECTION**
- Dosage made directly into bloodstream
- Useful for medications which are susceptible to effects of digestive system
- Permits extremely quick action, often used for drug administration in emergencies
- Permits extremely large dosages, for both medical and abusive dosages
- Called "mainlining" by addicts; permits the most extreme effects from certain drugs

**SUBCUTANEOUS INJECTION**
- Many of the same advantages of speed and avoidance of digestive system as are provided by intravenous injections
- Sometimes used to administer drugs which act specifically on muscle and nervous tissue, such as local anesthetics
- Called "skin popping" in common drug slang

INTRODUCING DRUGS INTO THE BODY

which is used in the treatment of diabetes, generally cannot be exposed to the digestive system's chemical action. Often, it is injected into the body.

After being taken into the body, drugs are distributed by the bloodstream to the many organs, tissues, and cells. The action or effect of a drug may be on the surface of cells, within the cell, or in the body fluids surrounding the cells. In most cases, the action takes place within the individual cells of the body and has either a direct or indirect effect on the central nervous system. Drugs enter the cells in the same way that water and other nutrients do, through the membranes of the cell. Many drugs include molecular parts similar to those found in the cell's normal "diet," and this permits the drugs to participate in a few stages of the cell's normal chemical processes. Ultimately, of course, the differences between the drug and the normal chemical will be detected by the systems of the cell. But by this time the drug's work has been done; the cellular processes are no longer normal; the cells, the organs, and the interrelated body systems have been altered—the drug has taken effect.

## DRUG ABUSE—
## POTIONS AND PREJUDICES

Most drugs which have come to the attention of mankind have legitimate and useful places in the treatment of disease and alleviation of pain and discomfort. This is the proper "use" of drugs. Theoretically, any drug can be abused; that is, used for purposes other than those intended by a physician. Drug abuse is defined as the self-administration of drugs in excessive or otherwise inappropriate dosages, which results in damage to an individual and/or society. Despite the usefulness of this definition, the term is still a difficult one to completely and adequately define. The spectrum of responsibility—from individual to social—frequently clouds important scientific and medical debates about drugs. Attitudes towards drug abuse have taken on political significance, again adding to the scientific confusion.

In the past, certain commonly abused drugs were said to be "habituating" or "addicting." The explanations of these terms most often quoted today are those of the Expert Committee on Addiction-Producing Drugs of the World Health Organization. But the terms "addict," "user," or "habitual user" can be ambiguous. In common usage, these words are defined in terms of the drug involved. For example, the addict has been described as someone who is dependent on the physically addicting drugs such as opium and its derivatives, synthetic narcotics, barbiturates, alcohol, and solvents. The user has been described as one who has an habituation to cocaine, amphetamines, marijuana, LSD, or other hallucinogenic drugs.

These terms have become obsolete because they fail to serve the needs of science, medicine, law, and society. Medically a physician needs to know if a person is addicted to a specific drug in order to prescribe proper treatment. Whether a drug is addicting or habituating makes no difference to the law and society. Addiction is a treatable personal problem of the individual. It has no significance in determining whether there are or are not social and legal problems associated with a specific drug. In place of the terms "habituating" and "addicting" these phrases are now being used: "psychological dependence," "drug dependence," "substance dependence," or "dependency." With the repeated use of any *substance* (food, tobacco, aspirin, alcohol, narcotics, and so on) some individuals develop a *dependence upon the substance*. The exact nature of this dependence varies with the type of substance being abused (narcotic, food, tobacco, sedative, hallucinogen); the social acceptability (degrees of acceptability of tobacco, alcohol, and heroin); and the individual's reasons (social, emotional, political) for dependence upon the substance.

Large amounts of food are consumed by individuals dependent upon food as an emotional stabilizer. Large amounts of mild pain relievers (analgesics) with aspirin or aspirin-like ingredients are consumed every day. Tranquilizers, sedatives, and hypnotics are the most widely prescribed and consumed drugs in the United States and the world. Many people believe they cannot get up, do their work, keep their nerves quiet, or go to sleep unless they have a drug to help them. There is sound medical basis for the temporary use of these drugs by some, and the permanent use by a few. But in general this is a form of "socially acceptable" drug dependence.

The drugs, whether socially acceptable or not, which cause problems for society are those that cause death (tobacco), marked personality changes, or abnormal social behavior. Such drugs may be called mood modifiers, *psychotropic, psychoactive,* or *psychotoxic* drugs. Most mood modifiers are abused because they cause euphoria (an extreme or exaggerated sense of pleasure or well-being), hallucinations (perceptions of objects with no relation to reality), or recognizable changes in personality or behavior. Drugs which are considered dangerous and unacceptable to society, when used for other than legitimate medical purposes, include narcotics, solvents, hypnotics, sedatives (including alcohol), tranquilizers, forms of cannabis, hallucinogens, cocaine and its derivatives, and amphetamines.

The term "mood modifying" points out the effects of a drug and is not a type of chemical or medical classification. Also, not everyone who explores the effects of mood modifying drugs will follow the same predictable pattern of behavior. Some may only experiment with such drugs because of social influences, curiosity about the pleasant effects, or because of short-range emotional problems. Such individuals should be termed "drug experimenters." Their action is unrelated to serious drug abuse because they have already made their decision not to abuse drugs. Too often they have been arrested during their experimentation and may carry a criminal record of their experiment for the rest of their lives.

Individuals who experiment and continue to use drugs find they need the gratification that mood-modifying drugs, or the accompanying social environment, give them. This is a form of psychological dependency. They use drugs infrequently, yet consistently, which is usually more than once a month but less than several times a week. (Individuals who use alcohol in a similar manner are called "social drinkers.") Such individuals use marijuana in relatively low dosages, and it is called a *social dosage.* These individuals should be termed "occasional" or "intermittent users."

Use of drugs daily or at least several times a week, extending over a long period of time, can be considered true drug abuse. These individuals often experiment with a wide variety of drugs and use the "in" drug. They function within society, but drugs are the central focus of their lives. It is not just an intermittent assist in the pursuit of a happy life but a part of a more general "turned-on" ideology and a membership in a life style or anticulture. These individuals are ranked as "regular," "moderate," or "heavy" drug users. A cigarette smoker who smokes more than eight cigarettes a day is a regular drug user. Persons who daily use tranquilizers for nervousness, amphetamines to lose weight, or barbiturates to sleep would be included also. Regular users of mood-modifying drugs are called heads, potheads, coke heads, acid heads, weekend drunks, or periodic alcoholics depending on the specific drug used. Often these users are the greatest defenders of the personal right to use drugs. They seldom have had bad experiences with drugs and have closed minds concerning drugs because of *street experimentation:* "I know because I have been there"—probably the most dangerous phrase in science.

The most dangerous aspect of regular drug use is the danger of lapsing into a *personality deficiency* that may restrict a user's ability to deal constructively with life. The self-destructive dependence of a smoker on cigarettes is a good example. Increased dependence upon mood-modifying drugs eventually will lead to compulsive drug abuse, very heavy drug use, addiction, or alcoholism.

Compulsive abuse (addiction, alcoholism) of mood-modifying substances is always associated with an abnormal personality. Whether this behavioral distortion is the cause or the result of the drug abuse is not known. The abnormal social behavior and modification of moods in such individuals is more of a problem to society than is the drug abuse itself, the responsibility for which lies solely with the individual.

In all cases of repeated drug abuse, the person who misuses such drugs chooses to do so. Once started, his abuse will lead to drug dependence, in response to his personality, or to drug addiction, according to the physical properties and physiological effects of the drug involved. On the other hand, the person who does not find a pleasurable experience in drug abuse, or whose only reason for experimenting was strong social pressure, will probably not continue to abuse drugs. His personality does not lack, or seek, what the drug has to offer and he therefore tends to reject it.

There must be recognition of the various patterns of drug abuse if our society is to reach a humane, just, and successful method of dealing with the serious problems posed by drugs.

## COMMONLY ABUSED MOOD-MODIFYING DRUGS

Today much research on drugs is concerned with how they work in altering states of mind. Researchers are attempting to discover how certain chemicals work in modifying people's moods, personality, and behavior.

Such studies are especially necessary in view of the widespread use and abuse of mood-modifying drugs. In the United States, over 20 million people use sleeping pills, over 10 million use amphetamines, and more than 50 million use tranquilizers. This includes those who have medical sanction for their use of drugs as well as estimated illicit users. By considering the sheer number of users, we can see that the medical, psychological, sociological, philosophical, and legal aspects of drug use and abuse are extremely important.

The abnormal social behavior of some drug abusers, moreover, causes other problems. One of these involves the issue of personal responsibility during times of drug-induced behavioral changes, which may be called "times out." During such an interval, a person might do things which represent a complete departure from rationality and morality.

In general, mood-modifying drugs act to increase or decrease the cellular activity of the cells of nerve centers and their conducting pathways. Depressant drugs have the ability to temporarily depress cellular, and consequently, body functions. Such drug-induced depression of the central nervous system is frequently characterized by a lack of interest in surroundings, inability to focus attention on a subject, and a lack of motivation to move or talk. The pulse and respiration become slower than usual, and as the depression deepens, the ability to use senses, such as touch, vision, hearing, smell, and taste, diminishes progressively. Psychological and motor activities decrease; reflexes become sluggish and finally disappear. Depressant drugs are often quite accurately called "downers." Literally, they slow down the cellular activity of an individual's nervous system. If a strong depressant is used, or if abusively large doses are consumed, depression progresses to drowsiness, stupor, unconsciousness, sleep, coma, and death.

A central nervous system stimulant is a drug that temporarily increases cellular processes which causes an increase in body or nerve activity. Stimulant drugs quickly produce a dramatic effect, but their medical usefulness is limited because of the complexity of their actions and the nature of their side effects. Such side effects may include hallucinations and delirium tremens. With repeated administration of abusive doses, convulsive seizures are often produced, alternating with periods of depression, coma, and exhaustion.

The degrees of depression and stimulation of drugs affecting the central nervous system are independent actions. The figure showing the continuum drug effects and responses was suggested and formulated by Dr. Robert W. Earle of the University of California at Irvine.

The continuum of drug effects reaches to overstimulation and death at one extreme, and to depression and death at the other. The neutral area of this continuum is the range of stimulation and depression an individual encounters normally. Often drugs in different groups have similar actions. For example, narcotics are used to relieve pain but they may also, as a side effect, induce sleepiness. Barbiturates are used for their ability to produce sleep but they do not have the ability to relieve pain. Thus, the sleep-producing effects of these two depressants,

narcotics and barbiturates, overlap on the continuum chart. In fact, many of the drugs that affect the central nervous system have similar actions.

As we progress along the chart from the neutral area outward, we can locate the specific points where the effects of drugs overlap. These points show where the continuum moves from the major effective area of one group of drugs into the area of another more powerful group of drugs. The weaker drugs are nearer the center, while the most powerful drugs are at the two extremes.

If dosages are increased, any of the drug groups listed may produce the complete range of effects of stimulation or depression. This overstimulation or extreme depression is the effect the drug abuser is seeking. Consequently, dosages used by drug abusers are far in excess of the dosages normally used in medical practice. The complete range of effects produced by increased dosages is represented in the next figure.

The drug continua in these two figures serve to point out the fact that the extreme effects the drug abuser seeks are nearly always the same. For example, any of the stimulants will produce hallucinations if the dosage is strong enough. This is why many individuals, while preferring one drug over another, will abuse any mood-modifying drug if it is available. As the specific actions of a drug become more familiar and less spectacular, the individual may experiment with new ways to use the drug. He may combine drugs of the same type—or of different types—to produce a more intense effect. He may progress from taking the drug orally to injecting it under the skin or into a muscle, to injecting it directly into a vein. Or, he may seek stronger and stronger drugs to produce more vivid effects, quicker actions, or longer-lasting experiences. Very few drug abusers are satisfied with experiences from only one drug at one consistent dosage. More

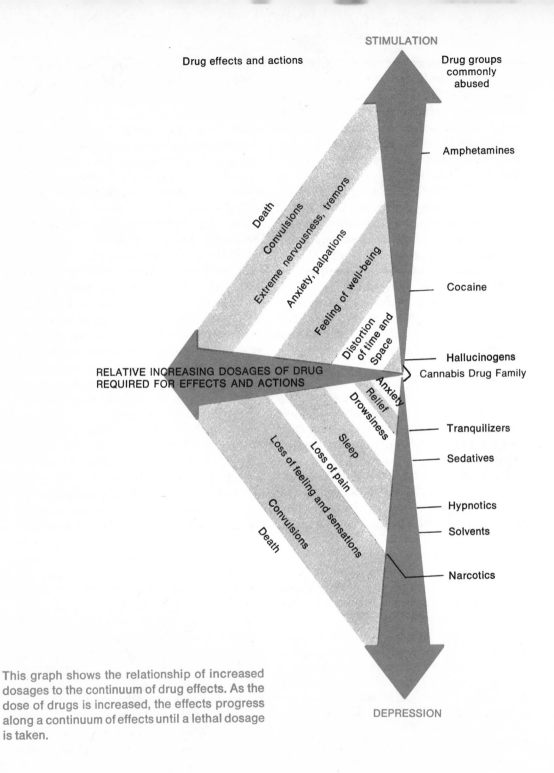

STIMULATION

Drug effects and actions

Drug groups
commonly
abused

— Amphetamines

Death
Convulsions
Extreme nervousness, tremors
Anxiety, palpations
Feeling of well-being

— Cocaine

Distortion
of time and
Space

— Hallucinogens
} Cannabis Drug Family

RELATIVE INCREASING DOSAGES OF DRUG
REQUIRED FOR EFFECTS AND ACTIONS

Anxiety
Relief
Drowsiness

— Tranquilizers

Sleep

— Sedatives

Loss of pain

Loss of feeling and sensations

— Hypnotics

Convulsions

— Solvents

Death

— Narcotics

DEPRESSION

This graph shows the relationship of increased
dosages to the continuum of drug effects. As the
dose of drugs is increased, the effects progress
along a continuum of effects until a lethal dosage
is taken.

often they will progress toward the extremes of the continuum.

The more commonly abused drugs, such as marijuana, barbiturates, and alcohol, are close to the center of the chart because of their mild effects when used in small dosages. The popularity of these drugs lies in the ability of the user to control the amount and, consequently, the relative effect of the drug. Many users of these drugs, particularly if they are not generally excitable or emotional, are contented with low dosages. On the other hand, highly emotional users or users seeking a specific "kick" are likely to increase the dosage and obtain a more intense effect. However, this ability to control drugs is offset when tolerance (increasing cellular resistance to the usual drug effects) to the drug develops, or when usage reaches addictive levels. Then, regardless of the individual's desire or emotional state, a small but increasing dose is regularly required to keep the individual from entering withdrawal. This increasing level must be reached daily to keep the individual functioning at approximately the same level. Or, with the tolerance-producing nonaddicting drugs, the individual must either increase the amount he is using to produce the desired effects or move up the continuum to a stronger drug. Thus, he finds himself locked into a pattern of constantly increasing dosage amounts.

Because the stimulant drugs and the milder depressant drugs do not seem to have the clear-cut addictive properties of the stronger depressants (some such as marijuana may show *reverse tolerance* where smaller dosages cause greater effects), many users never progress from these relatively mild drugs. They are able to control the effects they desire at a particular time. "Social drinking" of alcoholic beverages is an example of this kind of drug control. Others who start on the weaker drugs progress to stronger ones because they enjoy the slight differences of effects; some users, in seeking a more pleasurable reaction, eventually experiment with more dangerous drugs.

As already mentioned, each of these mood-modifying drugs either stimulates or depresses cellular functions. Caffeine, for instance, stimulates the nerve cells, while a barbiturate depresses them. Because of the complexity of the body's functions, drug action is often complex. At times, this makes it extremely difficult to place a group of drugs on a progressive continuum chart. Also, the complexity of a drug's action often leads to apparent paradoxes. For example, alcohol is a depressant and depresses nerve functions. If this is so why do people seem stimulated by a small-to-moderate amount of alcohol? The answer is that the brain contains a group of cells whose function is inhibition. These cells normally keep an individual from responding irresponsibly to every passing impulse. These inhibitory cells are more sensitive to alcohol and similar drugs (sedatives, hypnotics, and solvents) than the other brain cells. As the alcohol concentration in the blood begins to rise, the inhibitory cells are depressed and cease to function properly; many impulses, ideas, and actions which would otherwise be suppressed are acted out by the individual. Therefore, moderate amounts of alcohol, a depressant drug, can cause excitation by depressing a cellular inhibitory function.

If you are to deal with the mood-modifying drugs, or understand individuals who use them it is wise to learn something about the mind-altering or psychotropic effects of some of the more commonly abused drugs. We will group these drugs into eight classifications: (1) narcotics, (2) volatile solvents, (3) hypnotic sedatives (including alcohol), (4) tranquilizers, (5) cannabis drug family, (6) hallucinogens, (7) cocaine, and (8) amphetamines.

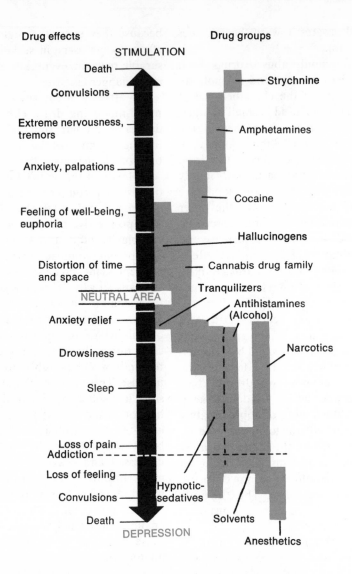

**Drug effects**  **Drug groups**

STIMULATION

Death — Strychnine

Convulsions —

Extreme nervousness, tremors — Amphetamines

Anxiety, palpations —

Cocaine

Feeling of well-being, euphoria —

Hallucinogens

Distortion of time and space — Cannabis drug family

Tranquilizers

NEUTRAL AREA

Antihistamines (Alcohol)

Anxiety relief —

Narcotics

Drowsiness —

Sleep —

Loss of pain —
Addiction – – – – – – – – – – – –

Loss of feeling —

Convulsions — Hypnotic-sedatives

Death — Solvents

DEPRESSION

Anesthetics

This illustration shows the continuum of drug effects and actions, as well as overlapping effects of drug groups.

### Narcotics

Narcotics, the most widely abused drug families throughout the world, include opiates (opium and its derivatives) and synthetic narcotics (drugs chemically similar to opiates, but made in a laboratory from materials other than opium).

Narcotics work by depressing specific cells of the body's central nervous system. Depending on which cells are depressed and to what extent they can produce *analgesia* (relief of pain), their first and foremost medical use, a number of other effects can result. These include sedation (freeing the mind of anxiety, relaxing the muscles, and calming the body), hypnosis (drowsiness to sleep), and euphoria.

The repeated consumption of some mood-modifying drugs, such as the narcotics, can produce biochemical and physiological changes which cause the user to keep increasing the dosage to maintain the same mood-modifying effect he desires. He is then said to have developed a tolerance for the drug. Tolerance is an acquired reaction to a drug that necessitates an increase of dosage to maintain a given action or effect. As his tolerance increases and he uses more of the drug, his body cells are gradually exposed to greater quantities of it. For a period of time the body will adjust to these slowly increasing amounts. However, it is always possible that the user may take a larger dose than his body can tolerate (an overdose) and he will become extremely ill or die.

An individual abusing narcotics may develop a physical dependence on the drug; that is, he may become *addicted* to it. Tolerance develops very quickly. Then, when a person whose body has developed a tolerance has his supply of the drug cut off, a condition called withdrawal illness (narcotic-solvent type abstinence syndrome) results. This is caused by the drug-tolerant cells trying to return to normal. The intensity and nature of withdrawal illness varies with the type and strength of the narcotic abused. The symptoms of withdrawal from opium and its derivatives include irritability, depression, extreme nervousness, pain in the abdomen, and nausea—all to an agonizing degree. After withdrawal, if he abstains from using the drug, his body will readjust to a relatively normal condition and he will lose the toler-

ance that has developed. Now even a relatively small dose of a narcotic can "overdose" and cause his death. Because of the relatively weak preparations sold illegally in the United States, some individuals can use narcotics intermittently without ever becoming addicted.

Recognition of a narcotics addict, especially when he is regularly obtaining an increasing daily dosage, can be extremely difficult. He certainly does not want to give away the fact that he is an addict, and he is often, through experience, very clever at disguising it.

Early in the process of addiction, before much tolerance has developed, the pupils of the eyes contract until they are "pin-pointed," even in a weak, dim light whenever the addict is under the influence of a narcotic. Unless he has also taken an antagonistic drug such as a stimulant, the addict's pupils will not react to light; that is, the pinpoint will not become smaller in a strong light, even when it is flashed directly into the eye, or larger (dilated) when the light is abruptly dimmed. In this condition, the eyes are said to be "frozen." After tolerance has begun to develop, the addict's pupils may begin to enlarge somewhat. When an addict has been without drugs for a short period of time (from 4 to 6 hours to overnight) and begins to enter withdrawal, his eyes become dilated and exhibit a sluggish reaction to light. Again, however, this condition may be disguised by the effects of antagonistic drugs.

Owing to the depressant effects of narcotics, a user who has been addicted for a long time is often pale and emaciated. He may suffer from severe constipation. His appetite is poor. His sexual drive is usually reduced. While under the influence of a narcotic, he may be lazy, in a semistupor ("on the nod"), and dreamy. He is not particularly dangerous and certainly not violent. But if an addict is deprived of a regular narcotics supply (and must have a "fix" every 5 to 12 hours), he may become dangerous and engage in petty thievery, mugging, or prostitution to support his habit.

Narcotics are used in medicine primarily for their analgesic effect—that is, their ability to relieve pain. Administered in controlled dosages, they cause insensitivity to pain without producing loss of consciousness or even excessive drowsiness. Doctors generally use anesthetics or members of the hypnotic-sedative group when they want to anesthetize patients for operations. They never use narcotics alone for this purpose, because narcotics used in dosages large enough to produce sleep or stupor could depress the respiratory center sufficiently to cause death.

A physician administering a narcotic usually gives a subcutaneous injection. This method produces too slow an action for most addicts, who prefer to have an intravenous injection. Because of the more rapid distribution throughout the body, an intravenous injection or "mainline" gives the desired effect immediately.

Some narcotics users start out by taking the drug orally. They will switch to injections when they learn—usually by associating with other users—that injections are more efficient. Then, less of the drug is needed to obtain the effect wanted. Also, the drug acts faster and its effect is more prolonged.

The following are the major narcotics abused throughout the world.

*Opium.* Opium is the juice obtained from cutting the unripe capsule of the oriental poppy *(Papaver somniferum)*. This drug is generally smoked in an opium pipe or eaten. Because it is difficult to obtain, American drug abusers seldom use opium today, but there is a great abuse of its derivatives, morphine, heroin, and codeine, which are the most important narcotic substances obtainable from opium.

*Morphine.* The major derivative of chemically refined opium is morphine. Morphine is the best analgesic available. It may be pure white, light brown, or off-white in color and comes in many forms: cubes, capsules, tablets, powder, or liquid solution. On the illegal market, morphine in a gelatine capsule is known as a "cap." The powder folded into a paper square is known as a "deck" or "package." Morphine is about ten times stronger than pure opium; it attacks the nervous system of the user more swiftly and with much greater intensity. Unlike heroin, very little morphine is sold on the streets. Rather, morphine addicts usually steal their supply from doctors' offices or pharmacies. Sometimes they obtain morphine by forging prescription forms that have been stolen from physicians.

*Heroin.* Heroin is produced from morphine. During this process the total amount of the drug is reduced in volume, which facilitates smuggling. This makes the heroin more potent per ounce than the morphine that went into the process. In studies carried out in England by Dr. J. H. Willis, nondrug users and drug users were unable to tell whether they were being given morphine or heroin. Heroin is able to enter the central nervous system more easily than morphine. Consequently, heroin seems to be a more potent drug. Pure heroin is a grayish-brown powder. Because of its strength and the economics of illegal drug traffic, heroin is diluted ("cut" or "hit") many times before it is sold on the "street." Usually heroin is cut with milk sugar (lactose), mannite (a substance from the ash tree used as a mild laxative), and quinine. Often unsafe chemicals (such as strychnine, LSD, and amphetamines) are used as diluents during this cutting process.

Street heroin ends up a white or off-white powder, usually containing no more than 1 to 4 percent pure heroin.

The main reason why laws controlling heroin have been unsuccessful is the tremendous amount of money made each year by the illegal sale of heroin in the United States. Heroin is a billion-dollar product on the streets. It passes through five or six levels of distribution before reaching the user. For example, one kilogram (2.2 pounds) of heroin can be purchased for $5,000 to $10,000 by someone who has a "connection" with the individuals preparing the heroin from morphine. This "importer" will have the heroin brought into the United States, have it diluted, and then sell it to a "wholesaler" for $18,000 to $20,000. The wholesaler dilutes it again, divides it into plastic bags containing about an ounce of cut heroin, and sells these to local "dealers" for about $700 a bag. The wholesaler obtains about $32,000 for his bags. The dealer dilutes it again and divides it into smaller portions called "pieces," "street ounces," or "vig ounces" (*vig* is a term used to describe the high interest charged by loan sharks). He packages these in folded squares of glassine paper ("papers"), or in clear or colored capsules ("caps") and sells these to the street "pusher." The dealer obtains about

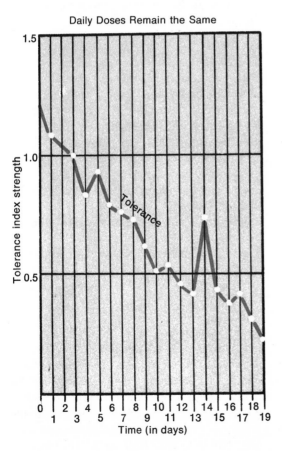

Daily Doses Remain the Same

Tolerance

Tolerance index strength

Time (in days)

At the National Institute of Mental Health Addiction Research Center in Lexington, Kentucky, a group of individuals were given an equivalent dose of heroin every day for 19 days. The euphoric effects were measured each day during the 19 days and graphed as the Tolerance Line. The effects of the standard dose decreased, and by the 19th day were almost nonexistent—even though the same chemically measured amount of heroin was given on day 19 as on day 1. Heroin users respond to the development of tolerance by progressively increasing their dosages of heroin. (Adapted from W. R. Martin and H. F. Fraser, "A Comparative Study of Physiological and Subjective Effects of Heroin and Morphine Administered Intravenously in Postaddicts," *Journal of Pharmacology and Experimental Therapeutics*, 1961, p. 397.) Copyright © 1961 by Williams and Wilkins Co., Baltimore, Maryland.

$70,000 for his product. The pusher will now sell to the individual user at the street price, after he has cut it or removed some for his own use. This practice varies from time to time or city to city. But, on the street the original one "kilo" of heroin can return $225,000. This single kilogram of heroin has produced $215,000 in profit.

Some individuals can use heroin off and on, on a nonregular basis, for years without becoming addicted. These individuals are called "joy poppers" or "chippies." Persons who use heroin regularly become addicted faster than users of any other narcotic. The body's tolerance to heroin builds up very rapidly. Thus, an addict requires increasingly larger doses to get the desired effect and to prevent himself from entering withdrawal. (See the graph showing the results of an experiment in drug tolerance.)

*Codeine.* Codeine is a relatively mild narcotic. The pure product is a white crystal powder which is sometimes taken in tablets for pain relief in combination with other ingredients (one such tablet is labeled "Empirin with Codeine"). Codeine is also widely used as an ingredient in liquid cough medicines.

In many states, medicines containing a small amount of codeine (not more than 1 grain per ounce) can be sold over the counter without a prescription, but the pharmacist must keep a record of the purchaser's name. In some states, such medicines will bear a label with the statement: "Contains codeine (opium derivative). WARNING—may be habit-forming. Do not give to children except upon advice of a physician."

Narcotics addicts sometimes resort to the use of codeine when deprived of their supply of stronger drugs, but codeine is not widely abused because it is too mild to give a "hard" narcotic user the high he wants. Still, codeine, especially that found in some cough medicines, is often abused by young people when they can obtain it. It is an addictive drug, particularly when used frequently and in large amounts.

*Synthetic Narcotics.* The synthetic narcotics differ from the opium derivatives and their compounds in that they are made synthetically in the chemical laboratory—not from opium, but from coal tar or petroleum products. Some of the more common synthetic compounds are Dilaudid, Percodan, Demerol, Perco-barb, Methadone, and Nalline. Their chemical properties resemble those of various opium derivatives; their narcotic effect (and addictive potential) varies. But all narcotics, including synthetic ones, are addictive.

### Volatile Solvents

The practice of inhaling vapors of volatile chemicals, chemicals that evaporate readily at room temperature, is also a major concern of society. The solvents in plastic or model-airplane cement are volatile chemicals and are often inhaled for their mood-modifying effects. These effects are primarily feelings of pleasantness, cheerfulness, euphoria, and excitement—feelings that closely simulate the early stages of alcohol excitement. As a person inhales more, he begins to appear "drunk," exhibiting disorientation and speaking in a slurred manner. Such behavior may continue for 30 to 45 minutes, followed by drowsiness, stupor, or unconsciousness. Unconsciousness may last for as long as an hour. If the person has inhaled too much glue vapor, or if his exposure to the vapors has been prolonged, he may die.

Several toxic solvents are used in the manufacture of airplane cements. Common to many brands are isoamyl acetate and ethyl acetate. Other toxic solvents used in many products include benzene, toluene, and carbon tetrachloride. High concentrations of these solvents are found in cleaning fluids, paints, and paint thinners. Also, the hydrocarbons in gasoline (such as butane, hexane, and pentane) may cause solvent intoxication when inhaled. Prolonged inhalation of the fumes of any of these fluids may cause death. Labels on many types of solvents and gasoline include the warning "Use only in a well-ventilated, open area."

Tolerance to solvents develops rapidly, and the user soon finds he must inhale the vapors from the contents of several tubes of cement to experience the effects he desires. By this time he will have become addicted to the solvents.

An addicted glue-sniffer often has a characteristic, unpleasant odor to his breath. He may salivate excessively and spit frequently. The salivary secretions result from the solvent vapors' irritation of the mucous membranes of the nose and mouth. A user of glue may also suffer insomnia (inability to sleep), nausea, and weight loss.

The toxic effects of solvents have been carefully observed. They include irritation of the mucous membranes, the skin, and the respiratory tract; alternate excitation and depression of the central nervous system; cellular injury in the heart, liver, and kidneys; alteration of bone marrow activity, which results in anemia (reduction in red blood cells), and leucopenia (reduction in white blood cells). There have also been reports of brain tissue deterioration, acute liver damage, and death from kidney failure.

The abuse of solvents leads to a strong drug dependence, including severe mood-modifying effects and a quickly developed tolerance. This is why solvents are placed at such an extreme position in the figure showing the continuum of drug effects.

In their quest to find volatile chemicals that have mood-modifying effects, some young people have tried to "sniff" anything that is in a pressurized can—from hair spray to the Freon gas used in refrigerators. Most of these spray cans either displace the oxygen in the air or coat the lungs with resins when "sniffed" in a closed area and have caused the deaths of hundreds of young people.

### Hypnotic-Sedative Drugs

This group of drugs is classified together because each drug has the ability to depress the central nervous system into a condition resembling sleep. This difference between a hypnotic action and a sedative action is one of degree of depression. A hypnotic drug, given in a moderate or even a small dose, will produce sleep soon after it is given. Such reduced dosages of sedative drugs, even when administered several times a day, will calm a person without producing sleep. With increasing dosages, all of the drugs in this group produce a continuum of effects from tranquilization, to sedation (the allaying of excitement), to the loss of psychomotor efficiency, to sleep, and then to coma and death.

For thousands of years the only hypnotic drugs man knew were alcohol, opium (actually now classified as a narcotic), and belladonna (a drug extracted from *Atropa belladonna,* or "deadly nightshade," a plant found in Europe and Asia.)

*Alcohol and Alcohol Derivatives.* The oldest hypnotic-sedative drug used in medicine is alcohol. Derivatives of alcohol have been used as hypnotics and sedatives for many years. The first alcohol derivative was *chloral hydrate,* developed in 1869; next was paraldehyde, introduced in 1882.

Both chloral hydrate and paraldehyde are very effective as sleep-producers, and both drugs also have an extremely disagreeable taste and odor. Consequently, they are usually made up into solutions into which spices and flavorings are added to disguise the unpleasant sensations. Even so, the odor

| COLOR AND SHAPE OF CAPSULE | TRADE (AND GENERIC) NAME | STREET NAME | CHIEF MEDICAL USE | DURATION OF ACTION |
|---|---|---|---|---|
| Blue-green | Amytal (Amobarbital) | "Blue dragons" | Sedative and hypnotic | Intermediate |
| Red | Seconal (Secobarbital) | "Reds" "Red birds" "Red devils" | Hypnotic | Short acting |
| Red-blue | Tuinal (Combination of amobarbital and secobarbital) | "Rainbows" | Hypnotic | Moderately long-lasting |
| Yellow | Nembutal (Pentobarbital) | "Yellow jackets" | Hypnotic, sedative and anticonvulsant | Short acting |
| Green | Luminal (Phenobarbital) | "Barbs" | Hypnotic | Long acting |

Barbiturates: About twenty of the several hundred barbituric compounds synthesized and tested are satisfactory for medical use. The barbiturates, which act on specific areas of the brain and induce sleep promptly, are effective in treating conditions of anxiety, muscular twitching, tremens, and convulsions. These compounds differ chiefly in the duration of their effects.

of these drugs lingers for hours on the breath and in the surrounding atmosphere of an individual who has taken them.

Occasionally these drugs are used to control patients who are hospitalized with delirium tremens, withdrawal illness, and convulsions. But their use decreases yearly, and they have been replaced largely by the barbiturates.

*Barbiturates.* The barbiturates are by far the most widely used and abused of all depressant drugs except alcohol. They were first used in the United States as hypnotic-sedatives in the form of barbitol, developed in 1903. Since that time, many new barbiturate compounds have been produced and put on the market. Doctors prescribe them mainly to help patients sleep. The figure showing some commonly used and abused barbiturates also gives trade and street names and chief medical use. On the illegal market, barbiturates are known as "sleeping pills," "goof-balls," "reds" (because of the usual capsule color), "downers," or "stumblers."

Barbiturates produce a surprisingly variable effect in the brain and nervous system of the person who uses them. After taking these drugs, many users undergo a short period of hyperactivity and excitement. Then, as the drug depresses their central nervous system, they become relaxed, euphoric, and sleepy. For some users, certain barbiturates produce a "truth serum" effect in which long-forgotten events are remembered. Also, a user may take a dose of barbiturates and discover that they seem to have no sedative or hypnotic effect at all because the period of hyperactivity and excitement has lasted throughout the night. With abusive dosages, drastic and sudden mood changes may occur—users are often described as friendly one minute, mean the next.

Barbiturates are addictive drugs when abused. Drug dependence and tolerance develops quickly. They are usually taken orally ("dropped"); however, users can dissolve the compound and inject it hypodermically, but it is very destructive to tissue when injected. Sometimes they are dropped in combination with a stimulant such as Benzedrine, Dexedrine, or Methedrine. This combination overcomes the depressing effects of the barbiturates and extends the excitement and euphoria. The use of a stimulant drug to antagonize the depressant effect of a barbiturate is extremely dangerous.

A risky practice indulged in by some persons who abuse barbiturates is to combine them with alcohol. Because the barbiturates interfere with the body's normal disposal of alcohol through the liver, the two drugs taken together have a total depressant effect far greater than the sum of their individual effects. Often, an overdose of either drug is taken unknowingly; the person is "too drunk" or "too doped up" to realize what he is doing. Because of this confused state it is difficult to tell whether a fatal drug overdose was suicide or accidental. The use of alcohol and barbiturates in combination, even in small amounts, is extremely dangerous and too often results in death.

Since both are hypnotic-sedative drugs, the effects of barbiturates and alcohol are very similar. A small amount of barbiturates makes the user feel relaxed, sociable, and good-humored. He is also less alert than he normally is. After taking more of the drug, he may become sluggish, gloomy, and quarrelsome. His tongue becomes "thick," he staggers, and then gradually slumps into a deep sleep. If he has had a large amount of the drug, or if he has taken it in combination with alcohol, he may suddenly lapse into a coma. At this point, only prompt medical attention can save him. (Such attention has saved the lives of persons who showed no sign of life after lapsing into a barbiturate-induced coma.)

The effects of barbiturates and alcohol may be similar, but barbiturates are by far the more potentially lethal drug. It is difficult for a person to consume enough alcohol to cause death; his stomach rejects large amounts of alcohol, and he vomits after he has consumed a certain amount. But barbiturates are seldom vomited; instead, all of the drug taken into the stomach will be absorbed unless the stomach is pumped.

The chronic user of barbiturates, who takes the drug for either its exciting and euphoric effects or to sleep at night, eventually finds that the dosage must be increased in order for the drug to be effective and to keep from going into withdrawal. Without a regular, daily dose, an addicted individual will experience *alcohol-barbiturate abstinence syndrome.* This includes hallucinations, mild-to-severe *delirium tremens,* and convulsive seizures that resemble *grand mal* epileptic convulsions. Often these are severe enough to cause death. Alcohol-barbiturate withdrawal is far more serious than narcotic-solvent withdrawal. A physician treating someone in barbiturate withdrawal must know the name of the drug (or combination of drugs) the individual was using to keep him alive.

*Other Hypnotic-Sedative or Anesthetic Drugs.* These drugs produce reactions similar to barbiturates. They are very strong depressants, and on the continuum of drug actions, their effects dip down to the level of the anesthetics. Some are naturally occurring drugs while others are synthetics. Many of these are used medically as anesthetics. Examples include *glutethimide* (Doriden or "Ciba"); *phencyclidine* (Sernyl), which is called PCP, "hog," "angel dust," or "the peace pill"; Ditran, and the JB and LBJ compounds.

### Tranquilizers

The tranquilizing drugs are a group of drugs able to relieve or prevent uncomfortable emotional feelings. They relieve tension and apprehension and promote a state of calm and relaxation. They are mild drugs but produce dramatic effects in calming an individual and in handling violent, overactive, psychotic individuals. These drugs are divided into two distinct groups, each with unique properties and uses.

The *major tranquilizers* do not cure mental illness, but they make it easier for psychiatrists to manage mentally ill patients. Consequently, the introduction of the major tranquilizers has had a great impact on psychiatry. This group is called *major tranquilizers* because they are strong drugs used by psychiatrists and other medical practitioners in helping persons with major mental illnesses. They are different from the minor tranquilizers, which are too weak to have much effect on psychotics.

*Minor tranquilizers* are widely used now among the general public. They are used mainly to combat anxiety and the symptoms that often accompany it, including fast heartbeat, tension headaches, gastrointestinal disturbances, restlessness, insomnia, and irritability. They have the specific ability to calm the emotions of an individual without producing extreme depression or upsetting his abilities to function physically.

Few of the minor tranquilizers are commonly used illegally because they do not produce exaggerated euphoria or marked mood-modifying effects. Some persons do use tranquilizers in larger quantities than their doctors prescribe, in which case sudden abstinence or unavailability can cause nervousness and symptoms of withdrawal. But individuals who use them in prescribed dosages usually experience no adverse effects, whether from the drugs themselves or from withdrawal.

### Cannabis Drug Family

Tetrahydrocannabinol (THC) is the mood-modifying substance obtained from the common hemp plant or hemp weed (*Cannabis sativa*), grown throughout the world. The leaves and flowering tops of the plant contain an amber resin containing many chemicals, one of which is tetrahydrocannabinol. The potency of the intoxicating drugs produced from the Cannabis plant varies widely, depending upon which plant variety, which part (stems, roots, and seeds do not contain tetrahydrocannabinol), method of preparation and storage are used.

This drug family, more than any other, cannot be described accurately without specifying dosage levels. Marijuana, as used in the United States, is probably the weakest preparation of the plant used in the world. Marijuana from plants grown in the United States often contains less than two-tenths of 1 percent THC. Marijuana from Mexican plants (which is 80 percent of the marijuana used in the U.S.) has a THC content of less

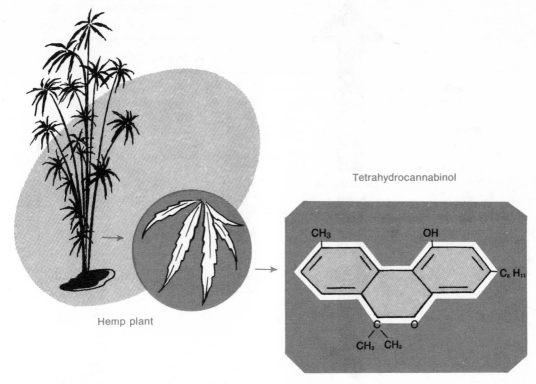

Tetrahydrocannabinol

CH₃   OH
C₅ H₁₁
C   O
CH₃   CH₃

Hemp plant

Most drugs produced by plants can be obtained only through some form of extraction technique. Marijuana plants are picked and processed. The potency depends on the available concentration of the active agent, tetrahydrocannabinol (THC).

than 1 percent. Marijuana from Jamaican plants or plants from Southeast Asia often have a 2 to 4 percent THC content. *Ganja,* a preparation containing flowering tops and the small leaves or bracts, may contain 4 to 8 percent THC if it comes from Jamaica. The most potent preparation of the hemp plant is *charas* (used mainly in India) or *hashish.* Charas is the unadulterated tetrahydrocannabinol resin obtained from the dried flowers of *Cannabis indica* (a specific variety of cannabis). Hashish, when used correctly, is a powdered and sifted form of charas. It is a chalky brown or black substance. Hashish generally contains between 5 percent and 12 percent THC.

Marijuana has been illegally imported into the United States for years. In 1972 marijuana sales in the United States were estimated at close to five billion dollars. Hashish or "hash" and "hash oil" extracts are now being illegally imported and sold in the U.S. A form of THC (Delta-3-tetrahydrocannabinol, Delta-3-THC) has been synthetically produced. It was found to be far less potent than the naturally occurring tetrahydrocannabinol, but is being sold on the streets. When tested, the street THC has been found to be mainly combinations of substitute drugs often containing hallucinogens and amphetamines. None of the liquid forms of THC is pure and often it is an unknown, broad

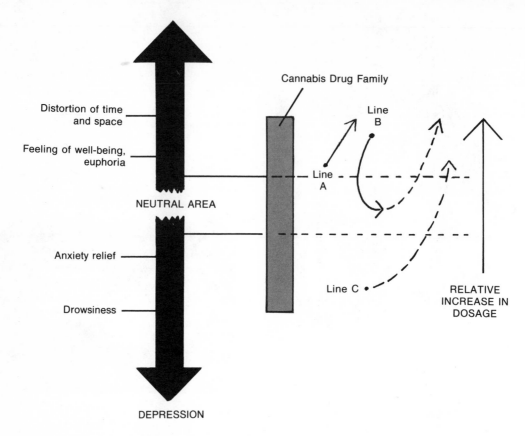

Distortion of time
and space

Feeling of well-being,
euphoria

NEUTRAL AREA

Anxiety relief

Drowsiness

DEPRESSION

Cannabis Drug Family

Line
B

Line
A

Line C

RELATIVE
INCREASE IN
DOSAGE

This continuum of drug effects and actions shows the relative effects of potency and drug dosage in the use of cannabis drugs.

mixture of chemicals that could be very dangerous. Cannabinol can be used in many ways; while marijuana and hashish are usually smoked, they are also baked into foods or added to drinks.

Taken in large, strong doses (hashish), the cannabis drug family bears many similarities to the hallucinogenic drugs. This is why, for the last few years, it has been classified as a *hallucinogenic drug* and will continue to be classified as such by many. The effects from a low dose or "social" use of marijuana are quite different and tend to approximate mild intoxication with some of the reactions similar to alcohol use. Because of these find-

ings and recent research and reports into the effects of cannabinol drugs (*Marihuana and Health* report to Congress in 1971, and *Marihuana: A Signal of Misunderstanding* in 1972), the authors of this book feel it should be given a classification distinct from all other drug families. The *Cannabis Drug Family* has been placed across the "neutral area" of the drug continuum because of its wide range of actions and effects depending upon the form of the drug used (marijuana to hashish), the amount used at one time, and the many "variables" (such as emotional state, "set," "setting," personality, and social factors) which affect the individual's response to tetrahydrocannabinol. Depending upon these factors cannabis intoxication can be similar to either hallucinogens (stimulants) or sedatives, such as alcohol (depressants).

The mood-modifying effects of cannabinol derivatives can only be described in terms of some important variables, of which dosage is the most important. As shown in the preceding graph (line "A"), if an individual uses a potent form (such as hashish) or consumes a large amount (a number of marijuana cigarettes) the physical and mental effects will continue to go toward the stimulant end of the continuum of drug actions. If a lower dosage is consumed (part of a cigarette to one or two cigarettes), often termed a "social dose," the reactions of the individual are more closely tied to the emotional and social variables present. As shown in the graph by line "B," if the individual is stimulated, or in a stimulating environment (music, colored lights), the reaction will be a slight depression causing him to relax and enjoy the situation. But if he continues to consume the drug he will start to progress up the continuum of drug actions toward the stimulating effects of the increased dosage. Also, as shown by line "C," if the individual is depressed at the beginning he will feel a stimulation with any intake of marijuana. This ability to control an individual's emotional reaction to his environment, the ability to change one's moods only slightly, is one of the main reasons people use marijuana in a social context.

*Hashish.* Individuals using potent extracts from cannabis plants experience distortions of auditory and visual perception, hallucinations, and a sense of depersonalization similar to that occurring with the use of LSD. Tolerance does develop when high dosages are used over prolonged periods, but there is no cross-tolerance with any of the hallucinogenic drugs such as LSD or mescaline. The effects of even large dosages of hashish are milder and more easily controlled than with hallucinogens. The differing "trips" or "highs" of the two classes of drugs are readily distinguishable by users; hashish users, even at high dosages, lack the major anxiety, panic, and stress reactions found in hallucinogen users. Since most hashish is actually powdered or in a liquid form the method of use becomes important. If injected directly into a vein the effect is rapid, maximal, and of a short duration (this is extremely dangerous because of the impurities commonly found in liquid THC). Smoking and inhalation cause rapid absorption into the bloodstream, but a certain amount is lost into the air and does not reach the lungs. Oral ingestion diminishes the effects of the drug, but prolongs its actions. THC capsules which are "dropped" and absorbed through the intestinal tract may cause a trip to last as long as 6 to 8 hours.

*Marijuana.* Marijuana is usually rolled into cigarettes and smoked. It cannot be confused with tobacco, being green rather than brown and having a different (alfalfa or tealike) smell. These cigarettes, "joints," burn hotter than do cigarettes made of tobacco, and the burning tip is brighter. Also, the lighted tip of a marijuana cigarette will go out easily unless an effort is made to keep it lit. Consequently, it would be difficult to imagine anyone smoking marijuana without knowledge of what he is doing.

A number of variable factors exert an important influence upon an individual's feelings and state of consciousness while under the influence of marijuana. The amount consumed is the most important variable. As with most mood-modifying drugs, the larger the dose, the greater the physical and mental effects and the longer the effects will last. Marijuana users prefer a relatively low dosage at any one time. The effects of the usual low "social" dosage, a moderate dosage, and a high dosage will be explained.

As mentioned previously, the *method of use* is important. Important variables in the individual's response to marijuana are the emotional environment ("set") and physical environment or "setting" in which the experience takes place. The emotional environment—personality, life style, philosophy, past drug experiences, mood at the time of drug use, and expectations of drug effects—is very important in determining the type and degree of response an individual will experience from a social dosage. These factors and the social setting—alone, with friends, at a party, or at a large event (such as a rock concert)—greatly account for the belief of a marijuana user that he is experiencing a "high" even when he has used a nonmarijuana substance (called a "placebo") but was told it was marijuana. Tolerance is also important in low dosage marijuana usage. There is little evidence that a tolerance develops, although it has been shown that with time and repeated consumption, the original level of satisfaction (or high) may last for a shorter period of time. The phenomenon of reverse tolerance has been observed; that is, the individual requires smaller doses to achieve the same high. However, this reverse tolerance has not been demonstrated in an experimental setting. Perhaps such reverse tolerance is related to one's *set,* especially the expectations of drug effects, and is actually the result of learning to get high and learning to recognize the more subtle mood-changes taking place at low dosages.

A person's reactions to marijuana are highly individualistic, and probably the closest analogy is the experience of daydreaming or the parade of passing thoughts, ideas, or feelings just prior to falling asleep. These effects are not constant and tend to cycle, periodically increasing and decreasing in in-

tensity. At low *social doses,* the marijuana user experiences an increased sense of well-being, some early restlessness and hilarity, followed by a dreamy, carefree relaxation (see line "B" on chart). Sensory perception is altered. There is an expansion and exaggeration of time and space relationships, cracks may look like rivers, and brief incidents may seem to take hours. The senses are heightened, intensifying smells, tastes, sounds, and sights. There are very subtle changes in thought formation and expression that often seem unusual to the unknowing observer. The individual finishes the experience, comes down feeling hungry, especially for sweets. To an unknowing observer, a person under the influence of this dosage of marijuana would not appear noticeably different from normal.

At moderate dosages, the physical and emotional reactions are intensified, but the intoxication of the individual would still be scarcely noticeable to an observer. At these higher levels of use, an individual may experience rapidly changing emotions, changing sensory reactions, lapses of attentiveness, altered thought formation, fragmented thoughts and sentences, flights of ideas, impaired short-term memory, inability to associate ideas and his physical senses, and an altered sense of self-identity. Some perceive an internal feeling of great insight.

At very high dosages, the marijuana experience closely resembles the "psychotomimetic" (or psychosis mimicking) reactions of the hallucinogenic drugs (such as LSD). These include distortions of body image, loss of personal identity, sensory and mental illusions, fantasies and hallucinations. Nearly all individuals who continue to use cannabis after experiencing these effects describe them as pleasurable. However, consistently unpleasant reactions may discourage further use.

When high dosages of cannabis (marijuana

or hashish) are used over a long term, causing constant tetrahydrocannabinol intoxication, *compulsive cannabis use* can develop. Compulsive, chronic use of cannabis might be compared with an alcoholic's preoccupation with alcohol. An individual may recognize the beginnings of a *compulsive use pattern* and a preoccupation with marijuana (or hash) by experiencing vague feelings that something is wrong and that they are functioning at a reduced level of efficiency. This is called "dropping out" or "dropping down." Individuals feel a loss of desire to work, to compete, to face challenges. Interests and major concerns become centered around marijuana. They may drop out of school, leave work, or ignore personal hygiene. The results of this reduced efficiency has been termed the "amotivational syndrome."

Controlled research studies to expand the available knowledge concerning marijuana are currently in progress. As time passes, additional information will become available to provide a more complete picture of the implications of cannabis use at various dosages and patterns of use.

### Hallucinogenic Compounds

Hallucinogens are drugs which create vivid distortions of the senses without greatly disturbing the individual's consciousness. Such distortions (hallucinations) may cause a person to see, hear, or smell things that aren't really there. Or, he may view the world much differently from the way it really is (or from the way he usually views it). Persons who abuse the hallucinogens may share with individuals who are mentally ill a tendency to experience hallucinations when they do not want to or when they are no longer under the influence of a drug. This is why some hallucinogens have been termed psychotomimetic (psychosis-mimicking) or psychotogenic (psychosis-producing) drugs. Such drugs, some authorities feel, are capable of temporarily turning a normal person into a psychotic. Users have often been hospitalized to prevent them from doing harm to themselves or others during what seems to be such a temporary psychosis.

During recent years, psychiatrists have been increasingly interested in hallucinogenic drugs. Some have taken doses of these compounds themselves in order to experience something of what their severely ill psychiatric patients must feel. Other researchers, influenced by colleagues who have defined these hallucinogenic drugs as "psychedelic," "mind-realizing," or "mind-expanding," have tried using them in an attempt to gain insight into their own minds. These drugs have also been given to alcoholics and other emotionally disturbed patients as part of therapeutic treatment. The results of these experiments have been contradictory, and in general they have not borne out the expectations of the investigators.

A large number of people acquire these drugs illegally and take them without medical supervision, sometimes while participating in group experiences. Occasionally a severe psychotic reaction or a prolonged delirious reaction follows the use of hallucinogens. Psychiatrists report that they are frequently called upon to give emergency help to persons who are suffering "bad trips" ("bummers") from these drugs. For its own protection, society has become involved in legislation against the abuse of all psychotogenic compounds.

*Mescaline* is named after the Mescalero Apaches, who developed a cult that involved using the drug in religious rituals. Mescaline is found in the small buttonlike cactus plant called peyote. This plant grows naturally in the watershed of the Rio Grande. Indian tribes in the southwestern United States chew the cactus in order to experience hallucinatory states as part of religious ceremonies.

Considerable controversy has developed in the past several years over whether the United States government should, or should not, permit such drug use. At present, the government feels that the constitutionally defined right of freedom of religion would be withheld if these Indians were forbidden use of peyote in religious ceremonies.

The buttonlike peyote plants are usually dried and then chewed. Sometimes they are boiled in water to make a broth. The effect of mescaline involves hallucinations and euphoria lasting for a period of between 8 hours and 2 days. These hallucinations may include the appearance of fantastic geometric patterns, distortions in the sense of time and space, and feelings of depersonalization.

Peyote itself is by no means convenient to use, a fact that limits its illicit use among persons who seek psychedelic experiences. The texture of the buttons is extremely unpleasant, and the juice from them is sickening. Persons who use peyote, even Indians experienced in its use, can expect to vomit several times while taking the drug. Besides an upset stomach, peyote causes sweating, elevated blood pressure, increased pulse rates, and muscle twitching. Pure mescaline, which is extracted from peyote buttons, is available on the illegal market in capsule form. The caps, of course, are much easier to take, although some users experience slight nausea at the beginning of their trip. Neither mescaline caps nor peyote buttons are physically addictive.

*LSD,* commonly referred to by users as "acid," is a tasteless, colorless, and odorless drug derived from lysergic acid diethylamide. The primary danger in taking LSD is that it may cause temporary psychosis, accompanied by a wide range of behavioral disturbances. Some users experience panic or depression, while others feel euphoria and a sense of great mental clarity or comprehen-sion. Visual hallucinations are commonly experienced.

An LSD trip lasts 8 to 16 hours. Afterward, users who have enjoyed their trip may describe a feeling of having been reborn, of having seen the world for the first time. This feeling is often accompanied by a sense of deep affection for others, particularly those who were present and participating in the trip.

Doses of LSD are measured in micrograms; an average dose can be anywhere from 150 to 250 micrograms. A user taking much larger doses may experience delirium and convulsions. After any dose, "flashbacks" may occur; that is, the psychotic effects of the drug may recur from time to time up to a year or more after the trip.

LSD dilates the pupils, raises the blood pressure, stimulates the brain's sensory centers, and blocks off its inhibiting mechanisms. It intensifies hearing, increases the ability to differentiate among textures, and may produce a tingling sensation and numbness of the hands and feet. Subjects often report crossovers of sensation; for example, they may seem to hear colors or smell the scent of music.

A user of LSD may experience minor physical discomfort, including nausea and abdominal pain. The possibility of much more serious, long-term effects of LSD has been reported, such as deformities among children born to women who took LSD while pregnant. There is evidence that the use of LSD has decreased in recent years.

### Cocaine

In criminal law, cocaine is classified as a narcotic. But it has a depressing effect only when it is used as a local anesthetic; its general effect on the body is to stimulate and induce excitement. Though not addictive, it produces a strong psychological dependence.

# COMMONLY USED AND ABUSED AMPHETAMINES

| COLOR AND SHAPE OF CAPSULE OR TABLET | TRADE NAMES | STREET NAMES |
|---|---|---|
| Red-pink | Benzedrine (spansule capsule) | "Bennies" |
| Pink | Benzedrine (tablet) | "Bennies" |
| Orange | Dexedrine (spansule capsule) | "Dexies" |
| Orange | Dexedrine (tablet) | "Dexies" |
| Green | Dexamyl (tablet) (contains dexedrine and amobarbital) | |
| White | Edrisal (tablet) (contains benzedrine, aspirin, and phenacetin) | |
| White | Biphetamine (capsule) | "Whites" |
| White | Methedrine (tablet) | "Meth" "Speed" "Crystals" "Whites" |

Amphetamines: The primary effects of the many brands of amphetamines — available in white or colored tablets or timed disintegration capsules — include an increase in confidence, euphoria, feelings of fearlessness, talkativeness, impulsive behavior, loss of appetite, and decrease in fatigue. Variously called "leapers," "uppers," "beans," "pep pills," and "diet pills," they produce strong psychological dependence.

Cocaine, or "coke," is prepared from the coca plant and processed into an odorless, white, fluffy, fine crystalline powder. On the criminal market, it is sometimes referred to as "snow" because of its appearance. It is sold in the same types of containers as heroin. But the price is always quite high because cocaine is more difficult to obtain than heroin.

Cocaine users usually sniff the drug into their nostrils. A few users take the drug by hypodermic injection. Sniffing is the more popular method but it is highly destructive to the tissues lining the nose and respiratory tract because, when the drug is absorbed slowly through the membranes of the nose, its effects last longer and are less violent than when it is injected. Advanced narcotic addicts may mix cocaine and heroin together. This combined injection is called a "speedball."

### Amphetamines

Included in the stimulant group are a large number of drugs which mimic the actions of adrenalin. In general, the physical reactions they produce are an increase in heart rate, a constriction of certain blood vessels, an increase in the breathing rate, an increase in perspiration, and a cottonlike dryness of the mouth. These side reactions are always combined with the primary actions of amphetamines on the brain—an increase in bodily activity and an elevation of mood. Feelings and behavior aroused by amphetamines include increased confidence, euphoria, fearlessness, talkativeness, impulsive behavior, loss of appetite, and a decrease of fatigue. The stimulating effects of amphetamines are often relied upon by criminals to increase their nerve.

There are on the market a large number of amphetamine drugs that are mainly used for weight reduction ("diet pills"). The most widely abused amphetamines, Benzedrine and Dexedrine, are prescribed for this purpose. On the illegal market they are known as "bennies," "dexies," "pep pills," or "whites" (because Benzedrine is often sold as a white tablet) or as "uppers" or "leapers" because of the mood elevation (see illustration). Several drug companies, without showing substantial evidence, make claims that their particular compound suppresses the appetite without causing central nervous system stimulation. No amphetamine or amphetaminelike compound has only one of these two effects on the body. Consequently, the usual circumstance is that while the user loses weight, he also loses sleep.

Actually, many chronic users of pep pills use a desire for weight loss as an excuse for taking these drugs. Amphetamines produce a weight loss by making people active and suppressing their appetites. If they continue to take more, they can keep going for hours or even days without sleep or rest. Consequently, these drugs are sometimes abused by those who want to work or play harder or longer than their normal capacities allow them to.

There are several ways in which these drugs can cause physical damage when they are used over long periods of time. The mechanism in the liver which activates amphetamines is destroyed or impaired quite quickly; therefore, users have to continually increase dosage levels to maintain the desired effectiveness. Prolonged use of increasing dosages causes long periods of sleep loss and mood and behavior changes, which may develop into a severe mental disorder or psychosis. The people suffering from this mental illness are usually characterized by extreme activity for long periods of time, feelings of superiority, bizarre forms of suspiciousness, hallucinations, and excitement—all to an exaggerated degree. Those that suddenly stop using amphetamines (often because these drugs have stopped being effective) usually go through a rather prolonged period of lethargy, depression, nightmares, and restlessness.

Young people particularly are abusing amphetamines for the mood-modifying qualities of these drugs. They frequently mix these drugs with either alcohol or barbiturates. Such abuse is extremely dangerous. It can cause death or lead to impulsive acts of poor judgment and to accidents. Especially abused is the amphetamine compound Methedrine (methamphetamine hydrochloride), commonly called "speed" or "meth." Some people swallow Methedrine pills, but the majority inject the compound into a muscle ("skin pop") or vein ("mainline") to get a quick euphoric flash or rush. With continued injections, they will stay awake for days and eat very little, until their bodies become completely exhausted ("strung out"). Then the worst part of a speed trip begins, the withdrawal from the drug, or "crashing." Heavy users stop their injections, slip between coma and sleep for days, then awaken and start their injections again.

A great danger from amphetamines is the effect they have on automobile drivers. When a number of pills are taken at one time, or if they are used for a long period of time without rest or sleep, they may produce hallucinations or delirium. Users may feel that someone or something in another automobile is following them. Or, they may black out suddenly while driving at high speeds. These effects are so dangerous that many states have made it a felony offense to drive while under the influence of amphetamine.

Beyond the chemistry and physiology of drug use is an extensive body of laws, attitudes, procedures, and treatments—as our society attempts to maintain some policy and method of dealing with these substances. This other side of drugs is explored in the next chapter.

# 6
# The Drug Problem

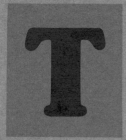

There are no proven techniques, procedures, or treatments that can be applied to the entire drug-abusing population. The basis of this problem is the lack of understanding of the causes of drug abuse. One popular theory holds that the persistent craving for drugs such as narcotics is the result of metabolic or other physiological changes caused by repeated narcotics use. Others believe that drugs are used by the emotionally disturbed as a reflection of their own psychological difficulties, by the economically deprived to escape the reality of their limited opportunity, or by those who, for other reasons, by repeated experimentation, have conditioned themselves to respond to stressful stimuli by additional drug use. At the other extreme of those holding to this theory are those who believe that drugs are abused purely for hedonistic purposes by delinquent, criminal individuals who are completely unconcerned with what society expects and are too immature to worry about possible long-term consequences.

Certainly some element of each of these causes can be identified in the extremely wide variety of drug abuse cases in the United States. There is no doubt that some patterns of drug abuse are specific to certain social, cultural, economic, and political segments of the population. The proportion of heroin addicts in urban areas, the amount of marijuana usage throughout society, and the excessive use of barbiturates and amphetamines in the suburbs are focusing attention on these areas and are prompting researchers to ask very specific cause-and-effect questions.

Yet, irrespective of these facts, all drug-abuse treatment programs are ultimately dependent on the motivation of the individual. By placing final responsibility and hope for "cure" on the will of the individual, we have also implied that the alteration of certain external factors will not be sufficient to reverse the tragic patterns of abuse which have occurred in recent decades.

## WHAT ARE THE GOALS OF TREATMENT?

At the present time, most research concentrates on determining which factors might be exercising a particularly strong influence in a certain type of drug-abuse syndrome. Then, when that one causative factor is isolated, psychiatrists, pharmacologists, and other specialists can seek to reverse its effects. Thus, the current methods of drug-abuse treatment in the United States are highly varied in their procedures and results.

As might be expected, the usual point at which the drug abuser and society as a whole first get together and really come to each other's attention is at the time that the user runs up against the law. Enforcement of the drug laws temporarily takes the user out of his environment, and, for the period of his jail sentence, forces him to do without drugs. Also, another beneficial effect of a jail sentence is that, for the moment, the innocent (the "forgotten man" in our laws) is protected from the compulsive drug user.

But emphasis solely on punitive confinement has never successfully helped any significant number of drug abusers. "Drunkards" have been jailed for centuries; opium eating was once a serious problem in the United States, but it was the elimination of the supply from China, rather than the early narcotics acts, which reduced its incidence; heroin addiction is demonstrably a consequence of factors that are evidently not affected by short-term detention.

Compared with the other possible modes of control—social, legal, and so on—self-control is the only one which can ultimately be relied upon for treatment. The environment or *setting* and the emotional *set* of the individual must be changed if he is to live a drug-free life. Development of an individual's self-control and changing his *setting* and *set*

are the aims of most drug treatment programs. Punishment alone will never work.

## TREATMENT LAWS AND FACILITIES

There are two agencies available for treatment of drug abuse: private and public. The private programs mainly emphasize treatment through family members or peer group populations. Individuals lacking the personal self-control to stay within the framework of a private program, and who would leave it against medical advice, will always be the ones who need to be placed within the legal controls of public programs. However, too often we commit people to public treatment programs out of anger and vindictiveness rather than humane concern. This is certainly emphasized by the penalties for drug possession. The predominant method of dealing with drug abuse has been to place the individual in jail. Following his release, he generally resumes using drugs. We still do not have effective methods of treatment for this kind of drug abuser.

The Federal Narcotics Addict Rehabilitation Act of 1966 is a law which helps states and local communities treat drug abusers. Many states have also passed legislation supplementing and defining the procedures of this act. In California, there is the Mental Health Act of 1969 (the Lanterman-Petris-Short Law). It defines in detail the conditions which permit voluntary and involuntary hospitalization for drug abuse. Under the Federal statute, an eligible person charged with a crime may be told by a judge that the criminal charge will be "held in abeyance" if he will submit to a medical examination to determine whether he is an addict and could be rehabilitated through treatment. The drug offender has 5 days in which to make a decision. If he elects to apply for

*131*

treatment he then is retained in a hospital for not more than 60 days for examination purposes. He will then be placed in a state hospital through a civil commitment procedure if he is found to be a suitable candidate for treatment.

The civil commitment is a legal mechanism utilized in place of a criminal commitment. This procedure ensures control over drug abusers during rehabilitation—first in a hospital or drug treatment institution, later in a halfway house, and still later in the community under the close supervision of a probation or parole officer. The significant step in this procedure is that the drug abuser does not establish a criminal record when seeking treatment and help.

An individual is limited to a 2-year maximum confinement, unless the judge renews the procedure at a later date. If, after release to the community, the individual resumes using drugs he may be returned for further treatment or the criminal proceedings may be started again. Should he be found guilty, any time served in the treatment program will be counted toward the time to be served under the criminal sentence.

If a person has been convicted of a non-violent crime, and a judge believes the criminal offender is an addict or in danger of becoming an addict, he may order him to be examined and then committed to a treatment program for an indeterminate period of time. This can not be more than 10 years but must be more than 6 months. He then may be released under the supervision of a probation officer. This is a criminal commitment procedure for drug abuse and does result in a criminal record.

There are two U.S. Public Health Service hospitals in the United States—one is at Lexington, Kentucky and the other is at Fort Worth, Texas. Under the Addict Rehabilitation Act of 1966, these hospitals were changed to research and limited treatment facilities because they were unsuccessful as treatment facilities. They are generally used as diagnostic and short-term treatment centers during commitment procedures.

Through federal legislation passed from 1968 to 1971, the states and communities have been given federal support, through the National Institute of Mental Health, to develop training programs: to construct, staff, and operate addiction treatment facilities. This support has helped the states expand their programs and facilities to meet their increasing needs.

Few states have proper or sufficient treatment programs. A handful have been instrumental in developing large-scale programs. The following are some of the more innovative programs at the state level.

In the state of New York, in 1962, the Metcalf-Voker Act placed arrested addicts in the state's Mental Hygiene Department hospitals for treatment instead of in jail. The milestone in this program was that medical rather than corrections personnel made the release decisions for the aftercare portion of the project. In 1965, New York initiated a Special Narcotic Project through which parolees with a history of drug abuse were given special supervision and help during their period of parole. In 1966, legislation amended the Mental Hygiene Law, establishing a comprehensive program for the treatment, rehabilitation, and aftercare of narcotics addicts. This program is conducted by the Narcotic Addiction Control Commission and now has wide control over treatment, control, prevention, and research into drug abuse in New York state.

As early as 1959, a Narcotic Treatment control project similar to the 1965 New York project was instituted in California. California's Civil Addict Program of 1961 provided hospital care and aftercare treatment and control for opiate (mainly heroin) users. Since the Mental Health Act of 1969 the civil commitment procedures used for addicts are identical to those used with other mental illness cases.

Effective mental hygiene legislation for drug abusers was enacted in New Jersey in 1964. The value of the New Jersey program is its approach of establishing a positive psychological position not directly connected with drug abuse. This program was under the direction of the Division of Mental Health and Hospitals, rather than the corrections facilities of the state. In 1967, a Bureau of Narcotic Addiction and Drug Abuse was established within the Division to carry out the treatment responsibilities for persons commited for treatment after being sentenced in New Jersey courts.

In 1965, Illinois created the Narcotic Advisory Council within the Department of Mental Health to make recommendations for the prevention, treatment, and rehabilitation of drug users. But, until 1968, the only actual treatment facility in Illinois was the House of Corrections in Chicago. In 1967, all treatment programs in Illinois were consolidated, and by 1968 a unified program began. Today it is a complete treatment program that includes research and evaluation.

## MODES OF DRUG ABUSE TREATMENT

Medical authorities feel that the compulsive drug abuser is a sick person. He is emotionally disturbed and physiologically ill. He needs treatment for the physical effects of the drug he is abusing and he needs psychological help to keep from going back to drug abuse when he leaves the hospital.

When an individual under the influence of drugs comes to the attention of a hospital staff or a private physician, it is usually in the context of an emergency situation. Some doctors in high drug abuse areas will see as many as 7000 drug users in one year.

The first information needed by the physician is the name of the drug or combination of drugs the individual is using. This is often difficult to determine because the user may be unconscious, semicoherent, disoriented, frightened, unreliable, and may often behave as an acute psychotic. Reassurance in a quiet and "cool" environment will often produce an accurate story of what happened and simplify this phase of treatment. Friends, the contents of the user's pockets, and the surrounding conditions under which the adverse reactions occurred might well help the doctor in his evaluation. During this acute phase of treatment, a well-established rapport between the physician and the patient can be a valuable tool.

During this "talk-down" phase little more than acceptance and reassurance is necessary. If definite signs of toxic complications occur, the physician will treat them as they appear, regardless of what the patient has told him.

A very important complicating factor in this procedure is the fear of legal incrimination. In addition to the aforementioned unpleasant feelings, the patient will probably fear the introduction of the police into the situation. He will try to cover-up potential evidence, will become wary of the doctor's questions, and might well have difficulty distinguishing medical from legal personnel. Though this is all very understandable, it will not do the patient any good.

Most drug prosecutions are based on evidence of possession. If the police obtained such evidence at the time they brought the patient to a health facility, his fears are simply too late. But even if they have not obtained the evidence, they will not pursue the search into the examining room. A doctor is not a law enforcement official. His goal is to help the patient come out of what was probably an extremely disturbing and dangerous experience. He needs the patient's greatest possible cooperation in order to succeed.

When treating a victim of addicting drugs, a doctor has a complicated task. Abrupt withdrawal, the so-called "cold turkey" is painful and can be fatal. Gradual withdrawal is usually done in a hospital. The American Medical Association suggests that a physician should not normally try to attempt withdrawal unless the individual is in a hospital.

During narcotics withdrawal, the drug abuser will suffer nausea, watery eyes, muscle spasms in the stomach and legs, and hot and cold flashes. The drug methadone may be substituted for any major opiate drug. This is called methadone detoxification. It tends to block the euphoric effects and relieves the craving for other narcotics.

In barbiturate withdrawal, *grand-mal* epileptic type convulsions and delirium tremens may occur. Here, the drug pentobarbital can be used as a substitute drug during detoxification withdrawal. Abrupt withdrawl from barbiturates is extremely dangerous and often has been fatal. Consequently, a physician must know both the quantity and nature of the barbiturates used before he can effectively treat the patient.

The first "chemical treatment" approach to drug abuse was the use of narcotic antagonists—drugs chemically and structurally so like narcotics that they can apparently occupy the "place" in the nervous system which is the object of narcotics action. Antagonists, when given to a person physically addicted to narcotics (usually heroin), will bring on withdrawal symptoms rather than prevent them. Even if the individual has taken only one or two doses of the narcotic within the last week, there are recognizable changes (such as effects on pupil size) that take place.

This way a physician can tell if an individual is currently using narcotics. Three of the most important narcotic antagonists are Nalline, cyclazocine, and naloxine.

Cyclazocine is the first of these to be used in treatment programs. While someone is taking several daily dosages of cyclazocine they will not feel the effects of a narcotic nor will they become addicted to it. Thus, during a treatment program, antagonists may provide a means of "unlearning" drug-abusing behavior. With these drugs people may keep from becoming physically addicted, making it possible for them to continue working and participating in a rehabilitation program. To be effective these drugs must be part of a broad program of psychological and social rehabilitation.

Nalline has been used as a diagnostic and testing drug for years. Usually, individuals must submit to weekly Nalline tests as part of parole procedures, but no other rehabilitation or psychological treatment is given him. True treatment programs using Nalline are relatively new.

Such uses of methadone, pentobarbital, and Nalline have certainly made possible some degree of progress in treating serious drug abuse cases. But these methods have also drawn a good deal of criticism. One reason for this criticism is the observation that these procedures succeed only with highly motivated individuals.

In 1965, Drs. Vincent Dole and Marie Nyswander, both of the Rockefeller University in New York City, developed the first systematic *methadone maintenance program.* This program is based on a slightly different use of methadone. The patient is given a quantity of the drug on a daily basis, thus having the opportunity to live a fairly normal life. Unlike the narcotics addict who is relying solely on illegal opiates, the individual being treated with methadone need not focus his entire existence on obtaining his drug. Methadone thus permits the individual a more immediate, responsible view of self and society.

Methadone is an addicting opiate. When given in sufficient dosages (about 100 milligrams per day) methadone blocks the effect of heroin (if an individual tries to continue using heroin), relieves the craving for heroin, and also does not alter the mood or behavior of the individual. Since 1965 the success of methadone maintenance programs throughout the United States can be demonstrated by remarks from the New York Academy of Medicine. The Academy has stated that while methadone maintenance is not the ultimate cure for heroin addiction, "No other regimen currently available offers so much to the chronic addict." By 1972, 25,000 heroin addicts were in methadone programs. This number is now doubling. Such programs are limited, not by the number of addicts willing to enter them (they all have waiting lists), but by a lack of funds, trained staff, and public officials willing to expand the programs.

Many physicians, politicians, and others feel that the use of methadone is based upon a morally and ethically imperfect scheme of substituting one addictive drug (methadone) for another (heroin). But one of the advantages of methadone is that it is addicting. The patient must take the drug day after day, year after year, just as a diabetic must continue to take insulin. Both situations are unfortunate but it continues to remind the individual that he has a unique problem that requires ongoing treatment and concern. A continuing treatment program is the basis of all successful drug treatment programs (for example, A.A., Teen Challenge). Several nonaddicting drugs have been tried, without a great deal of success, to treat heroin addiction. Among them are the narcotic antago-

nists cyclazocine and Nalline. Because they are not addicting, the poorly motivated patient can drift away from the program and, in time, return to heroin.

Here are two reasons why methadone maintenance programs have been so successful. First, methadone is legal, and the individual can view himself in a different light than when he dealt in illegal heroin. For this reason, the term *addict* should be dropped when someone enters a methadone program. The public, staff, friends, family, and the individual himself should view him as a *methadone patient*. This avoids the stereotyped image of an addict, and also shows respect to someone who is trying to change his complete *set* and *setting*. Second, methadone is cheap. Illegal heroin is expensive to everyone—the addict, the police (attempting to enforce the law), the medical profession and society (lost productivity, theft, and abnormal social behavior by the drug user). The average cost of heroin to an addict is $20 a day or more. Methadone costs about 10 cents a day. In programs it is either supplied free or at $10 to $14 a week. At either rate, the cost to society is small, compared with illegal heroin use. Unlike heroin, methadone does not present the tolerance problem; while using methadone, the patient does not crave larger doses once he has reached the stabilization point.

Two other advantages of methadone are that it blocks the euphoric effects of heroin and is also long-acting. Often a patient, to his own amazement, will shoot some heroin after he has taken methadone and finds that the heroin has no effect. This blocking effect is due to *cross-tolerance* among opiates and synthetic narcotics. Any opiate or synthetic narcotic, in a specific dose, will block the effects of any other opiate or synthetic narcotic given at a smaller dose. Thus, the methadone dose is set at whatever level is necessary to block the largest heroin dose a patient is likely to take. An important condition to this blockage is that the methadone be taken orally, usually dissolved in orange juice. When methadone is mainlined, however, it is possible to get the same euphoric reaction as from heroin. Consequently, an illegal market dealing in methadone has sprung up in recent years.

The long-acting effect of methadone is important. An oral dose taken in the morning will keep an individual stable until the next morning. He does not have to "shoot up" several times a day and "ride the roller coaster," "high" (up), "on the nod" (sedated, drowsy), or "sick" (going into withdrawal) periodically throughout the day. The patient does have to go to a clinic daily or, in the case of patients who have been on a program for a number of years, be given a week or two supply of methadone (an abusive amount if injected). This problem may be eliminated with the use of new, even longer-acting drugs similar to methadone. One being tested is acetylmethadol (acetyl-alpha-methadol), which may be effective for three days or longer. Such drugs would require the patient to visit the clinic only once a week or twice a month, which would be sufficient for emotional and psychiatric reinforcement to remain heroin-free.

Another distinct approach involves the establishment of complex social systems, houses, homes, or communities that are directed almost exclusively by ex-addicts. These are called therapeutic communities. Such organizations as Synanon (California), Daytop House, Phoenix House, Odyssey House (New York), Gateway House (Illinois), and the federally sponsored Tacoma Narcotics Center (Washington) are some of the better known therapeutic communities. Individuals are not required to remain at these centers continuously, and are free to leave

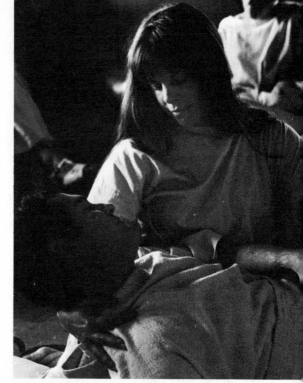

Synanon—An experiment in interpersonal communication. *Photo by R. Foothorap.*

permanently at any time. However, in order to remain at the center, they must participate in the center's programs and must conform to the strict community rules.

Therapeutic communities are designed to provide care through three mechanisms: (1) encounter group therapy, (2) a highly structured community organization, and (3) a reward-punishment system based on simple behavioral psychology. The key to the therapeutic process is the group encounter, usually called the "Synanon game," "attack therapy," or the "verbal street fight." The second phase consists of a complete behavioral dissection through the encounter therapy and scaled program of house jobs, starting with dishwashing or garbage control, and progressing to ordering supplies and leading group therapy sessions (this phase can last for years).

These communities are designed to develop and reinforce the standard middle-class norms of behavior and attitudes. Theoretically, the community tries to make the individual goal-oriented—willing to work hard and sacrifice in order to obtain eventual security and success. Men and women's roles are carefully defined and sexual behavior is subject to the censure and influences the individual would encounter outside the community (homosexual relationships are prohibited; heterosexual relationships are permitted only after an extended period of time in the community).

The black and brown communities criticize this type of program because of the personality and identity destruction that goes on in encounter therapy. These people feel that they have been stripped of their identity by the white society long enough and that the reconstruction of black and brown identity is a valid concern of these programs. Also, almost all of these programs are conducted exclusively in English, so that the Spanish-speaking person is always at a disadvantage. The middle-class norms do not take into consideration the poverty backgrounds of most black and brown addicts. A program based on positive racial identification and self-help has been started in New York (The Community Thing).

In the past, reentry into society was the desired last stage of a successful therapeutic community treatment program. But very few ever achieved full-time employment in positions unrelated to addictive programs. Also, therapeutic communities do not make people independent. The communities provide a life that is better than "real life." This encourages addiction to "community life" rather than to

hard drugs. Experience now indicates that many addicts require the permanent support of a therapeutic community in order to prevent the resumption of their drug-taking behavior. This seems to be the case with alcoholics; they must continue their association with Alcoholics Anonymous. And narcotics addicts must remain on methadone maintenance.

The most successful people within the communities are those who are articulate and capable of assuming leadership. In the beginning there was very little emphasis on education within the communities because it interfered with the therapeutic process. In recent years, with entire families becoming permanent residents, therapeutic communities have become strongly education-oriented. Synanon operates its own elementary and secondary schools and encourages colleges and universities to hold classes in its facilities.

Both the therapeutic community and the maintenance programs tend to reduce compulsive drug abuse and addiction to the level of an individual problem. This may well be the key to drug abuse treatment. After an individual has been treated for drug abuse and returns to society he faces many personal problems, which may be social, legal, economic, and medical. Often, with drug problems, the offender and the victim are the same person and the social pressures that encourage him to abuse drugs in the first place are still present in this environment when he returns.

If there are facilities available to provide for a gradual reentry into society, or if he has not established a criminal record (civil commitment rather than criminal conviction) because of drugs, he has a much better chance of adjustment. Short visits home should be made at first, then a halfway house, work camp, parish house, or a day-night hospital may help beyond phase three of the therapeutic community. Any of these settings is potentially useful in providing the abuser with social, therapeutic, educational, and vocational services; these give him controlled contacts with the community.

But all too often, the treated drug abuser leaves the hospital (or more often, the jail) and literally is "dumped back on the street." Consequently, it is a very short time before he is again abusing drugs and is back or beyond where he was when treatment was initiated.

Drug treatment programs can only succeed when they deal with the basic fact that the compulsive user or addict has no ability to combat the ordinary stresses in life. He has relied for months, or perhaps years, on the external solace provided by drugs. A cure of his addiction must help him redirect his attitudes toward his own weaknesses.

The cure of the confirmed drug user is simply not a reliable prospect. A great deal more research will be necessary in order for our society to maintain a consistent level of cure and rehabilitation. The damage done by drug abuse is so powerful and so widespread that the only practical long-range "cure" is prevention.

Obviously, the trend is away from purely punitive measures and toward rehabilitation and treatment. There is no doubt that rehabilitation and planned prevention hold much greater promise for both the individual and society than does punitive confinement.

A person who has been rescued from a possible life of drug abuse has saved society a good deal more than the cost of his future treatment. The more our nation's policy-makers become convinced that the cost of ambitious, well-planned, humane programs is money well spent, the more progress we can expect to witness.

## DRUG CONTROL AND LAW ENFORCEMENT

Control of drug use in the United States has had a mixed and confused history, and few guidelines are clearly revealed. Prohibition of alcoholic beverages during the 1920s has generally been considered an overwhelming failure. It most probably did not discourage drinking (in fact, quite the contrary), nor did it produce a generation of nondrinkers. Yet, control-by-prescription laws of certain other drugs has certainly determined that these substances will not be routinely abused on a wide scale. A person cannot simply walk into a drug store and purchase morphine without a prescription; a 5-year-old child cannot purchase even aspirin by himself. Surely the legal requirement that certain substances be dispensed only upon the approval and under the direction of a physician has affected most people's attitudes toward drugs.

One of the most interesting aspects of the problem is the current argument centered on the possible legalization of marijuana. Reflected against the history of drug control in our country, this debate highlights some interesting points. The pressure for legalization of marijuana is hardly universal and the eventual change of status of this substance is certainly not a foregone conclusion at this time. But some recurring themes can be found in the arguments of the legalization proponents. Mainly, the analogies to the prohibition of alcohol demand some attention.

Proponents of legalization have insisted that prohibition during the 1920s did not work and that the restrictions on the cultivation, sale, use, and possession of marijuana are not working either. Marijuana does little to the body that alcohol does not do, given these same arguments, and yet society has hypocritically banned one and permitted the other. A driver "stoned " on grass is a potential danger on the highways, but the major cause of serious automobile accidents in the United States is alcohol. To those who say that we need more information and more time to understand the effects of marijuana—before we can confidently legalize it—proponents respond that we know little about certain major aspects of alcohol use. The nature of the damage alcohol does to the metabolism, the causes of alcoholism, and the cure for a hangover are still relative mysteries, yet alcohol is permitted a controlled but important place in our society.

The major conclusion to be drawn from the present marijuana legalization argument is that our society has the most difficulty in developing useful policies toward those substances which occupy a middle ground in the public consciousness. Alcohol, tobacco, and marijuana have attained such an undefined position primarily because their effects are not readily predictable, and their use does not necessarily interfere with normal functioning in our society.

As Prohibition went headlong against the attitudes of many Americans and thus failed, so has the outlawing of marijuana use come into conflict with the viewpoints and life style of a generation.

### The Public Attitudes

Laws are functional representations of what a society believes in. We have laws against forms of conduct we condemn and laws designed to encourage conduct of which we approve. Between generations the body of laws, along with other factors, provides new and young members of the society with guidelines for their behavior and attitudes.

Helen H. Nowlis, Professor of Psychology, University of Rochester, outlined nine points that help explain how attitudes toward drugs develop (Nowlis, 1968).

1. *Ignorance* of the actions of chemical substances upon the complex, delicately balanced chemical system that is the living person can be a large factor. There is also a lack of knowledge about the relationship of variations in human behavior and human behavior itself. Here drug abuse is a problem of opinion, emotions, and beliefs in the absence of knowledge.

2. *Semantics* plays an important part because every term can be entangled in myth, emotions, assumptions, beliefs, and attitudes that too often turn the dialogue into a futile argument.

3. *Communication* between scientists themselves and with the public has been a significant problem in our society for decades. Technical jargon, scientific precepts, and assumptions are frequently very difficult for the layman to comprehend. Too, there is a communication problem between a generation brought up before, and during the development of automation, television, jet travel, nuclear energy, large urban centers, cramped schools, and an affluent social order with a generation that has known no other conditions.

4. *Lack of understanding of scientific method and concepts* refers to the lack of understanding that there are no simple cause and effect relationships when we deal with human behavior. The term "proof," which people seek in determining their attitudes, cannot always be used reliably. The design and execution of experiments might be open to bias; conclusions might be colored by the scientist's own viewpoint.

5. *Living a life in a world of constant and dramatic change* has contributed toward a disorientation of the traditional beliefs and

assumptions of society. The future seems unpredictable and people have become increasingly centered on the "here and now."

6. *The philosophy of social control* has become an increasingly difficult aspect of the problem. What can society prevent a person from doing to himself? How does the entire social structure suffer when an unjust or unenforceable law continues to diminish public respect for the judicial and legislative processes?

7. *Education* is both a major key to and an important part of the difficulties of determining social attitudes toward drugs. Our educational institutions and the information media have an obligation to inform citizens of new developments in scientific research, but our institutions of learning then become vulnerable to short-sighted attacks when people disagree with these conclusions and the institutions that produced them.

8. *Our society is a "pill society."* This well-advertised proposition states that there is a chemical solution for any problem of unpleasantness, strain, or discomfort. This pill society spends more on alcohol, tranquilizers, sleeping pills, and tobacco than it does on education or on solving its social and economic problems.

9. *Increasing retreat in the face of complex problems* is the end point of the process. As our society becomes more complex, less fixed and definite people seek more absolutes and find themselves less and less able to relate to the society and to understand their own role. For many people, "black-and-white" choices seem easier than careful, deliberate decisions based on information and sound judgment.

Set against these important psychological and social viewpoints of drug abuse and drug attitudes is the criminal philosophy of drug abuse. This philosophy suggests three ways of controlling or eradicating drug abuse:

1. Complete control of drug supplies
2. Elimination of "pushers"
3. Isolation and elimination of drug users

This plan does not attack the problem but just jails the offenders. The proper control of drug abuse lies in resolving the nine basic problems mentioned above, but the problems are complex. D. P. Ausubel, in his book *Drug Addiction,* lists a fourth approach to drug abuse control:

4. Research into the nature, causes, treatment, outcome, and epidemiology of drug addiction.

Our society is seeking sound solutions to the basic causes of drug abuse. It presently relies on a certain body of laws to protect itself. Laws can be preventive measures, but the current controls now available are not meeting present needs. Some type of control is needed for the treatment of drug abuse. This may be legal, social, or self-control, but it must be present. More control than is necessary becomes punishment, but less control than is necessary is useless. Up until the middle 1960s the major laws were established to control illegal possession, manufacture, and sale of drugs rather than their abuse. Treatment programs were left out completely. As described earlier, during the middle 1960s laws were established that governed research into the effects and actions of drugs that permitted greater flexibility in the treatment and control of drug abuse and the rehabilitation of drug abusers. This trend separated treatment laws from those governing the possession and sale of drugs.

### The Drug Control Laws

The federal government's control of the sale and possession of drugs is based on laws which have been enacted over the last 60 years. In tracing the history of these laws, we will be recapitulating the record of drug abuse in this country.

During the 1800s, narcotics were taken as constituents of patent medicines and cure-alls. This use increased greatly with the invention of the hypodermic needle and syringe just before the Civil War. Doctors actually encouraged their patients to buy this device and to use narcotics on a "do-it-yourself" basis. The "miracle medicines," "elixirs," and "tonics," which contained large amounts of narcotics—usually opium preparations—were easy to obtain and were reputed to be cures for everything.

By the end of the Civil War, thousands of soldiers had received injections of narcotics to relieve their suffering from wounds and sickness. Many became addicted to these drugs. A much greater percentage of the population was addicted at this time than is today. Then, with the growth of advertising and the promotion of patent medicines containing narcotics, great numbers of people took such medicines and became addicted to them. Some, having discovered the fact that these medicines contained opium, bought and used "straight" opium. Narcotic abuse climbed steeply even after 1914, when the first effective drug-control laws were enacted. There was very little actual reduction in the abuse of narcotics until the Federal Bureau of Narcotics was established in 1930 to enforce the earlier narcotics laws and apprehend violators. The name of this agency has since been changed to the Bureau of Narcotics and Dangerous Drugs (BNDD).

The first federal measure seeking control over drugs was enacted by Congress on February 9, 1906. The *Federal Pure Food and Drug Act* prohibited the importation of opium, its preparations, and its derivatives, except for medicinal purposes. A second law was enacted December 17, 1914, the *Harrison Narcotic Act,* which further restricted the importation, manufacture, sale, and dispensing of opiates. It required the keeping of accurate records and inventories of narcotics and made the possession of narcotics a criminal (felony) offense. It established the legal definition of a narcotic as *any drug that produces sleep or stupor and relieves pain.* Certain specific drugs were legally labeled narcotics regardless of their medical nature. Opium, its derivatives, coca leaves and their derivatives (such as cocaine), marijuana, peyote (mescaline), and any synthetic drug that produces sleep or stupor and relieves pain was declared a "habit-forming narcotic drug."

The Harrison Act required physicians to dispense opiates only "in the course of their professional practice" for bonafide medical purposes. It limited the selling of narcotics to licensed druggists and only after they receive a lawful written prescription issued by a qualified medical or dental practitioner.

The next federal statute, approved in 1922, was an extensive revision of the Harrison Act. It is known as the *Narcotics Drugs Import and Export Act.* This revision and subsequent minor revisions are considered the official position of the federal government with regard to the legal and illegal possession, importation, manufacture, and exportation of narcotics. It authorizes the importation of specific quantities of crude opium and coca leaves needed to provide for the medical and legitimate scientific needs of the United States. It prohibits the importation of any form of narcotic drugs, except the prescribed limited quantities of crude opium and coca leaves. It specifically prohibits the importation of opium for smoking or for the manufacture of heroin. This law made it illegal to possess heroin in any form in the United States.

Another principal federal statue controlling narcotics was approved in 1942; it is known as the *Opium Poppy Control Act.* This act was passed when World War II cut off the supply of opium to the United States from

Asia. The law requires that a license be issued by the federal government for the cultivation of the opium poppy in the United States. The issuance of this license is conditioned by a determination of the necessity of supplying the medical and scientific needs of the country. The development of synthetic narcotics has minimized the likelihood that a scarcity will occur.

From 1951 to 1956 intensive studies were conducted by congressional committees on the rising narcotic problem among young people in the United States. These committees recommended that heavier penalties be imposed as a more effective deterrent to narcotic traffic and abuse. Consequently in 1956 Congress passed the *Narcotics Control Act,* which set forth a range of stringent, mandatory minimum sentences and fines for violation of federal narcotics laws.

The law known as the *Marijuana Tax Act* was patterned after the Harrison Act and was enacted in 1937. This act later became part of the Internal Revenue Code and is really a tax, rather than a narcotics control law. The statute requires the registration and payment of a tax by all persons who import, manufacture, produce, compound, sell, deal in, dispense, prescribe, administer, or give away marijuana. This catalog of possible illegal actions is interesting for two reasons. First, like other drug-control laws there is no functional reference to the use of the proscribed drug. Second, the law, by specifying a wide range of actions, seeks to cover all aspects of the drug abuse with the same legal umbrella.

The need for more stringent controls over the manufacture, distribution, and illegal abuse of the dangerous drugs became a point of focus in the early 1960s. In 1965, the *Drug Abuse Control Amendments* to the 1938 Federal Food, Drug, and Cosmetic Act were enacted by Congress. This law applies not only to barbiturates and amphetamines, but

it established the current definition of a dangerous drug. Under the 1965 amendments all wholesalers, jobbers, and manufacturers of dangerous drugs are required to register annually with the Food and Drug Administration and keep records of sales of these drugs. Pharmacists, hospitals, researchers, and doctors who regularly dispense and charge for the controlled drugs must maintain records that are available for inspection by the Food and Drug Administration. Prohibitions include refilling a prescription more than five times or later than six months after the prescription is originally written, and requiring the registration of drug firms that manufacture, process or sell controlled drugs.

In 1970 a new scheduled of federal drug penalties was established (*Comprehensive Drug Abuse Prevention and Control Act*). This law established five classes of drugs whose illegal manufacture, distribution, possession for use, possession for sale, and sale are controlled by the federal government. The following table is an outline of these five classes. Also, the law does away with the term "dangerous drugs" by defining drugs as either *narcotics* or *nonnarcotics.*

Class 1 drugs are considered to have the highest potential for abuse because of their mood-modifying qualities. They carry the most severe penalties, are regarded as the most dangerous, and are outlawed in any form (even for medical use) in the United States. Class 2 drugs are medically used drugs that have the same potential for abuse as Class 1 drugs. Class 3 drugs are considered to have a potential for abuse but not as high a potential as Class 1 and 2 drugs. Class 4 drugs have a lower potential for abuse and Class 5 drugs have the lowest potential for abuse, and the penalties are the mildest.

A very controversial aspect of this federal act is the so-called *no-knock provision* that allows police to enter and search a home or room without the ordinary warrant or without

# SCHEDULES AND PENALTIES FOR VIOLATION OF THE COMPREHENSIVE DRUG ABUSE PREVENTION AND CONTROL ACT OF 1970[a]

| DRUG SCHEDULE | POTENTIAL FOR ABUSE | MEDICAL USE | PRODUCTION CONTROLS | EXAMPLES OF DRUGS IN EACH CLASS | MAXIMUM PENALTIES FOR MANUFACTURING AND DISTRIBUTION | MAXIMUM PENALTIES FOR SIMPLE ILLEGAL POSSESSION |
|---|---|---|---|---|---|---|
| Class 1 | High | None | Yes | Opium derivatives, cannabis drugs, and hallucinogens Examples: heroin, marijuana, THC, LSD, and mescaline | *Narcotics* First offense: 4 to 15 years; $15,000 fine Second and subsequent offenses: 6 to 30 years; $50,000 fine | |
| Class 2 | High | Yes | Yes | Medically utilized narcotics and injectable metamphetamines Examples: morphine, cocaine, and methadone | *Nonnarcotics* First offense: 2 to 5 years; $15,000 fine Second and subsequent offenses: 4 to 10 years; $30,000 fine | First offense: up to 1 year (probation possible); $5,000 fine Second offense: up to 2 years; $10,000 fine |
| Class 3 | Moderately high | Yes | None | Mild narcotics Examples: codeine, amphetamines, and barbiturates | First offense: 2 to 5 years; $15,000 fine Second and subsequent offenses: 4 to 10 years; $20,000 fine | |
| Class 4 | Low | Yes | None | Mild barbiturates Examples: chloral hydrate and some tranquilizers Example: meprobamate | First offense: 1 to 3 years; $10,000 fine Second and subsequent offenses: 2 to 6 years; $20,000 fine | |
| Class 5 | Quite low | Yes | None | Low percentage narcotic mixtures and tranquilizers | First offense: up to 1 year; $5,000 fine Second and subsequent offenses: up to 2 years; $10,000 fine | |

[a]Schedules and penalties may be changed by the U.S. Attorney General at any time.

knocking, if there is a reason to believe that drugs may be on the premises.

Individual possession of nonnarcotic drugs (such as marijuana) is now a misdemeanor. Minimum mandatory penalties for such possession have been eliminated, and a maximum penalty of 1 year for possession (first offense) and 3 years for subsequent offenses were established. Also, for a first offense, an individual under 21 years of age who is convicted of possession may be placed on probation (without sentencing), and if he successfully completes the probation, the official arrest, trial, and conviction can be erased from his record. The law also gives the U.S. Attorney General the power to decide to which class a new drug belongs on the basis of its "potential for abuse."

State laws dealing with drugs are highly variable. In 1932 a model uniform state narcotics law, patterned after the Harrison Narcotics Act, was submitted to several states. Since that time most states have enacted laws similar to this act. It also became the basis of the laws controlling the nonnarcotic or dangerous drugs. Some states enacted legislation with even heavier penalties. For example, in 1955 Ohio provided a 25-year minimum penalty for the unlawful sale of narcotics.

Legislation was passed in California in 1968 which allows a judge the option to sentence an individual after a conviction for possession of marijuana or restricted dangerous drugs (first offense) to either 1 year or less in county jail (a misdemeanor sentence) or to a state prison for 1 to 10 years (a felony sentence). But with the passage of the federal Comprehensive Drug Abuse Prevention and Control Act in 1970, there has been a trend toward strengthening laws and increasing penalties for possession for sale.

In 1972 California established five classes for narcotics and "restricted dangerous drugs," bringing California's drug laws into conformity with the federal act. New York passed laws in 1972 which provide for penalties which are even more severe than the federal penalties. Only time will tell where the trend will go in the future.

## FOR FURTHER READING

Birdwood, George, *Willing Victim: A Parent's Guide to Drug Abuse.* New York: International Publishers, 1970. *A good reference to help parents to understand drug abuse among young people.*

Brean, Herbert, *How to Stop Smoking.* New York: Vanguard Press, 1958. *Summary of smoking problems and suggested methods for stopping smoking.*

Brecher, Edward M., *Licit & Illicit Drugs.* Mount Vernon, New York: Consumers Union, 1972. *The most complete volume concerning the use and abuse of drugs available.*

Brenner, Joseph H., Robert Coles, and Dermot Meagher, *Drugs and Youth.* New York: Liveright, 1970. *Describes the chemical and legal aspects of contemporary drug abuse.*

Child Study Association of America, *You, Your Child and Drugs.* New York: Child Study Press, 1972. *A small reference for school children and their parents.*

Diehl, Harold S., *Tobacco and Your Health.* New York: McGraw-Hill, 1969. *A popularly written book explaining the health consequences of tobacco.*

Fast, Julius, *How to Stop Smoking and Lose Weight.* New York: Newspaper Enterprise Assoc., 1969. *This book offers the most data available on diet and weight control while stopping smoking.*

Fort, Joel, *Pleasure Seekers: The Drug Crisis, Youth & Society.* Indianapolis, Indiana: Bobbs-Merrill, 1969. *Traces the drug abuse patterns among young people today; written by a pioneer in drug treatment programs.*

Fort, Joel, *Alcohol: Our Biggest Drug Problem.* New York: McGraw-Hill, 1973. *A popularly written book showing how alcohol is the major drug problem in the United States.*

Hentoff, Nat, *Doctor Among the Addicts.* Chicago: Rand McNally, 1968. *An account of a physician who treated addicts during the height of drug problems in the United States.*

Jones, Kenneth, Louis Shainberg, and Curtis Byer, *Drugs, Alcohol, and Tobacco.* San Francisco: Canfield Press, 1970. *An overview of the abuse of drugs and a discussion of the medical, social, legal, and therapeutic aspects of drug abuse.*

Jones, Kenneth, Louis Shainberg, and Curtis Byer, *Drugs and Alcohol,* 2nd. ed. New York: Harper & Row, 1973. *A scientific report on the sources and effects of drugs, and drug abuse. Alcohol is treated in its proper context as a mood-modifying abusable drug. It is written in easily understandable language.*

Lingeman, Richard, *Drugs from A to Z: A Dictionary.* New York: McGraw-Hill, 1969. *An annotated dictionary of drug terms, containing interesting notes on the derivation of some common drug terms.*

National Commission on Marihuana and Drug Abuse, *Marihuana: A Signal of Misunderstanding.* Washington, D.C.: U.S. Government Printing Office, March, 1972. *The latest and most accurate findings on marihuana and its abuse.*

Nowlis, Helen, *Drugs on the College Campus.* Garden City, New York: Doubleday, 1968. *Includes an excellent section describing the reasons for drug abuse.*

Oakley, Ray S., *Drugs, Society, and Human Behavior.* St. Louis, Missouri: C.V. Mosby Co., 1972. *A medical explanation of the relationships between drugs, society, and behavior. Written in the layman's language.*

Phillipson, R., *Modern Trends in Drug Dependence and Alcoholism.* New York: Appleton-Century-Crofts, 1970. *Shows the interdependence between all types of drug dependence and the changing nature of modern society.*

Terry, Luther, chairman, *Summary: World Conference on Smoking and Health.* New York: American Cancer Society, 1967. *A collection of papers presented during the world conference in New York City in 1967. There are also two updates of this report available (1968, 1969).*

Wesley, Sesley C., *The Drug Epidemic: What It Means and How to Combat It.* New York: Dial Press, 1970. *Includes a glossary of terms and a list of referral services in the United States for drug abuse victims.*

# 7
# Alcohol—
# A Socially
# Acceptable Drug

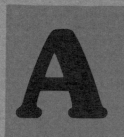t a time when there is great public interest in the mood-modifying drugs, which have become substantially identified with the "youth culture" in our country, it is important and useful to remember that the most prevalent and potentially dangerous mood-modifying drug consumed in the Western world is alcohol. Yet alcohol occupies a very distinct place in our society—its use, manufacture, advertisement, and sale are major parts of our environment.

Alcohol use has many different facets. Most Americans find it a pleasant and generally enjoyable part of dinner parties, social gatherings, celebrations, and so on. Unlike most of the hallucinogens and opiates, the use of alcohol in our society is not *necessarily* questioned or condemned; nor is it illegal. It becomes a legal or social problem for individuals and society only under specific conditions—driving while under the influence of alcohol, public intoxication, the tragic per-

sonal consequences of excessive drinking. The effects of alcohol are part of a complex web—some are definitely due to problems of body chemistry, some relate more to social control and responsibility; often severe psychological problems are involved. In this, alcohol is the same as the drugs mentioned previously—it is difficult to directly predict all its effects, or to understand how it affects different individuals.

Ironically, because of the generally freer attitudes toward alcohol use, we are able to see and understand more of its harmful results. With the possible exception of heroin addiction, we know more about the damage done by alcohol than we know about any other drug mentioned so far.

Yet, at the same time, millions of people derive great enjoyment from the delightful alcohol products available without ever seriously threatening the well-being of themselves or society. The reasons for the differences between these two groups are not all clear, but in this and the following chapter, we will consider those facts known to science and medicine.

## KINDS OF ALCOHOL

Among the many varieties of alcohol is *methyl alcohol,* commonly called "wood alcohol," which is used in many commercial products, such as antifreezes and fuels. *It must never be consumed,* since even small amounts can cause blindness and death. "Bootleg liquor," liquor sold illegally to avoid payment of taxes, is occasionally found to contain wood alcohol and is therefore potentially extremely dangerous.

A second common type of alcohol—also poisonous—is isopropyl alcohol. While it is usually called "rubbing alcohol," it is also used as a disinfectant and a solvent.

The only kind of alcohol that can be consumed safely in alcoholic drinks is ethyl alcohol, or grain alcohol. Denatured alcohol is ethyl alcohol to which poisonous chemicals have been added to prevent human use. The removal of these poisons requires complex laboratory procedures, so there is no household way to make denatured alcohol safe for drinking. Ethyl alcohol is produced from various forms of starches and sugars. Each type of carbohydrate produces a particular type of alcoholic beverage. Beer, for example, is made from fermented malted (sprouted) barley. Wine is fermented grape juice. The hard liquors are made from the distilled products of the fermentation of various grains and other plants. Because distillation greatly concentrates the alcoholic percentage of a beverage, the distilled liquors are much stronger than beer or wine and are often made into highballs, i.e., diluted with water or soft drinks. The table on alcoholic content shows the percentage, distillation processing, and source of the alcohol in various common beverages.

The alcoholic content of distilled beverages is expressed as the "proof," a figure which is exactly double the alcoholic percentage.

Thus 86 proof whiskey is 43 percent alcohol. The alcoholic content of wine is usually expressed directly as a percentage.

In addition to alcohol and water, drinks contain flavoring and coloring agents. Alcoholic beverages have almost no food value. As shown in the table on the nutritional values of alcoholic beverages, there are no vitamins, minerals, fats, proteins, or usable carbohydrates in alcohol. The one exception is beer, and the amounts present are nutritionally insignificant.

Calories, however, are abundant in all alcoholic beverages. Most of the caloric value of alcoholic beverages is derived from the alcohol itself. These are "empty calories"—providing nothing towards good nutrition, but displacing potentially nutritious foods from the diet.

Thus, alcohol can be described as a mood-altering drug with a significant caloric value. As a food, alcohol can be consumed with meals and will go a long way towards providing one's daily calorie requirement. But as a drug, alcohol can have serious effects on the normal functioning of the mind and body.

## THE EFFECTS OF ALCOHOL ON THE HUMAN BODY

Alcohol's effects can be viewed as either specifically short-range, or specifically long-range. A person who is neither an alcoholic nor a heavy drinker will go through a definite pattern of physiological and psychological experiences when he has had something to drink. If he has had too much to drink, he might also go through a period of discomfort, a "hangover," the next day, and then will return to his old self—feeling only slightly worse for wear. In all probability, his body will show no permanent effects.

## SOURCE AND ALCOHOLIC CONTENT OF ALCOHOLIC BEVERAGES

| BEVERAGE | SOURCE | DISTILLED | PERCENT OF ALCOHOL BY VOLUME |
|---|---|---|---|
| Beer | Malted barley | No | 4–6 |
| Ale | Malted barley | No | 6–8 |
| Wine | Grape juice | No | 12–21 |
| Whiskey | Malted grains | Yes | 40–50 |
| Brandy | Grape juice | Yes | 40–50 |
| Rum | Molasses | Yes | 40–50 |
| Vodka | Various sources | Yes | 40–50 |
| Gin | Various sources | Yes | 40–50 |

Alcohol is a mood-modifying substance and can temporarily produce a state of euphoria and an apparent stimulation. This, undoubtedly, is the basis of its attraction. The stimulant effect of alcohol is an illusory one, however. Actually, alcohol is a *depressant;* it slows down the functions of the brain and central nervous system. The first part of the brain to "go" is the center that controls judgment and inhibitions. Thus, paradoxically, alcohol stimulates the drinker for a brief period by depressing the restraining factors of his personality. He becomes talkative, happy, and assumes that he is being witty and charming. Frequently, the stimulation will cause him to say and do things he would prefer, if sober, were left unsaid and undone.

The best quantitative measure of what is happening as a normal healthy person drinks is the blood-alcohol concentration. After a drink, alcohol shows up in the bloodstream very quickly. At first, in small amounts, al-

## NUTRITIONAL VALUES OF ALCOHOLIC BEVERAGES

| FOOD NUTRIENT | QUANTITY CONTAINED | | |
|---|---|---|---|
| | BEER (12 OZ) | WHISKEY (2 OZ) | WINE (8 OZ) |
| Calories | 171 | 140 | 275 |
| Calories from alcohol | 114 | 140 | 240 |
| Protein, gm | 2 | 0 | 0 |
| Fat, gm | 0 | 0 | 0 |
| Carbohydrate, gm | 12 | 0 | 8.5 |
| Thiamine, mg | 0.1 | 0 | 0 |
| Nicotinic acid, mg | 0.75 | 0 | 0 |
| Riboflavin, mg | 10 | 0 | 0 |
| Ascorbic acid, mg | 0 | 0 | 0 |
| Folic acid, mg | 0 | 0 | 0 |

cohol is absorbed into the blood through the lining of the stomach, but this process slows and then stops just as quickly. The presence of food in the stomach impedes absorption; this is the reason many people prefer a light snack at cocktail parties—it helps modify the effects of the alcohol. Unlike the stomach, the intestinal lining absorbs alcohol rapidly, regardless of the amount of alcohol or the presence of food. Consequently, moderate and high blood-alcohol concentrations are controlled by the emptying time of the stomach. Anything that increases the emptying time of the stomach reduces the blood-alcohol concentration by spreading its absorption over a long period of time. Carbon dioxide ($CO_2$) is one such factor; it speeds up the passage of alcohol into the intestines. A carbonated mixer with a whiskey drink is more potent than a whiskey and water highball. Dissolved $CO_2$ is what gives champagne its extra kick.

The table on blood-alcohol levels shows the relationship between body size, number of drinks, and resultant blood-alcohol concentration. Body size is a factor because the larger the bloodstream into which the alcohol passes, the more dilute it will be. Blood-alcohol concentration levels are the basis of drunk driving determinations in almost all states. The appearance and demeanor of a suspected drunk driver has no bearing on whether he can be found guilty of driving while intoxicated. Alcohol is believed to be a contributing factor in 25 to 50 percent of all fatal traffic accidents. Although alcohol is not officially listed as the actual cause in many of these cases, it is believed that many accidents blamed on "high speed" or "failure to negotiate a curve" are actually due to excessive drinking. Research has shown that alcohol starts to be a factor in accidents at blood levels as low as 0.03 percent.

Because all the voluntary muscles are under the control of the brain and nervous system, muscle control is impaired at all blood-alcohol levels. This results in a loss of coordination and a lengthened reaction time, and, of course, these changes are especially detrimental to automobile drivers. Some people feel that their driving ability is improved by small amounts of alcohol, but the truth is that alcohol only makes these people *think* they are driving better. The drinking driver seldom realizes how much his driving ability has deteriorated, because the same effects on the brain that cause him to be a dangerous driver also make him unaware of how poor his driving has become.

At low blood-alcohol levels, the main effect on driving is a reduction in the level of judgment and care used. The person can still drive straight enough, but he may take chances he might otherwise not risk. With higher blood-alcohol levels, there are the additional factors of poor vision and slowed muscular reactions. As the drinker takes in more alcohol, more primitive or lower parts of the brain are depressed progressively. If extremely high levels of alcohol are in the blood, the primitive reflex centers that control breathing and other body functions may be depressed to the point that the person dies. Such high blood-alcohol levels are seldom reached through normal drinking, however, because a person usually vomits or becomes unconscious first. Nevertheless, a fatal dose of alcohol could be consumed if a person very rapidly drank a large quantity of straight distilled liquor.

Sight is the first sense affected by alcohol. Although small amounts of alcohol increase a person's sensitivity to light, he is less able to distinguish between two different intensities of light, and focusing becomes more difficult. Increasing amounts of alcohol cause a great loss of vision. Hearing is affected less than sight, but is still significantly impaired at higher blood-alcohol levels.

Alcohol interferes with both the storage

## BLOOD-ALCOHOL LEVELS (PERCENT ALCOHOL IN BLOOD)

| BODY WEIGHT | DRINKS[a] | | | | | | | | | | | |
|---|---|---|---|---|---|---|---|---|---|---|---|---|
| | 1 | 2 | 3 | 4 | 5 | 6 | 7 | 8 | 9 | 10 | 11 | 12 |
| 100 lb | 0.038 | 0.075 | 0.113 | 0.150 | 0.188 | 0.225 | 0.263 | 0.300 | 0.338 | 0.375 | 0.413 | 0.450 |
| 120 lb | 0.031 | 0.063 | 0.094 | 0.125 | 0.156 | 0.188 | 0.219 | 0.250 | 0.281 | 0.313 | 0.344 | 0.375 |
| 140 lb | 0.027 | 0.054 | 0.080 | 0.107 | 0.134 | 0.161 | 0.188 | 0.214 | 0.241 | 0.268 | 0.295 | 0.321 |
| 160 lb | 0.023 | 0.047 | 0.070 | 0.094 | 0.117 | 0.141 | 0.164 | 0.188 | 0.211 | 0.234 | 0.258 | 0.281 |
| 180 lb | 0.021 | 0.042 | 0.063 | 0.083 | 0.104 | 0.125 | 0.146 | 0.167 | 0.188 | 0.208 | 0.229 | 0.250 |
| 200 lb | 0.019 | 0.038 | 0.056 | 0.075 | 0.094 | 0.113 | 0.131 | 0.150 | 0.169 | 0.188 | 0.206 | 0.225 |
| 220 lb | 0.017 | 0.034 | 0.051 | 0.068 | 0.085 | 0.102 | 0.119 | 0.136 | 0.153 | 0.170 | 0.188 | 0.205 |
| 240 lb | 0.016 | 0.031 | 0.047 | 0.063 | 0.078 | 0.094 | 0.109 | 0.125 | 0.141 | 0.156 | 0.172 | 0.188 |

| Under 0.05 | 0.05 to 0.10 | 0.10 to 0.15 | Over 0.15 |
|---|---|---|---|
| Driving is not seriously impaired[b] | Driving becomes increasingly dangerous | Driving is dangerous | Driving is *very* dangerous |
| | 0.08 legally drunk in Utah | Legally drunk in many states | Legally drunk in any state |

[a]One drink equals 1 oz of 100-proof liquor or 12 oz of beer.

[b]There is substantial evidence from recent studies that drivers below the age of twenty-five may experience serious impairment of their driving skills even if their blood alcohol level is below .05 percent. Also, studies show that some persons with a blood alcohol level below .05 percent are involved in accidents. Figures in the table are "average" figures based on the "average" person under "average" conditions. Individual differences—both physiological and psychological—must be considered.

SOURCE: The New Jersey Department of Law and Public Safety, Division of Motor Vehicles, Trenton, New Jersey.

and retrieval of information. When a person is under the influence of alcohol, his ability to learn and to recall past events and information is decreased. His problem-solving ability is also greatly diminished. Even simple puzzles and arithmetic problems may be difficult or impossible for the intoxicated person to solve.

The steady, heavy drinker and the alcoholic (a distinction we will discuss in a later section) show additional, and in some cases different, effects of drinking from those mentioned here.

For example, alcohol frequently damages the stomach of the heavy drinker. High concentrations of alcohol are definitely irritating to the stomach lining and may lead to chronic gastritis. The irritating effect of alcohol on the stomach lining is also the reason that persons who drink too much may vomit. Vomiting is a reflex action that relieves the stomach of irritating substances.

Probably the most serious organic damage caused by alcohol abuse is to the liver and its auxiliary systems. The liver is the primary chemical unit of the body. Almost 90 percent of the alcohol taken into the body is metabolized by the liver; at the same time, the liver's health is essential to the normal functioning of the entire digestive and nutritional process. Alcohol abuse can thus have two effects on good nutrition; it can displace useful calories in the diet and can interfere with the body's ability to digest the available nutrients properly.

The liver is the basic mediator of the chemical process by which alcohol is removed from the body—oxidation of the alcohol, which converts it to carbon dioxide and water, which can then be exhaled and excreted. The ability of the liver to handle this process determines the speed at which a person will "sober up." Generally, the oxidative process can handle one drink per hour; during a 4-hour party, drinking at the rate of one drink per hour will probably not cause excessive intoxication.

Every individual has a rate at which he can oxidize alcohol. This rate varies among different people, but it cannot really be affected by such factors as drinking black coffee or walking in cold night air. Only time can sober up an individual.

Evidence indicates that for a long period of time, during the progression of alcoholism, prolonged drinking of more alcohol than the liver can comfortably metabolize (about a quart a day) leads to the development of a supplemental system for alcohol metabolism in the liver. Under these circumstances, the ability of the liver to metabolize alcohol may double. But, this tolerance is reversed later, greatly reducing its ability to metabolize alcohol.

Liver ailments are especially common among alcoholics. One such ailment is fat deposition, which is a measure of the degree of malnutrition present in the individual. Often abnormal liver tests show alcoholic hepatitis, a result of liver cell death. The lesion produced is fatal to about one in ten or it heals as cirrhosis (occurring in one of two cases), a hardening of the liver. This development requires both excessive alcohol and poor nutrition. Cirrhosis is six times as common among alcoholics as among the general population.

Another relative mystery is the chemistry of the hangover. There is considerable evidence that hangovers result in part from the overactivity characteristic of excessive drinking. Alcohol itself plays less of a part. The nausea of a hangover (or during drinking) is apparently due to congeners (chemicals other than alcohol), which determine many of the characteristics of alcoholic beverages. Vodka, which is almost pure alcohol, is low in congeners. Bourbon whiskey, on the other hand, is high in congeners and apparently produces more nauseous hangovers than vodka or gin. Alcohol speeds up excretion of water through the kidneys, thus causing the intense thirst usually associated with hangovers. The alcohol-induced changes in kidney function can also include a shift of water from inside the body's cells to the intracellular fluids. Over a long period of time, this shift of body water can cause the bloated look common to heavy drinkers and alcoholics.

The predictability of many of the unpleasant side effects of excessive drinking is usually instrumental in helping people control their use of alcohol. After a few years of alcohol use, most people do learn how much alcohol is "enough" for mild, pleasant stimulation; how certain drinks affect their ability to function sensibly and responsibly; what combination of beverages might be harmful or unpleasant to them. These last few pages have presented a substantial portion of what science can contribute on the subject; a large part of the task of developing sensible and enjoyable attitudes toward alcohol thus rests on the individual. Undoubtedly, the people who really enjoy alcohol the most are those who use it properly.

## ALCOHOLISM—A DRUG ABUSE ILLNESS

Alcoholism is probably America's number one "hidden" health problem. Behind the public attitudes and condemnation, alcoholism does extensive damage to individuals, families, and to society as a whole. The alcoholic has difficulty holding a job, continuing his education, and maintaining a stable family life. An important factor in bringing a formerly hidden disease out into the open is the potential for cure. To many people, the available treatment methods seem nebulous and difficult to understand. There is no one method, no one drug, which can provide a cure. Since it appears to people that there is little to gain from open discussion of the problem, many people will choose to spare themselves the pain.

### What Is Alcoholism?

There is no clear-cut, widely accepted definition of the word "alcoholism." Some people would suggest so simple a definition as "an alcoholic is someone who drinks too much." But what is "too much" drinking? Probably everyone has a different opinion. A better general definition might be, "an alcoholic is someone whose drinking interferes with a useful life." An important point is suggested here: the way to determine if someone is an alcoholic is not to measure how much he drinks, but to observe what effect his drinking has on his life. This is the central problem in any drug abuse illness.

There are also more restrictive definitions of alcoholism, such as that given by Doctors Chafetz and Demone in their book titled *Alcoholism and Society* (New York, Oxford University Press, 1962):

[alcoholism is] a chronic behavioral disorder manifested by undue preoccupation with alcohol to the detriment of physical and mental health, by a loss of control when drinking has begun (although it may not be carried on to the point of intoxication), and by a self-destructive attitude in dealing with relationships and life situations.

Despite years of research efforts at a cost of millions of dollars, the causes of alcoholism are still not definitely known. Many theories have been presented, some of which are backed by extensive scientific evidence while some are pure speculation. It has not been clearly determined whether alcoholism is caused by physical factors, psychological factors, or a combination of the two. Each theory has strong supporters. There is certainly reason to believe that personality problems are a facet of alcoholism. Yet there is also evidence that some people simply respond differently to alcohol; this is probably related to some metabolic problem such as the lack of an enzyme which prohibits the normal processing and removal of alcohol from the body; possibly, some factor in brain action is involved. All authorities today do agree that alcoholism should be thought of as a disease, regardless of its cause, and that the alcoholic should be treated as an ill person, rather than condemned as a sinner or a good-for-nothing. Public acceptance of other drug abusers as "ill" individuals is taking a longer period of time. If alcoholism, like other abuse problems, were solely a problem of self-discipline, it would be possible for the reformed alcoholic to return to controlled, social drinking. But this is almost never the case. A cured alcoholic who has a single drink might well return to a completely alcoholic pattern of behavior, no matter how strong his resolve.

Certain personality traits are commonly found among alcoholics. The alcoholic typically has a low opinion of himself. Having little sense of his own worth, he feels insecure and isolated from other people. These feelings cause him emotional pain, and he drinks to wipe out this pain. These feelings are also found among drug abusers and overeaters.

The difficulties in finding a suitable definition of, and treatment for, alcoholism are related to the quantitative problems of determining how many alcoholics there are in the United States. Those who try to estimate incidence of alcoholism must use as a primary statistic the number of alcoholics who come to the attention of the police or who require medical care for their alcoholism, and this means that most estimates are probably on the low side. A typical estimate is that about one in every twenty adults in the United States is an alcoholic.

The role of alcohol consumption in a family is influenced by the religious, ethnic, and social affiliations of that family. Interestingly, among those ethnic groups which are traditionally associated with the use of alcoholic beverages in the home and as part of religious observances, the incidence of alcoholism is low. As long as the drinking practices of the family members are in accord with those of the social groups to which the family belongs, drinking usually does not lead to alcoholism.

When drinking does become associated with family problems, it is of prime importance to determine whether the drinking is the cause of the family problems or a symptom of a deeper personal emotional problem. In the past, alcohol was automatically held responsible for family poverty, divorce, child neglect, juvenile delinquency, and most other family problems. Today alcoholism is often recognized as being one of several complex emotional problems. However, a vicious circle often develops in which personal and

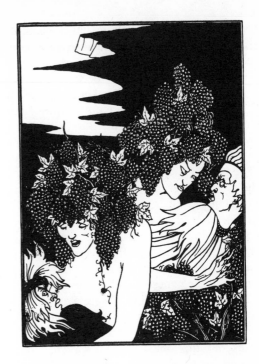

The Snare of the Vintage by Aubrey Beardsley. Reproduced by permission of Messrs. Lawrence and Bullen. *Courtesy of Dover Books.*

family problems lead to excess drinking, which leads to further family problems, which leads to the eventual destruction of the family unit.

The police spend much of their time and effort in handling problems associated with the abuse of alcohol. Many of these cases involve relatively minor offenses, such as drunkenness in a public place, being drunk and disorderly, or "vagrancy." But others have become involved in much more serious offenses, such as assault, murder, or felonious traffic violations.

### Stages of Alcoholism

In trying to deal with the consequences of alcohol abuse, society has been forced to rely on the consistent patterns and few predictable sides of the problem—in the absence of definite knowledge of causes and cures.

No one ever decides to become an alcoholic. Almost every new drinker assumes that he will always be able to handle liquor—and he is almost always right. But there is no way to predict which drinker will be the one who does develop the disease of alcoholism. The great majority of those becoming alcoholics do not even realize what is happening to them until it is too late to stop.

Fortunately, there are ways in which a person can observe signs of developing alcoholism. Recognition of the incipient problem requires both knowledge of the warning signals and the honesty to admit the seriousness of what is happening. There is only one remedy—to stop drinking, and it requires a good deal of strength and determination to seek out this one cure. No way has been found for an alcoholic to return to normal, controlled, problem-free drinking.

As they become dependent on alcohol, many people learn to appreciate and rely on the feelings of relief from tensions and escape from reality that alcohol can provide. The first step toward alcoholism occurs when a person starts to drink specifically for these effects. About one-fifth of all drinkers can be classified as occasional escape drinkers. These people are not yet alcoholics, but they should be aware of the possible development of the condition. In those who are progressing toward alcoholism, escape drinking becomes more and more frequent. It may quickly develop into a pattern of heavy drinking every night or every weekend.

Another pattern of developing alcoholism which should not be ignored is the "binge" pattern. The binge, or periodic, drinker may go for weeks or months without drinking any alcohol, but then goes on a drinking spree that lasts for days or even weeks. The periodic drinker may be just as much an alcoholic as the regular drinker. He is even more likely to lose his job, due to his habit of staying drunk for days at a time.

An *alcoholic blackout* is a period of temporary amnesia. It should not be confused with passing out, which involves unconsciousness. Anyone who drinks too much will pass out. He will then be unconscious or asleep. Passing out is not a sign of alcoholism; it merely indicates the drinker's own poor judgment or lack of experience with alcohol—or, of course, his desire to reach a state of temporary oblivion.

A blackout is something else entirely. It may occur after the drinker has taken just a few drinks. The drinker remains conscious and appears fully aware of what he is doing. He may appear normal to others, and he may seem fully capable of walking, talking, driving, dancing, and drinking as usual.

But after he has finished drinking, the drinker who has had a blackout will have no memory of what took place while he drank. He will remember neither the major events nor the minor details. His memory will have blacked out everything that happened after those first few drinks. A blackout usually lasts for several hours; during a binge, however, it may last for several days.

Anyone who has had such a blackout either *is* an alcoholic or is very nearly so. Blackouts usually occur after several months or years of drinking, but some alcoholics report that they experienced blackouts from the very beginning of their drinking.

The most important symptom of alcoholism is *loss of control*. This means that the alcoholic cannot stop at a reasonable number of drinks once he starts drinking, but must continue until he is drunk or sick. Depending on the drinking pattern of the individual, such drinking will continue for hours, days, or even weeks.

Loss of control does not mean that the alcoholic can't choose whether or not to drink on a certain day. But if the alcoholic does take a single drink, he then cannot really determine when he will stop.

Alcoholism is a progressive disease. Every case of alcoholism develops at its own speed. Some alcoholics reach an advanced state in just a few months; others take many years to reach a pattern of problem drinking.

The alcoholic has several defense mechanisms which partially deal with the guilt resulting from his or her drinking problem. He might appear extremely jovial, but the remorse he feels will show itself in crying jags and serious periods of depression.

Most alcoholics have problems with employment and finances. Intoxication on the job is usually grounds for dismissal from any position. Once a person has been fired for drinking, it becomes very difficult for him to find another job. In the face of such seeming failure to earn a living and support his family, the alcoholic might go on spending sprees, making investments and purchases he really can't afford. As his self-esteem sinks lower, he might try to prove what a "good guy" he is, buying drinks for total strangers.

The female alcoholic generally reaches the extreme stages of the syndrome faster than a man. In previous years, a woman with a drinking problem could hide her illness in the home. But like many aspects of alcoholism, the problem among women is now subject to more examination and treatment. Boredom, dissatisfaction with a life bound to the home, and marital difficulties are frequently cited as causes of alcoholism among women.

Many of alcoholism's effects on marriage are the results of the financial strains just described. Money problems always place a strain on a marriage, but when these problems are the direct result of the excessive drinking of one spouse, the other spouse is likely to be highly resentful.

Other problems in the alcoholic's marriage result from the family's loss of his companionship and, in some cases, the abuse of family members while he is under the effects of alcohol.

The alcoholic's family tends to become socially isolated. They no longer bring friends home because they fear embarrassment by the alcoholic's actions. This fear is an especially painful problem for the children of an alcoholic mother. They know that she is likely to be at home and intoxicated at any time of the day or evening.

Another problem in the alcoholic's marriage is jealousy. This is one of the many cause-and-effect dilemmas of alcoholism. Some alcoholics give their spouse's infidelity as a reason for their drinking problem, while others recognize that their drinking problem has ruined their marriage and driven their spouse into an extramarital relationship.

The alcoholic often suffers a loss of sexual drive. As the sexual relationship in the marriage deteriorates and intercourse becomes less frequent, the alcoholic tends to blame the deterioration on anything but the real cause—alcohol-induced reduction of sexual drive. Very often, the alcoholic's spouse is then accused of having extramarital love affairs. And it is this suspicion and jealousy which can lead to the eventual end of the marriage.

### True Alcohol Addiction

The basis of the physical addiction in alcoholism seems to be altered metabolism which is alcohol-induced and produces chemicals in the body similar to those produced in opiate addicts. Alcoholism and drug addiction are similar processes, the major differences are the length of time and the dosage required for development of physical dependence. In 1970, the Expert Committee on Alcohol and Alcoholism of the World Health Organization stated: "that recent evidence makes it appear that there is more resemblance between the responses of the withdrawal from alcohol and from opiates than was previously realized . . . when serious symptoms follow the withdrawal of alcohol they persist almost as long as do those following the withdrawal of opiates." Consequently, the World Health Organization now defines physical addiction as either *narcotic-solvent abstinence-syndrome type addiction* or *alcohol-barbiturate abstinence-syndrome type addiction.*

When a physically addicted alcoholic is suddenly withdrawn from alcohol, extreme hypersensitivity to all external stimuli usually appears within a week after the alcohol blood levels return to normal. Such hypersensitivity in its most extreme form (delirium tremens or convulsions) is *alcohol-barbiturate abstinence syndrome* and requires emergency medical treatment. This is caused by a return of function to previously anesthetized neurons, aggravated by prolonged magnesium and potassium deficiency. Many physicians believe that magnesium deficiency is responsible for the alcohol-withdrawal syndrome and often treat it with magnesium compounds.

After several attacks of delirium tremens, a very serious condition called "wet brain" may develop. This is a chronic or long-term condition, seldom curable, and often fatal. The alcoholic's thought processes are completely disrupted. All functions of his nervous system are impaired. The alcoholic who reaches this stage will either die or spend the rest of his life in an institution.

### The Treatment of Alcoholism

Most chronic, long-term alcoholics do not voluntarily stop drinking. Even if an alcoholic could stop, he would risk serious or even fatal withdrawal symptoms. He must, therefore, have intensive medical treatment during his sobering up ("drying out") period. He may require hospitalization during this time. Such drugs as tranquilizers, insulin, thiamine, magnesium compounds, and caffeine may be used in this treatment. Once he has passed through the more serious parts of the withdrawal period, he must never take another drink and generally should seek continuing treatment. Some of the current approaches to the long-term treatment of alcoholism are discussed below.

Since alcoholism is at least partly the result of emotional sickness, it is understandable that one approach to its treatment is psychotherapy. The success of psychotherapy depends greatly on the amount of understanding the therapist has of the personality of the alcoholic. It is very difficult for someone who has never been an alcoholic to understand what it means to be one. Group psychotherapy is becoming increasingly important, because a group of alcoholics do understand each other. This approach has some similarity to that of Alcoholics Anonymous.

Aversion therapy involves the use of drugs that make a person sick if he drinks alcohol. These can be administered in two ways. One is by a daily dosage of a drug such as Antabuse (Disulfiram), which causes unpleasant bodily reactions if any alcohol—even a small amount—is consumed. Breathing becomes difficult, the heart pounds, and nausea and vomiting occur. As long as a person is taking Antabuse, he is not likely to drink. This drug is sometimes taken for months or years. For Antabuse to be successful, the patient must want to stop drinking; otherwise he will simply stop taking the drug.

Another type of aversion therapy that sometimes works is to give the alcoholic a drink of alcohol along with a drug which makes him sick. After several of these treatments, he may develop a conditioned reflex so that alcohol alone makes him sick.

The problem with either type of aversion therapy is that severe psychotic symptoms may occur if the alcoholic is suddenly deprived of his escape. Most alcoholics have become dependent on alcohol as an escape from life; if no effective psychotherapy is given or if it cannot provide replacement, he may undergo severe emotional stress and disintegration.

One of the most successful approaches to the treatment of alcoholism has been that of *Alcoholics Anonymous* (commonly called A.A.). It is believed that A.A. has the greatest recovery rate—75 percent of those who want to stop drinking—of all methods of treatment for alcoholism.

Alcoholics Anonymous is an organization whose only purpose is to help its members stay sober. Today, almost every city has regularly meeting A.A. groups ranging in size from a handful of members to over a hundred. A large city might have groups meeting every night of the week. There are even special groups for teenage alcoholics and for spouses and children of alcoholics.

The approach taken by A.A. is that of group therapy. Like the "dope fiends" of Synanon groups, which to some extent are patterned after A.A. meetings, alcoholics often find a deep personal, emotional, and spiritual experience through close association and conversation with others who have shared their addiction. An evening's program usually consists of several members telling informally how miserable their lives were during their drinking years and how they have changed since joining A.A. The new member often finds that these admitted alcoholics have had experiences similar to his own. He can identify with the older member, who "speaks his language." As they tell of their past experiences, the older members are helped too. The stories serve as a constant reminder of the unhappiness of their periods of drinking; they help him to prevent a return to drinking.

Alcoholics Anonymous does not claim to cure the alcoholic; rather it helps him to stop drinking and regain his sobriety. It emphasizes that an alcoholic is always an alcoholic, even when he doesn't drink; if he starts drinking again, he would still drink in an alcoholic manner. For this reason, members always begin their personal stories by stating "I am an alcoholic."

There have been many cases where members of Alcoholics Anonymous decided, after years of sobriety, to try a return to social drinking. These attempts are never successful. Alcoholics Anonymous can only help those who have a strong desire to stop drinking forever, because their drinking is a problem.

# 8

# Tobacco and Its Effects

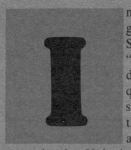

**I**n 1972 the U.S. Surgeon General Jesse L. Steinfeld stated that "cigarette smoking is deadly." Consequently, tobacco smoking is probably the most widespread and dangerous drug usage in the United States. More people smoke, and show the harmful effects, than is the case with any of the substances mentioned previously. To challenge the smoking habit is to challenge a habit of nearly 48 million Americans; however, this has not always been the case. The cigarette consumption in the United States has generally been subject to certain predictable factors. For example, the greatest increases in smoking have occurred during wars. As shown by the graph on cigarette consumption, a brisk rise began in 1915. World War II produced another jump; the rise between 1942 and 1946 (the actual war years) was extremely sharp.

The main reason for this periodic increase is that during a time of national crisis the population in general experiences increased tension. Facts that might ordinarily go unquestioned, moreover, such as the impressive evidence that smoking is harmful, no longer seem important when the whole nation is under such stress. Another reason for this increase during wartime is that young servicemen are introduced to smoking as a tension reliever and morale booster. Many of today's habitual smokers were first introduced to cigarettes with the gift packages donated by charities and cigarette companies during the war. Only in recent years have military hospital administrators stopped the practice of gift cartons being given to ill or convalescing soldiers. Many cigarette companies have long encouraged the development of the smoking habit by giving away cigarettes through their "representatives" on college campuses.

Certain government actions have substantially changed this picture. In 1970, Congress passed the Public Health Cigarette Smoking Act which prohibited cigarette commercials to be broadcast on TV or radio after January 2, 1971. It has long been suspected that cigarette advertising serves two purposes. First,

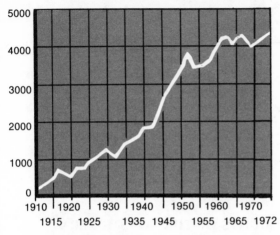

A profile of the growth of cigarette consumption in the United States between 1910 and 1972. These figures include nonsmokers and smokers 15 years old and over. Compiled from United States Department of Agriculture, Economic Research Service Publications.

this time from 16 million dollars in 1969 to between 50 and 75 million dollars; magazine advertising rose from 10 million dollars to about 40 million dollars; and billboards went from 2 million dollars to 6 million dollars. In 1970, anticigarette campaigns of the United States Public Health Service National Clearinghouse on Smoking and Health spent about 500,000 dollars. The American Cancer Society spent some 700,000 dollars in its efforts, and other voluntary health agencies and public service groups were only able to spend an additional 500,000 dollars. Consequently, only about 1,700,000 dollars could be spent to counteract a campaign of between 96 and 121 million dollars to promote cigarette smoking.

Another sad commentary on our times is that at the same time the government was launching its antismoking campaign, the government continued its multi-million dollar subsidy programs for tobacco. This included 27.9 million dollars to subsidize exports of tobacco to other nations, 240,000 dollars for advertising American cigarettes in Australia, Japan, and Thailand alone, and 31.3 million dollars for tobacco donated to hungry nations under the Food for Peace Program. The U.S. Agriculture Department provides the tobacco industry with free grading and inspection of its products (a service paid for by the producers of fruits and vegetables), which is estimated to cost us (as taxpayers) about 2.9 million dollars a year. Former Surgeon General Luther Terry urged an end to tobacco industry supports, saying "the expenditure of 73.2 million dollars of taxpayers' funds in the support of the tobacco industry is inconceivable in the face of known health facts."

The use of tobacco by Americans has increased tremendously since the turn of the century. In 1900 the per-person (both smokers and nonsmokers, 18 years of age and over) consumption rate was less than 50 cigarettes

it definitely helps develop brand loyalties, and it emphasizes the differences between basically similar tobacco products. This is accomplished mostly by the creation of a certain image of the product and the type of people who choose a particular brand. In addition, cigarette advertising encourages young people to take up smoking in the first place, and this is the reason the government sought to control cigarette advertising. TV presented smoking as part of a way of life most young people found attractive and exciting—full of beautiful people, enjoyable times, interesting places. Physical appeal, success in business, and other positive attributes were consistently associated with particular brands, and with smoking in general.

The cigarette advertising industry is an immense and powerful target. Through 1970 and into 1971, the cigarette companies strengthened their campaigns in the printed media. Estimated newspaper ads rose during

per year. By 1930 this had risen to 1389 cigarettes consumed per person per year, and then to 4345 in 1963, ending this continual increase. Reports from the Internal Revenue Bureau's statistics from cigarette sales taxes show that in late 1967 and early 1968 there began a drop in per-person consumption of cigarettes. According to figures published by the National Clearinghouse for Smoking and Health, 33.8 percent of men smoking in 1966 had quit by 1970. 25.4 percent of the women smoking in 1966 had quit during that same period. This trend reversed and smoking started to rise in 1971 (3960 cigarettes consumed per person), during the first year of the TV cigarette commercial ban. Contributing to this rise is the increase in smoking by women and teen-agers promoted by aggressive advertising in magazines. The consumption rose again in 1972 (4060 cigarettes per person) and has continued to rise since then. During 1970–71 the percent of women in the United States who smoke increased from 8 percent to 12 percent. While 25 percent of male smokers who stopped stayed off cigarettes, only 15 percent of females have continued to give up cigarettes. Also, during this period individuals in the 14- to 18-year-old range have increased along the same lines as the women. If this trend continues through the 1970s the heaviest smoking population will be the 25- to 34-year-olds, especially females.

Despite public information campaigns on the subject, too few smokers realize the degree and extent of damage to their bodies associated with cigarette smoking. Early morning hacking and smoker's cough are so common that millions of Americans consider these "normal," rather than signals that warn of damage to the body. Each day in the United States, 271 people die of heart attacks, 200 of lung cancer, and 150 from other cigarette-related diseases. Minor ailments directly related to smoking compete with the common cold as major causes of time lost from work and school.

It is very disturbing that the greatest number of smoking women (40 percent) is in the age groups 25 to 34 and 35 to 44—the critical childbearing years (25 to 34) and when a mother can influence the health of her children the most (35 to 44). Remember, women who smoke during pregnancy affect two lives—mother and child. They also have more spontaneous abortions, stillbirths, and premature babies than do nonsmokers.

## RIGHTS OF THE NONSMOKER

Studies have shown that exposure of anyone to a "smoking environment" causes measurable effects in their body. These include increased heart rate, blood pressure, and amount of carbon dioxide in the blood. Other possible effects individuals may feel include eye and nose irritation, headache, sore throat, cough, hoarseness, nausea, and dizziness. Because of the uncomfortable feelings of nonsmokers air carriers have agreed to set aside nonsmoking areas. The American Medical Association went as far as to ask member doctors to keep people from smoking in their waiting rooms. In 1971 the Interstate Commerce Commission issued a regulation requiring separate seating on all interstate buses for smokers and nonsmokers.

Smoking in the presence of a nonsmoker should be considered "an act of aggression." Cigarette smokers in a crowded, ill-ventilated room or automobile can raise the level of carbon monoxide to a point dangerous to one's health. Experiments show that in a small room a smoker can raise the level of carbon monoxide to 50 parts per million. At this level, after an hour and a half, a nonsmoker can have trouble discriminating time intervals and visual and auditory cues. The right of smokers to enjoy their habit is frequently cited in opposition to antismoking regulations. However, the rights of nonsmokers to a clean, smoke-free environment must also be recognized. Nonsmokers definitely should feel free to discourage smoking in their homes. They should also have the option to avoid contact with cigarette smoke in restaurants, airplanes, and theaters.

## THE SMOKING HABIT

As early as 1967 the World Conference on Smoking and Health concluded that the individuals who exhibit a continuing need to smoke show a dependence which is similar to all other major forms of drug dependence. The evidence seems to indicate that there are two basic groups of dependent smokers. In one group the dependence is more psychosocial and giving up smoking is relatively easy, involving little physical discomfort. The other group of smokers seems to be physically dependent on tobacco. In this case the dependence is harder to eliminate, and withdrawal symptoms are definitely present. Because of the large number of deaths linked directly to cigarettes, smoking is the most dangerous form of drug abuse in the United States today.

Of all the substances known to be present in tobacco smoke, only nicotine has effects that could produce the dependence associated with smoking. This statement is based on established scientific facts concerning the properties of nicotine, the descriptions of symptoms given by those who smoke (or try to stop smoking), and comparisons made with other drug abuses.

A person's first experiences with smoking tobacco are usually tied to psychological and social pressures. A person with this extent of dependence falls into the psychosocial category, and he can smoke or not at will.

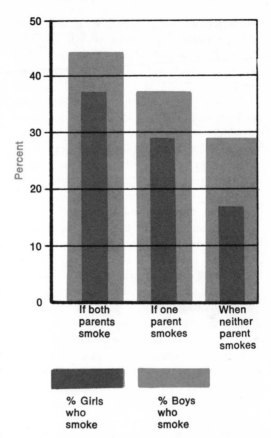

Smoking habits of teenagers and their parents. A large majority of teenage smokers come from homes where one or both parents smoke. *(Courtesy American Cancer Society, Profile 1970.)*

As a result, he may have periods of smoking and abstention throughout his lifetime. The smoking periods will be in response to peer, social, or psychological pressures. But the continued use of tobacco is encouraged, reinforced, and then made habitual by the dependence-producing effects of nicotine. The effect of tobacco on the smoker seems to be that of a stimulant and can be followed by depression, depending upon the person's real or imagined reaction to smoking. But whatever the particular reaction, nicotine-free tobacco, or cigarettes made from other plant materials (such as lettuce), do not satisfy smokers.

As mentioned earlier, the years from the early teens to the early twenties are the years in which a majority of people begin to develop the habits and social patterns that will cause them to start to smoke or to become smokers later. Two factors help explain why young people begin smoking: (1) the desire to imitate those around them, and (2) the wish for adult status. In many cases there is a relationship between smoking and a need for status among friends and peer groups, an increase of self-assurance, and a desire to feel or appear more mature. Psychiatrists see smoking behavior as an accelerated striving for social status in the sense that the beginning smoker is often trying to show an adultlike need for personal and social standing.

A strong relationship has been found to exist between parents' and youngsters' smoking habits. Apparently, parents' smoking habits influence the age at which children take up smoking more than it influences whether the children will be smokers or nonsmokers. Consequently, many authorities believe that the most effective way to cut down smoking among young people is to decrease smoking among their parents.

It should also be noted that many studies reveal that the health damage is greater among individuals who start cigarette smoking early in life than among those who start later. Also, the ability of an individual to stop smoking whenever he desires is clearly related to how long he has been smoking.

There have been a few scientific studies of the personal and social reasons for smoking. Evidence suggests that early smoking is linked with self-esteem and status-seeking in ambitious young people. The pattern or style

of living an individual seeks within his family, community, and peer group seems to have a strong influence on his smoking behavior. A permissive cultural climate (one in which smoking is readily permitted) results in an increase of smoking among young people, especially those who tend to conform to the society's liberal standards.

Although no "smoker personality" has been shown to exist, certain common personality traits have been reported among smokers. Smokers tend to be extroverted (outgoing) people who perhaps place too strong an emphasis on immediate pleasure. Because smokers often take a large part in various social activities, they are placed in situations that reinforce their smoking habits. They are also more open to suggestions from social influences and friends.

Generally, it seems that different personality types tend to establish specific smoking habits. The pipe and cigar smokers often look for sedation in smoking; the cigarette smoker more often wants stimulation. Consequently, very few cigarette smokers can change to pipes or cigars and be as satisfied as they were with cigarettes.

Stress seems to be conducive to smoking, as it is to so many other habits. Tense or challenging situations contribute to the beginning of the smoking habit, its continuation, and to the number of cigarettes a person smokes. Increased experiences of stress among young people, together with social situations favorable to smoking, may set off experiments with smoking. Later, tense or strained situations tend to reinforce or strengthen the habit. By the time a smoker has developed the habit, he may respond to even the slightest tension by reaching for a cigarette.

Intelligence does not seem to be a factor in whether or not individuals take up smoking. But evidence indicates that smokers tend

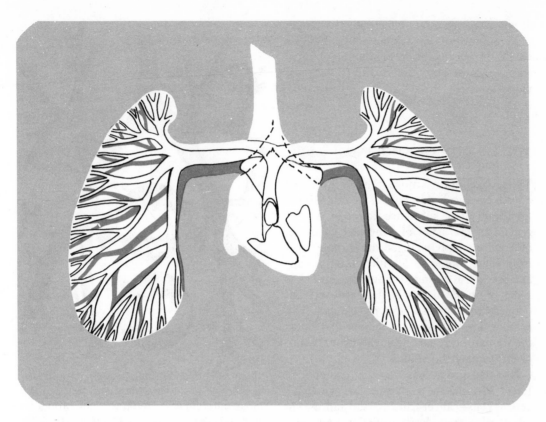

The respiratory system. The bronchial tube begins at the windpipe (trachea), then divides into two tubes (bronchial tubes). Each tube in turn divides as many as 22 times. Because of the tree-like structure of the tubes they are sometimes known as the "bronchial tree." The deeper a cigarette smoker inhales, the further along the bronchial tree the smoke moves. Dotted lines represent the bronchial tubes as they pass behind the heart.

to achieve less in schoolwork than non-smokers. The reason for this tendency is extremely hard to determine. It is unlikely that smoking, in itself, is responsible for unsatisfactory schoolwork. But it is possible that whatever causes an individual to smoke may also reduce his interest in school—for example, the increased social activity that smokers seek at this age. Smoking might also result from frustration or might be a reaction to failure.

Tobacco is not legally classified as a dangerous drug, for the most part because it does not cause the drastic mood-modifications or behavior changes found among those who abuse the more potent drugs. However, smokers do exhibit mood-modifications when without cigarettes. These are not dangerous enough to society to warrant legal controls of the severity of those used against heroin. But tobacco should be classified as a "socially acceptable" mood-modifying drug. Also, although the immediate effects of tobacco are mild, the overall, long-range physical effects are drastic because of the continuing physical damage to the body and health of the individual—enough, in fact, to classify its use as drug abuse.

## THE EFFECTS OF SMOKING

Tobacco contains more than a hundred known chemical compounds, including nicotine. Some of the substances found in tobacco remain in the ashes of a burned cigarette; others are greatly changed during the burning process. Moreover, additional compounds are produced during combustion, and it is some of these materials that are of great concern to scientists and physicians. The composition of the cigarette smoke that enters the human body has been the primary aim of most analytical studies.

Nicotine and at least 15 other compounds found in cigarette smoke are known to be carcinogens—cancer-causing substances. In addition to these known carcinogens, cigarette smoke also yields substances that have not yet been tested to determine their cancer-causing properties. Also present are hydrocarbons—chemicals closely related to the chemicals in gasoline. As explained earlier in the section on "Solvents" the long-term effects of hydrocarbon inhalation may also cause death.

When a person inhales cigarette smoke, the smoke passes down the trachea (windpipe) to the bronchial tubes and into the lungs. The drawing of the lungs shows that each bronchial tube is wider at each fork. The air or smoke slows down as it enters this region of greater width and deposits particles it may contain. This process is much the same as that of a river that deposits its sediment in the form of a delta where the river broadens

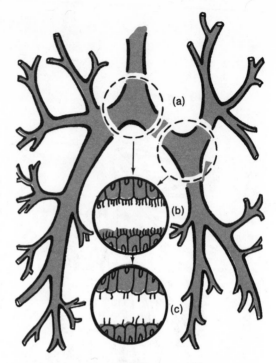

Effects of smoking on the protection mechanisms of the bronchial tubes and lungs.[a] The smoke entering these regions of the bronchial tubes is slowed down by the greater width. This is where changes leading to cancer are most likely to occur.[b] The surface of the bronchial tubes contain cilia which propel irritating substances out of the lungs.[c] In response to the smoke, the cilia gradually disappear altogether, thus depriving the tubes of this protective mechanism.

into a lake or ocean. The exposure of the bronchial tubes to the particles (including carcinogens) contained in cigarette smoke is thus greatest at the points where the tube is widest. Autopsies of hundreds of human lungs have shown that it is precisely in these areas of maximum exposure that precancerous changes are most likely to take place—and where lung cancers are most likely to appear.

Smoking also causes damage to the protective mechanisms of the lungs. The lining of the bronchial tubes is normally moist. It is covered with mucus that is produced by cells along the surface of the tubes. Many of the surface cells also contain small whiplike fringes called cilia which, with a back-and-forth waving motion, propel the mucus upward and outward toward the throat. Any irritating or poisonous particles or dust entering the bronchial tubes or lungs are trapped in the mucus and propelled by the cilia out of the lungs and bronchial tubes into the throat. This protective mechanism removes the unwanted and irritating foreign materials from the easily damaged lungs. Cigarette smoke paralyzes the action of the cilia in the bronchial tubes. It also causes changes to occur in the lining of the tubes, so that the cilia eventually disappear altogether. Thus, some relationships between smoking, lung cancer, and many other respiratory conditions, at least in part, are due to the effects of smoke on the cilia rather than to the direct carcinogenic action of the chemicals in the smoke. Furthermore, cigarette smoke is itself an irritant. Heavy smokers can feel this irritation in their throats and very often develop "smoker's cough" after a few years of smoking.

All of the effects of cigarette smoke on the tissues of the body are damaging. The actual role of cigarettes in the production of diseases is great because there is a combination of harmful factors. Any one of them could be responsible for damage, but together they are deadly.

The relationship between smoking and health has received a great deal of attention. Research brought to light by the 1964 Surgeon General's report *Smoking and Health* has shown definite links between smoking and the occurrence of a variety of diseases, some of which we will discuss. This report and subsequent revision through 1968 *(The Health Consequences of Smoking)* continue to confirm previous findings and suggest additional mechanisms that may cause diseases such as cancer in smokers. Section Two of *Progress Against Cancer 1970* (Research on Chemical Carcinogenesis) reaffirms these previous findings, establishing more links between smoking and disease. These links have become stronger every year since then.

In fact, such a tremendous body of information had been accumulated as early as 1967 that in September of that year, a World Conference on Smoking and Health was held in New York. In the opening address, Dr. Luther L. Terry, former Surgeon General of the U.S. Public Health Service, set the theme of the conference and summed up the case against cigarettes when he said:

We have come to the end of one era in the smoking and health field. The period of uncertainty is over. While science will continue to probe the reason why, there is no longer any doubt that cigarette smoking is a direct threat to the user's health. . . . There was a time when we spoke of the smoking-and-health "controversy." To my mind, the days of argument are over.

Dr. Terry was the U.S. Surgeon General who issued the historic 1964 report.

Through to the 1970s evidence was accumulated that explained the processes and chemicals in tobacco smoke which cause the many disease problems associated with smoking. The amounts of carcinogenic chemicals in tobacco are very small, in some cases they are measured in fractions of micrograms. But the normal functioning of the cell is a very delicate process. Constant irritation over long periods of time allows these carcinogens to change normal cells into cancerous cells. The chances of cancer for nonsmokers and smokers, verified by scientific investigations, are described and summarized in the table on expected and actual deaths

## EXPECTED AND ACTUAL DEATHS FOR SMOKERS OF CIGARETTES

| UNDERLYING CAUSE OF DEATH | EXPECTED NUMBER OF DEATHS IN THE GENERAL POPULATION | ACTUAL NUMBER OF SMOKERS DYING IN GENERAL POPULATION | INCREASED RATIO OF SMOKER DEATHS |
|---|---|---|---|
| Cancer of lung | 170.3 | 1,833 | 10.8 to 1 |
| Bronchitis and emphysema | 89.5 | 546 | 6.1 to 1 |
| Cancer of larynx | 14.0 | 75 | 5.4 to 1 |
| Oral cancer | 37.0 | 152 | 4.1 to 1 |
| Cancer of esophagus | 33.7 | 113 | 3.4 to 1 |
| Stomach and duodenal ulcers | 105.1 | 294 | 2.8 to 1 |
| Other circulatory diseases | 254.0 | 649 | 2.6 to 1 |
| Cirrhosis of liver | 169.2 | 379 | 2.2 to 1 |
| Cancer of bladder | 111.6 | 216 | 1.9 to 1 |
| Coronary artery disease | 6,430.7 | 11,177 | 1.7 to 1 |
| Other heart diseases | 526.0 | 868 | 1.7 to 1 |
| Hypertensive heart disease | 409.2 | 631 | 1.5 to 1 |
| General arteriosclerosis | 210.7 | 310 | 1.5 to 1 |
| Cancer of kidney | 79.0 | 120 | 1.5 to 1 |
| All causes of death[b] | 15,653.9 | 26,223 | 1.7 to 1 |

[a]This table shows the expected and actual deaths for smokers of cigarettes only and the ratios of such deaths to expected deaths in the general public.

[b]Includes all other causes of death as well as those listed above.

SOURCE: Adapted from U.S. Department of Health, Education, and Welfare, *The Health Consequences of Smoking,* Washington, D.C., 1968.

for cigarette smokers. This table also shows the increased death rates from cancer expected of heavy smokers in any one year.

The most common type of cancer found in smokers is lung cancer; more people die of lung cancer than of any other type of cancer—the majority of them being male smokers. The number of victims has risen sharply during the past thirty years, and lung cancer now exceeds automobile accidents as a significant cause of death.

The first symptoms of lung cancer—a cough, wheeze, or vague chest pain—are so commonplace in smokers that they rarely cause a person to consult his physician and suspect that he might have cancer. Thus, lung cancer is seldom diagnosed in its early stages. The smoker's familiarity with these symptoms increases the likelihood the disease will continue to its most dangerous stages. Yet, lung cancer is the most preventable and one of the most treatable forms of cancer. The relationship between it and smoking is clearly and irrefutably established. Although lung cancer is not unknown among nonsmokers, it is many times more common among smokers. Cigarette smoking is more likely to result in lung cancer than is cigar or pipe smoking, since an individual is more likely to inhale cigarette smoke than pipe or cigar smoke, but cigar and pipe smokers are substantially susceptible to lip, tongue, mouth, throat, and larynx (voice box) cancer. These cancers are associated with all forms of tobacco usage (cigarettes, pipes, cigars, and chewing tobacco), but the risk of lip, tongue, and mouth cancers is greater among pipe and cigar smokers than among cigarette smokers.

Smoking does not make these cancers inevitable. They are not even the greatest hazard associated with smoking (heart disease is more common). But the chance of getting lung cancer and the other forms of cancer just mentioned is greatly increased by heavy smoking.

Recently, studies of large groups of people have shown that cigarette smokers are more likely to die of certain cardiovascular disorders than nonsmokers. Such diseases of the heart and blood vessels are the most common causes of death in our population. A cause-and-effect association has theoretically been established between cigarette smoking and the incidence of coronary attacks in humans, especially among men between 35 and 55 years of age. The risk of death in male cigarette smokers in relation to nonsmokers is greater in middle age than in old age. Statistics indicate that smokers are often struck down with disease when they should be most active and enjoying life. They also imply that men who stop smoking have a lower death rate from coronary diseases than those who continue to smoke.

Smoking is increasingly linked to the development and progression of respiratory diseases, such as bronchitis and emphysema. Air pollution and respiratory infections as well as smoking cause and aggravate chronic bronchitis and emphysema. Any pollutant, condition, or infectious agent that can cause permanent damage to the respiratory system can be linked with these diseases. However, smoking causes an increased irritation above and beyond the pollutants and irritants commonly encountered.

In the past 10 years, the cigarette companies represented by the American Tobacco Institute (ATI) have attempted to present the "other side" of the smoking-cancer debate. The studies on which the Surgeon General's 1964 report was based were statistical ones. They included massive evidence of a *statistical correlation* between smoking and cancer. There are also many reports of animal cancers induced by application of cigarette residues to exposed portions of tissue.

But the ATI repeatedly emphasizes that no *human* case of cancer has ever been demonstrably induced by cigarette smoke in the laboratory. The industry insists that the studies simply have not proven that cigarette smoking causes human cancers. The cigarette companies put a good deal of faith in this assumption. They suggest the possibility that both smoking and lung cancer are "caused" by the same third, unknown factor which results in their being linked statistically. And though it seems nonsensical, there is at least the theoretical possibility that cancer causes smoking—this would also yield the same statistics.

At the same time that they protest the government's reliance of the Surgeon General's reports of 1964 and 1968, the cigarette companies do see what is coming for them.

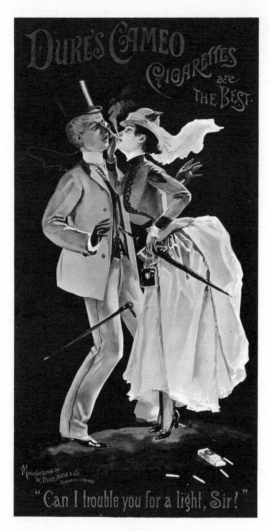

There have been suits brought against the companies by victims or survivors of emphysema, lung cancer, and heart disease. There is currently a trend among these cigarette corporations to diversify and minimize their dependence on this dangerous trade. The advertising agencies which had relied heavily on cigarette-promotion revenue are also seeking other sources of income. Despite the tobacco industry's dismay, the public is not coming to realize the significance of the dangers of smoking. But the smarter Americans are "kicking the habit."

## HOW PEOPLE ARE BREAKING THE SMOKING HABIT

As is true of all other cases of drug abuse, the smoking habit can only be controlled by prevention. The antismoking commercials on TV and radio have had a tremendous impact on the public by placing cigarettes in an unfavorable light. They have been so effective that similar antidrug abuse commercials are being seen more and more frequently.

The antismoking commercials were the outcome of a 1967 ruling by the Federal Communications Commission requiring broadcasters who were accepting cigarette advertising to provide a "significant" amount of time warning of the smoking risks. These warnings were supplied by both public agencies, such as the National Interagency Council on Smoking and Health, and voluntary agencies, such as the American Cancer Society, and the American Heart Association. The content of these messages has moved, over the years, from a simple warning of the risks to an emphasis on the benefits of giving up smoking and tips on how to quit.

Since cigarette advertising has been removed from TV and radio, the status of the antismoking commercials, generated in response to the industry's advertisements, is now in question. Many stations have already indicated that they will continue to run these commercials as part of their regular public service broadcasting.

After an individual has started smoking, there is good evidence that the ability to stop is related to the forces which led to the smok-

# TAR AND NICOTINE CONTENT OF CIGARETTES

| BRAND | TYPE | TAR (MG/CIG) | NICO-TINE (MG/CIG) | BRAND | TYPE | TAR (MG/CIG) | NICO-TINE (MG/CIG) |
|---|---|---|---|---|---|---|---|
| Alpine | King, M | 18 | 1.2 | Herbert | | | |
| Belair | King, M | 17 | 1.3 | Tareyton | King | 29 | 1.8 |
| | 100 mm, M | 19 | 1.4 | Home Run | Reg., NF | 19 | 1.3 |
| Benson & | | | | Kent | Reg. | 10 | 0.6 |
| Hedges | Reg., HP | 18 | 1.3 | | King, HP | 17 | 1.0 |
| | King, HO | 20 | 1.4 | | King | 17 | 1.0 |
| | 100 mm | 21 | 1.4 | | 100 mm | 19 | 1.2 |
| | 100 mm, M | 21 | 1.4 | | 100 mm, M | 19 | 1.1 |
| Bull Durham | King | 30 | 1.9 | King Sano | King | 6 | 0.3 |
| Camel | Reg., NF | 25 | 1.5 | | King, M | 6 | 0.2 |
| | King | 20 | 1.3 | Kool | Reg., NF, M | 21 | 1.3 |
| Carlton | Reg. | 3 | 0.2 | | King, M | 18 | 1.4 |
| | King | 4 | 0.4 | | 100 mm, M | 19 | 1.4 |
| Chesterfield | Reg., NF | 25 | 1.5 | L & M | Reg. | 16 | 1.0 |
| | King, NF | 29 | 1.7 | | King, HP | 17 | 1.1 |
| | King | 19 | 1.2 | | King | 19 | 1.3 |
| | King, M | 19 | 1.1 | | 100 mm | 19 | 1.3 |
| | 101 mm | 19 | 1.3 | | 100 mm, M | 19 | 1.2 |
| Domino | King, NF | 27 | 1.4 | Lark | King | 17 | 1.0 |
| | King | 21 | 1.3 | | 100 mm | 18 | 1.2 |
| | King, M | 20 | 1.3 | Life | King | 10 | 0.6 |
| Doral | King | 14 | 0.9 | Lucky Strike | Reg., NF | 29 | 1.7 |
| | King, M | 14 | 1.0 | Lucky Filters | King | 22 | 1.6 |
| DuMaurier | King, HP | 18 | 1.2 | | 100 mm | 22 | 1.6 |
| Edgeworth | | | | Mapleton | Reg., NF | 25 | 1.0 |
| Export | King, HP | 18 | 1.2 | | King | 23 | 1.1 |
| | 100 mm | 19 | 1.3 | Marlboro | King, HP | 19 | 1.3 |
| | 100 mm, M | 18 | 1.3 | | King | 20 | 1.3 |
| English Ovals | Reg., HP | 25 | 1.8 | | King, M | 18 | 1.1 |
| | King, HP | 30 | 2.2 | | 100 mm, HP | 21 | 1.5 |
| | 100 mm | 17 | 1.2 | | 100 mm | 22 | 1.5 |
| Eve | 100 mm | 17 | 1.2 | Marvels | King, NF | 23 | 0.8 |
| | 100 mm, M | 17 | 1.1 | | King | 5 | 0.2 |
| Fatima | King, NF | 32 | 1.9 | | King, M | 4 | 0.2 |
| Frappe | King, M | 10 | 0.3 | Maryland | 100 mm, M | 20 | 1.3 |
| Galaxy | King | 20 | 1.4 | Montclair | King, M | 17 | 1.3 |
| Half & Half | King | 24 | 1.7 | Multifilter | King, PB | 16 | 1.1 |

NOTE: This is an alphabetical listing by brand names. NF—Nonfilter (all other brands possess filters). M—Menthol. PB—Plastic box. HP—Hard pack.

| BRAND | TYPE | TAR (MG/CIG) | NICO-TINE (MG/CIG) | BRAND | TYPE | TAR (MG/CIG) | NICO-TINE (MG/CIG) |
|---|---|---|---|---|---|---|---|
| | King, M, PB | 12 | 0.9 | | King | 17 | 1.2 |
| New Leaf ......... | King, M | 19 | 1.3 | | 100 mm | 18 | 1.3 |
| Newport ......... | King, M, HP | 19 | 1.1 | Salem............. | King, M | 19 | 1.3 |
| | King, M | 20 | 1.1 | | 100 mm, M | 20 | 1.3 |
| | 100 mm, M | 21 | 1.2 | Sano ............. | Reg., NF | 15 | 0.5 |
| Oasis ............ | King, M | 18 | 1.1 | | Reg. | 4 | 0.2 |
| Old Gold | | | | Silva Thins ...... | 100 mm | 16 | 1.1 |
| Straights........ | Reg., NF | 22 | 1.2 | | 100 mm, M | 16 | 1.1 |
| | King, NF | 28 | 1.5 | Spring ............ | 100 mm, M | 22 | 1.1 |
| Pall Mall......... | King, NF | 29 | 1.8 | Tareyton............ | King | 19 | 1.3 |
| | 95 mm, HP | 19 | 1.3 | | 100 mm | 19 | 1.3 |
| | 95 mm, M, HP | 17 | 1.2 | Tempo ........... | King | 12 | 0.9 |
| | 100 mm | 19 | 1.3 | True ................. | King | 12 | 0.6 |
| | 100 mm, M | 18 | 1.4 | | King, M | 13 | 0.7 |
| Parliament ...... | King, HP | 16 | 1.0 | Vantage ......... | King | 12 | 0.8 |
| | King | 16 | 1.0 | Viceroy............ | King | 17 | 1.2 |
| | 100 mm | 19 | 1.3 | | 100 mm | 18 | 1.3 |
| Peter | | | | Virginia Slims.... | 100 mm | 17 | 1.1 |
| Stuyvesant.... | King | 19 | 1.4 | | 100 mm, M | 18 | 1.2 |
| | 100 mm | 20 | 1.5 | Vogue | | | |
| Philip Morris...... | Reg., NF | 24 | 1.5 | (Black) ......... | King, HP | 27 | 0.9 |
| Philip Morris | | | | Vogue | | | |
| Commander.. | King, NF | 29 | 1.8 | (Colors) ........ | King, HP | 18 | 0.7 |
| Picayune ......... | Reg., NF | 19 | 1.3 | Winston ......... | King, HP | 20 | 1.3 |
| Piedmont ......... | Reg., NF, HP | 24 | 1.3 | | King | 19 | 1.3 |
| Players............. | Reg., NF, HP | 33 | 2.4 | | 100 mm | 20 | 1.3 |
| Raleigh........... | King, NF | 26 | 1.6 | | 100 mm, M | 21 | 1.5 |

SOURCE: U.S. Department of Health, Education, and Welfare, Federal Trade Commission, *Chart Book on Smoking, Tobacco, and Health*, Washington, D.C., January 1973.

ing habit in the first place, the number of cigarettes smoked per day, and the number of years he has smoked. An ability to stop smoking has consistently been found to be highest among those who started late in life and whose average cigarette consumption is low.

If a person is unable or unwilling to quit, he should at least try to reduce his consump-tion of cigarettes as a means of decreasing the harmful effects of smoking. The National Clearinghouse on Smoking and Health rec-ommends the following five steps to reduce one's intake of cigarette smoke:

1. *Choose a cigarette with low tar and nic-otine.* The U.S. Department of Health, Edu-cation, and Welfare publishes a current list of the tar and nicotine contents of cigarettes

every 6 months. (A recent example is shown at the end of this list.) See how your brand compares and find out how much you can reduce your tar and nicotine intake by switching to another brand. Will such a switch result in your smoking more? Probably not. Most smokers who make such a change either continue to smoke at their previous rate or even smoke less. One possible reason for the lower rate is that nicotine and tar contribute to the taste of a cigarette. Lower tar and nicotine cigarettes will not seem as flavorful to a smoker who is used to high tar and nicotine concentrations. This can result in his finding smoking in general less enjoyable.

2. *Don't smoke your cigarette all the way down.* No matter what cigarette you smoke, the most tar and nicotine is found in the last few puffs. The sooner you put your cigarette out, the lower your dose of harmful ingredients. This same fact also points up the added risk of the new longer cigarettes. Their extra puffs are really extra perils for you.

3. *Take fewer draws on each cigarette.* With practice, some people find they can substantially cut their actual smoking time without really missing it.

4. *Reduce your inhaling.* Easier said than done? Perhaps. But remember it is the smoke which enters your lungs that does most of the damage. It is this smoke that causes lung cancer and creates the cardiovascular changes that can bring on heart attacks.

5. *Smoke fewer cigarettes per day.* Pick a time of day when you promise yourself not to smoke. It may be before breakfast. Or while driving to school or work. Or after a certain hour each evening. It's always easier to *postpone* a cigarette if you know you will be having one later. Maybe you're a pack-a-day smoker. Buy cigarettes one pack at a time. Try buying your next pack an hour later each day. It may also help to carry your

cigarettes in a different pocket. Or, at work, keep them in a drawer of your desk or in your locker—any place where you aren't able to reach for one automatically. The trick is to change the habits you have developed over the years. Make a habit of asking yourself, "Do I really want *this* cigarette?" before you light up. You may be surprised how many cigarettes you smoke you don't really want.*

In August 1968 the newsletter of the National Interagency Council on Smoking and Health reported that one-fourth of all American men and one-fifth of all American women who have ever smoked have quit. But, there are still 48 million smokers in this country. Of this number, an estimated 40 million feel some concern about their continuing smoking habit. Many of these people find it too difficult to overcome the smoking habit.

In the September 1968 issue of *Diseases of the Chest*, Lawrence Stross, M.D., Menninger Clinic, Topeka, Kansas, stated:

In the face of the overwhelming medical evidence about the inevitable dangers and harmful effects of cigarettes, as a psychiatrist I would categorically say that anyone who continues smoking or begins smoking is acting in an irrational way and denying reality. I think cigarette smoking can properly be described as a kind of masochistic perversion in which people get pleasure out of hurting themselves and making themselves sick.

Thus, for a person to stop smoking he must first stop ignoring the health dangers of smoking and accept his smoking as a personal problem he must conquer. Breaking the habit is now being accomplished in a number of ways, but the most successful methods fall into the following categories: (1) individual medical care provided by physicians or psy-

*Adapted from *If You Must Smoke*, Public Health Service publication number 1786, U.S. Government Printing Office, Washington, D.C., 1968.

chologists; (2) self-help programs based on books, magazines, lectures, and pamphlets (such services are available from such organizations as the American Cancer Society, the American Heart Association and others); and (3) withdrawal clinics or "smoker's clinics," often conducted by hospitals or medical and health organizations.

Withdrawal clinics, which are quite successful, are actually group therapy sessions in which physicians and health professionals conduct a series of sessions that explain the health hazards of smoking. They often have a psychologist who conducts part of the session to help reinforce the individual and suggest methods of stopping or reducing smoking. The participants are encouraged to explain how well they are doing and to make suggestions to other members of the group. Also, past participants may conduct part of a session with small groups who identify with the problems this individual had when he stopped smoking.

Once the group has been established there are three goals to accomplish to successfully stop smoking: (1) to assist the individual in building a strong motivation for stopping smoking; (2) to constructively confront the individual's attitudes toward smoking, especially those relating to events and feelings associated with the withdrawal experiences taking place with the group; and (3) to provide support and guidance during and immediately following the period of withdrawal from tobacco.

Preparations containing lobeline, a drug with actions similar to those of nicotine, are now sold over the counter at drugstores. The smoker takes such lobeline compounds in decreasing doses once he has cut down on his consumption of tobacco. While these drugs claim to help the smoker to break his dependence on nicotine, they do not replace the habit of smoking. Thus the smoker may find, when he tries to stop, that he acquires new habits to replace smoking. To keep his hands busy, he may become a "fiddler." To satisfy what has been called his "oral need," he may overeat or become a nailbiter. But because these habits are seldom as satisfying to him as smoking, he more often than not returns to tobacco.

Little is known of the relationship between not smoking and normal health. The main areas of study have so far been confined to the relationships between smoking and disease. These studies are just beginning to show which body changes in response to cigarettes are transitory and which are permanent.

Based on 12 years of experience in conducting smoking withdrawal clinics, Dr. Borje E. V. Elrup, Clinical Associate Professor of Medicine, Cornell Medical Center, New York, has been able to demonstrate the following anatomical and physiological changes in ex-smokers.

Digestive and eating patterns start to change even during withdrawal from cigarettes. Soon after a person stops smoking, intestinal motility decreases—often causing constipation for a short time. The absorption of food is greater, the appetite is better, and both the taste of food and the sense of smell are improved—all contributing to a weight gain.

Patterns of circulation also change. The ex-smoker is less tired. He often arises earlier in the morning and is more alert during the day. Skin circulation improves. The complexion of the face can be seen to change for the better, even during the process of stopping. Increased circulation helps to slow the pulse rate, reduce blood pressure, and increase heart efficiency—both at rest and after exercise.

Responses from the respiratory tract show a decrease in breathing rate, as well as an increase in maximal breathing capacity, and a better exchange of oxygen between the lungs and the circulatory system. Such respiratory conditions as chronic bronchitis improve and coughing disappears during withdrawal. Emphysema patients are able to breathe more easily and many asthma conditions improve substantially.

The age at which one stops smoking has a lot to do with the benefits. The younger a person is when he stops, the greater the benefits. There have been studies showing increases in death rates for smokers as young as 11 years of age. An individual between 35 and 54 shows a marked decrease in the chances of dying from diseases associated with cigarettes if he stops smoking. However, a person between 55 and 74 shows only a slight decrease in his chances of dying as a result of such diseases.

In conclusion, although quitting smoking is seldom easy, the effort required may be handsomely rewarded in added years of good health. If you smoke—quit now. If you do not smoke—*do not start!*

Andrews, George, and Simon Vinkenoog (eds.), *The Book of Grass.* New York: Grove Press, 1967. *A collection of writings tracing marijuana's history and uses; tends to present only the positive side of this important controversy.*

Birdwood, George, *Willing Victim: A Parent's Guide to Drug Abuse.* New York: International Publishers, 1970. *A good reference to help parents to understand drug abuse among young people.*

Brean, Herbert, *How to Stop Smoking.* New York: Vanguard Press, 1958. *Summary of smoking problems and suggested methods for stopping smoking.*

Brenner, Joseph H., Robert Coles and Dermot Meagher, *Drugs and Youth.* New York: Liveright, 1970. *Describes the chemical and legal aspects of contemporary drug abuse.*

Byrd, Oliver, *Medical Readings on Drug Abuse.* Menlo Park, California: Addison-Wesley, 1970. *A collection of medical papers on drugs and drug abuse.*

Chayet, Neil, "Old Laws for New Junkies," *Emergency Medicine,* Vol. 3, No. 4 (April, 1971), pp. 216, 217, 221. *An excellent article concerning the legal implications of drug abuse by young people.*

Diehl, Harold S., *Tobacco and Your Health.* New York: McGraw-Hill, 1969. *A popularly written book explaining the health consequences of tobacco.*

Fort, Joel, *Pleasure Seekers: The Drug Crisis, Youth & Society.* Indianapolis, Indiana: Bobbs-Merrill, 1969. *Traces the drug abuse patterns among young people today; written by a pioneer in drug treatment programs.*

Gay, George, David Smith, and Charles Sheppard, "The New Junkie," *Emergency Medicine,* Vol. 3, No. 4, (April, 1971), pp. 116-216. *An excellent article explaining the differences between the drug abuser of today and the classical "dope addict" of the past.*

Hentoff, Nat, *Doctor Among the Addicts.* Chicago: Rand McNally, 1968. *An account of a physician who treated addicts during the height of drug problems in the United States.*

Jones, Kenneth, Louis Shainberg, and Curtis Byer, "Drugs: A Personal Perspective," *Age of Aquarius.* Pacific Palisades, California: Goodyear Publishing, 1971. *A collection of articles that set the current drug abuse problem into a meaningful context.*

Jones, Kenneth, Louis Shainberg, and Curtis Byer, *Drugs, Alcohol, and Tobacco.* San Francisco: Canfield Press, 1970. *An overview of the abuse of drugs and a discussion of the medical, social, legal, and therapeutic aspects of drug abuse.*

Kaplan, John, *Marijuana: The New Prohibition.* Cleveland, Ohio: World Publishing, 1970. *An excellent reference showing the trends in marijuana's acceptance in society, posing a number of valuable questions.*

Lingeman, Richard, *Drugs from A to Z: A Dictionary.* New York: McGraw-Hill, 1969. *An annotated dictionary of drug terms, containing interesting notes on the derivation of some common drug terms.*

Nowlis, Helen, *Drugs on the College Campus.* Garden City, New York: Doubleday, 1968. *Includes an excellent section describing the reasons for drug abuse.*

Phillipson, R., *Modern Trends in Drug Dependence and Alcoholism.* New York: Appleton-Century-Crofts, 1970. *Shows the interdependence between all types of drug dependence and the changing nature of modern society.*

Shafer, Raymond R., chairman, *Marihuana: A Signal of Misunderstanding.* Washington, D.C.: United States Printing Office, March, 1972.

Terry, Luther, chairman, *Summary: World Conference on Smoking and Health.* New York: American Cancer Society, 1967. *A collection of papers presented during the world conference in New York City in 1967.*

*The Health Consequences of Smoking* (1968 Supplement). Washington, D.C.: Department of Health, Education, and Welfare, 1968. *An updated treatment of the 1964 Surgeon General's Report on Smoking.*

*The Non-Medical Use of Drugs: Interim Report of the Canadian Government's Commission of Inquiry.* New York: Penguin Books, 1971. *Examines in detail many dimensions of drug abuse behavior, offering a thorough account of the use of law enforcement in response to drug abuse.*

Wesley, Sesley C., *The Drug Epidemic: What It Means and How to Combat It.* New York: Dial Press, 1970. *Includes a glossary of terms and a list of referral services in the United States for drug abuse victims.*

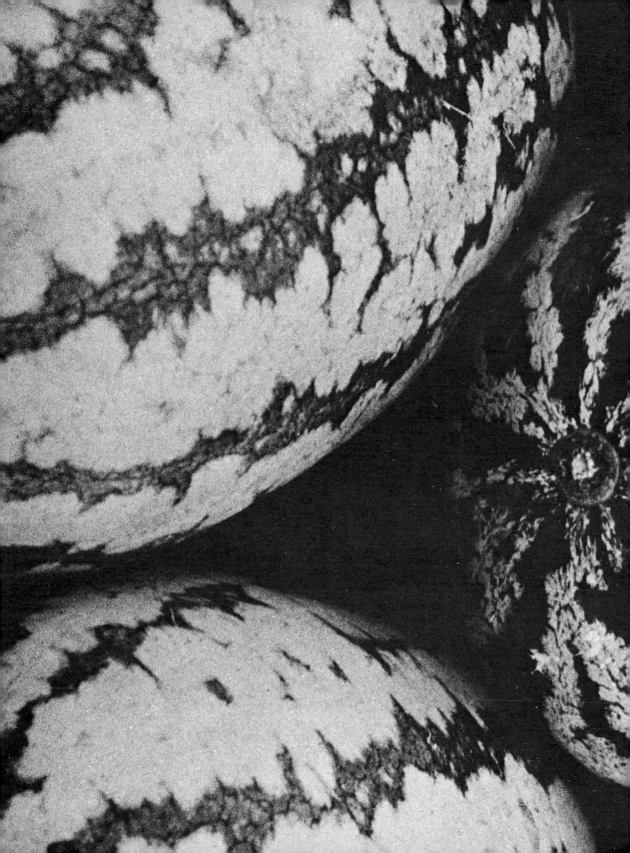

# 4 Good Health in the Marketplace

# 9

# Food —
# The Basis
# of Good Health

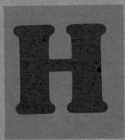

**H**uman nutrition can best be understood if life is thought of as a complex series of physical and chemical reactions. Maintaining these reactions requires a constant supply of energy and chemical building blocks. Food provides both of these factors.

The problem is to match the food needs of individuals with the chemicals found in foods—both in quality and quantity. International food organizations (Food and Agriculture Organization of the United Nations) as well as many national and private groups (Food and Nutrition Board, National Research Council of the National Academy of Sciences) continue to investigate and recommend sound practices of food consumption.

## THE CHEMISTRY OF FOOD

All food is not alike. Nor is man able to synthesize all of those chemicals that he fails to get through his eating. Supplying known physiological requirements demands eating a balance of certain foods in kind and amount. The well-fed person is not necessarily the well-nourished person. Balance is the key—balance not only in vitamins and calories, but also in protein, minerals, essential fatty acids, and water.

### Metabolism

The human body is an efficient machine, and like any machine, it needs energy to function. The body converts certain types of food into the energy it needs. Such food contains *potential energy*, or energy in a form that can be set into action. The body is able to convert this potential energy into heat, movement, growth, and all the processes that take place in the body. Energy that is being used or is working is termed *kinetic* energy.

The conversion of potential energy into kinetic energy takes place through chemical reactions in every cell of the body. The term metabolism refers to the total of all the chemical processes that make up the functions of life. The extent of metabolic functions in the human body can be viewed as existing on two levels. The body requires energy just to stay alive; this energy is used for those processes which sustain the living system—breathing, heartbeat, and glandular secretions. This basal metabolic rate (BMR) is a useful measure of the healthy function of the body, and can be measured while a person is awake, as long as he is relaxed and reclining. The basal metabolic rate is most directly under the influence of the thyroid gland, through its secretion of the hormone thyroxin.

The quantity of energy released from a given quantity of food is measured in Calories (the upper-case C designates this unit as equaling one thousand "small" calories, an impractical unit when considering human metabolism). One Calorie is the amount of heat energy required to raise 1 kilogram (approximately 2.2 pounds) of water 1 degree centigrade. In nutrition, this large calorie (C) is sometimes not capitalized or is referred to as a *kcal* (kilocalorie).

The energy released from food, though measured in a heat energy unit, is readily converted into those forms of energy needed by the system—electrical energy (for nerve impulses), light energy (as in the glow of a fire-fly), mechanical energy (for movement of the body and of internal muscles such as the heart), and sound energy.

An individual can calculate the approximate amount of energy he needs for his basal metabolism by allowing 1 calorie per hour, 24 per day, for each kilogram of body weight. For example, an adult male weighing 154 pounds (70 kilograms) requires 1680 (24 x 70) calories per day for his basal metabolism; besides varying with a person's weight, it also varies with a person's sex (the basal metabolic rate of females is typically lower than that of males), body build, thyroid level, and age. The basal metabolic rate is highest in child-

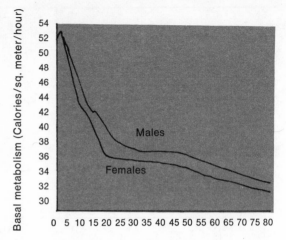

Normal basal metabolic rates at different ages for each sex.

hood and drops gradually throughout life, requiring a gradual decrease in the amount of food a person consumes to avoid excess weight in later years.

In addition to the energy needed for basal metabolism, a widely varying quantity of energy is needed for everyday activities. The inactive person may utilize as few as 500 additional calories, whereas a man doing heavy manual labor may need several thousand additional calories per day. Thus the total energy requirements of an individual may range from slightly more than the energy needed by him for his basal metabolism to more than double that amount.

## WHAT'S IN YOUR FOOD?

Food supplies the materials for growth and replacement of worn or damaged cells, as well as for the manufacture of cellular products, such as enzymes and hormones. The overall composition of the body is about 59 percent water, 18 percent protein, 18 percent fat, and 4.3 percent minerals. At any one time there is less than 1 percent carbohydrate in the makeup of the body. These substances which make up the body are not distributed equally in all organs. For example, the percentage of water varies from 90–92 percent in blood plasma to 72–78 percent in muscle, 45 percent in bone, and only 5 percent in tooth enamel. Proteins are found most abundantly in muscle. Fat tends to concentrate in the adipose (fat) cells under the skin and around the intestines. Carboyhydrates are found mainly in the liver, muscles, and blood. As for the minerals, high levels of calcium and phosphorus form part of the bones and teeth, sodium and chloride are found mainly in the body fluids (blood plasma and lymph), potassium is the main mineral in muscle, iron is essential to red blood cells, and magnesium is general throughout the body. These are the main minerals supplied to the body as food, but many other minerals are essential to the human body in proportionately smaller amounts. These minerals are termed "trace elements," and they too must be ingested with our food. Other chemicals (vitamins) are needed in very small amounts for various functions of the body to take place.

Although the hundreds of substances we consume as food (hamburgers, steak, salads, ice cream, etc.) show little similarity, the nourishing materials they provide fall into only six chemical classes of substances.

### Carbohydrates

The carbohydrates consist of sugars and starches. For the majority of people in the world today, carbohydrates are the most important source of energy. It is estimated that, of the total calories consumed in the United States, about 45 percent come from carbohydrates. If the diet is low in carbohydrates, fats or proteins will be converted into glucose (blood sugar) as a source of energy. If there is a surplus of carbohydrates in the diet, the surplus is converted into human fats and stored in the adipose tissues for possible future use. Foods high in carbohydrates include rice, corn, grains (and grain products), potatoes, and all sugar products.

Carbohydrates consist of one or more simple sugar units. The simple sugars are glucose (also known as dextrose) and fructose, found in many fruits and honey; and galactose, found in milk. Examples of carbohydrates consisting of two simple sugar units connected together (compound sugars) are sucrose, which is table sugar (cane and beet sugars are identical); maltose, produced by germinating grains; and lactose, found only in milk.

Carbohydrates consisting of long chains of simple sugar units connected together are called starches. One starch, cellulose, although present in most of our foods that come from plants, is not converted into energy by humans, because we lack the digestive enzymes necessary for its breakdown. Cellulose is useful, however, in stimulating intestinal activity.

It actually matters little whether carbohydrates are consumed as simple sugars, compound sugars, or starches, since the process of digestion reduces all of them to their simple sugar units before they are absorbed into the blood. The simple sugars other than glucose are further converted by the liver into glucose. Glucose is the only carbohydrate that can be used as a source of energy by the cells of the body. The liver and muscles store some carbohydrates in the form of glycogen (an animal starch), which is then available for rapid conversion into glucose when extra energy is needed.

Thus, glucose, irrespective of the source, is the energetic medium of exchange in the human body. The table on energy values compares the three basic energy-yielding food groups (carbohydrates, fats, and proteins).

As shown, each pound of carbohydrates consumed yields 1860 calories of energy.

### Fats

In addition to being a high calorie source, fats serve as the body's energy storage, form a part of the membranes of cells, act as carriers for the fat-soluble vitamins A, D, E, and K, and provide both insulation and protection for the body.

A fat is made up of one glycerol molecule connected to three fatty-acid molecules. (Through digestion fats are broken down into the four components.) The human body is able to produce most of the fatty acids it needs through the conversion of carbohydrates. Fatty acids that the body needs but is unable to produce itself in sufficient amounts are called "essential fatty acids"; they must be obtained from our food. Fortunately, these essential fatty acids are widely and abundantly distributed in foods such as meats, whole milk, cheese, nuts, olives, and fish. Such food products as butter, margarine, oils, and shortenings are almost pure fat.

Some fats are designated as "saturated" fats and others as "unsaturated" fats according to the amounts of hydrogen in the molecule—the more hydrogen, the more saturated the fat. Although there has been some suggestion that too high a ratio of saturated fats in the diet can have a direct influence on atherosclerosis (fatty deposits in the bloodstream), this idea is not an established fact. For certain types of conditions, physicians may recommend substituting unsaturated fats for saturated ones, but it appears that normal bodies need both kinds of fats. In an effort to reduce intake of saturated animal fats some people have used "imitation milk" products. In imitation milk the butterfat is replaced with coconut oil, an unfortunate choice of fats, because it is one of the few fats from plant sources that is highly *saturated*. Thus imitation milk would be a poor choice for someone who was trying to decrease the intake of saturated fats.

### Proteins

Proteins in the diet are a source of nitrogen, both in its elemental form (uncombined with other chemicals) or in the form of amino acids (simple nitrogen compounds found in nature). There are twenty-three amino acids, some of which cannot be synthesized by the body—the eight "essential" amino acids must be derived from the proteins consumed in food. The other amino acids can be made from molecular pieces and other substances in the body.

Proteins containing all eight essential amino acids in significant amounts are *complete*. Proteins low in one or more of these amino acids are *incomplete*. Most animal proteins are complete while most plant proteins are incomplete. This is why it may be more difficult for a vegetarian to obtain all the essential amino acids. Two incomplete proteins may be used to complement each other, if they are deficient in different amino acids. The combination of a whole grain and a legume (beans, peas, peanuts) serves this purpose and plays an important dietary role in many parts of the world (for example, beans and rice or beans and corn).

From the constituent amino acids, the body makes the enzymes (chemical catalysts), hormones, secretions, and tissues it needs. These

| ENERGY VALUES OF BASIC ENERGY-YIELDING FOOD GROUPS | | |
|---|---|---|
| TYPE OF FOOD | CALORIES PER GRAM | CALORIES PER POUND |
| Carbohydrates | 4.1 | 1860 |
| Fats | 9.3 | 4220 |
| Proteins | 4.1 | 1860 |

are highly complex substances, made possible by the literally millions of possible combinations of amino acids that the body can prepare.

In contrast to fats and carbohydrates, amino acids are not stored in the cells. Thus, a person needs a daily supply of protein in his diet. An individual should eat at least 68 grams (about 2¼ oz) of protein a day. (The average American eats about 125 grams of protein per day.)

### Minerals

Many mineral elements are found in the body. They may occur as simple compounds or be incorporated into very complex materials. Many of these elements (such as calcium, phosphorus, sodium, potassium, chlorine,

## MINERALS LIKELY TO BE DEFICIENT IN AMERICAN DIETS

| MINERAL | RICH SOURCES | FUNCTION | DEFICIENCY SYMPTOMS |
|---|---|---|---|
| Calcium | Dairy products, leafy vegetables | Building material for bones and teeth; necessary for blood clotting and nerve function | Rickets; poor bone and tooth structure; stunted growth; cramps, twitching and other symptoms of increased nerve irritability |
| Phosphorus | Milk, liver, meat, beans, whole grains, cottage cheese, broccoli | Essential in cell metabolism; building material for bones and teeth; serves as buffer to maintain proper pH of blood; important in many enzyme systems including energy release | Poorly developed teeth and bones, stunted growth, rickets, weakness, loss of weight |
| Iron | Liver, meat, shellfish, egg yolk, legumes, dried fruits | Ingredient of hemoglobin, the oxygen-carrying pigment in red blood cells; necessary for enzymes of cellular respiration | Anemia (low oxygen-carrying capacity of blood) |
| Iodine | Iodized salt | Basis of thyroid hormone | Low metabolic rate; goiter |
| Fluorine | Drinking water in some areas of U.S. | Strengthens bones and teeth | Tooth decay |

magnesium, iron, sulfur, iodine, manganese, cobalt, copper, and zinc) perform essential functions in the body—they make up vital parts of cells, bones, teeth, and the blood. Other mineral elements make up important parts of hormones and secretions.

As is true of all nutrients, there are specific patterns of deficiency and abundance in the distribution of minerals in the American diet. The table on deficient minerals lists some of these and shows their deficiency symptoms.

## Vitamins

Vitamins are a group of important compounds that are found in very small proportions in food. They are needed in trace amounts for the proper functioning of the body. Vitamins function along with enzymes to carry out very specific, important chemical reactions in the body. Like enzymes, vitamins act by helping a reaction take place (in some cases, enzymes and vitamins make reactions possible that could not occur in their absence), but vitamins are neither changed nor incorporated into the products of the reaction. Because of this action, vitamins are also called co-enzymes.

Except for vitamins D and K, vitamins cannot be synthesized directly in the body; they must be obtained from the diet. And even though vitamins D and K are synthesized within the body, the chemicals from which they are synthesized still must come from what we eat. Consequently, they also depend upon a proper diet. As shown in the vitamins table, whether a vitamin will dissolve in water or in fat (or oil) is important. This can tell you the source of a vitamin, how it is absorbed into the body, and what happens to it inside the body. The water-soluble vitamins are not stored in the body and should be taken in each day. In general, fat-soluble vitamins are stored within body

tissues and can cause toxic effects in large overdoses. Excessively high intake of fat-soluble vitamins, especially in infants where the body is small, should be avoided. On the other hand, their absence has serious consequences. An entire class of diseases called vitamin deficiency diseases (see vitamins table), can result from a lack of these vital chemicals in the diet. However, a well-balanced, carefully selected diet easily provides all the required vitamins in more than sufficient amounts.

## Water

No food serves the body in as many vital functions as water. The importance of water to the body is so great that a loss of only 10 percent can result in an individual's death. The body is over 50 percent water, and many of the tissues of the body (such as blood) are as much as 90 percent water. Digestion, absorption, and the secretion of materials must take place in water. All chemical reactions of metabolism also require water. It provides the moisture in the cells of the lungs that enables the membranes to exchange oxygen and carbon dioxide; it is important in distributing heat uniformly throughout the body; it transports many vital substances throughout the body; and it also serves as a cushion for the brain and spinal cord.

How much water a person requires each day depends largely on the air temperature around him and the kind of physical activity he is engaged in. Water loss may range from 2½ quarts for a moderately active person to several times that much for a person working vigorously in the hot sun. The loss occurs primarily through the kidneys, lungs, digestive tract, and skin.

This water loss can be replenished by liquids and foods of all kinds. All foods—even dry bread—contain some water. Some water is produced within the body through the

## VITAMINS

| VITAMIN | RICH SOURCES | PROPERTIES | FUNCTION | DEFICIENCY SYMPTOMS |
|---|---|---|---|---|
| **FAT-SOLUBLE VITAMINS** | | | | |
| Vitamin A | Cheese, green and yellow vegetables, butter, eggs, milk, fish liver oils; carotene in vegetables converted to vitamin A by liver | Lost through oxidation during long cooking in open kettle; overdose possible | Necessary for growth, tooth structure, night vision, healthy skin | Slow growth, poor teeth and gums, night blindness, dry skin and eyes (lack of tears) |
| Vitamin D | Beef, butter, eggs, milk, fish liver oils; produced in the skin upon exposure to ultraviolet rays in sunlight; no plant source | One of the most stable vitamins; large doses may cause calcium deposits, poor bone growth in children, congenital defects | Necessary for metabolism of calcium and phosphorus; essential for normal bone and tooth development | Rickets; poor tooth and bone structure; soft bones |
| Vitamin E | Widely distributed in foods; abundant in vegetable oils and wheat germ | Lost through oxidation during long cooking in open kettle; overdose not known | Not definitely known for humans. May help oxygen content of blood | Not definitely known for humans |
| Vitamin K | Eggs, liver, cabbage, spinach, tomatoes; produced by bacteria of intestine | Destroyed by light and alkali; absorption from intestine into blood depends on normal fat absorption | Necessary for blood clotting | Slow blood clotting; anemia |
| **WATER-SOLUBLE VITAMINS** | | | | |
| Vitamin B$_1$ (thiamin) | Meat, whole grains, liver, yeast, nuts, eggs, bran, soybeans, potatoes | Not destroyed by cooking, but being water-soluble, may dissolve in cooking water; not stored in body; daily supply needed | Necessary for carbohydrate metabolism, normal nerve function; promotes growth | Beriberi; slow growth, poor nerve function, nervousness, fatigue, heart disease |
| Vitamin B$_2$ (riboflavin) | Milk, cheese, liver, beef, eggs, fish | Not destroyed by cooking acid foods; unstable to light and alkali | Essential for metabolism in all cells | Fatigue, sore skin and lips, bloodshot eyes, anemia |

| Niacin (nicotinic acid) | Bran, eggs, yeast, liver, kidney, fish, whole wheat, potatoes, tomatoes; can be synthesized from amino acid tryptophan | Not destroyed by cooking, but may dissolve extensively in cooking water | Necessary for growth, metabolism, normal skin | Pellagra; sore mouth, skin rash, indigestion, diarrhea, headache, mental disturbances |
|---|---|---|---|---|
| Vitamin B₆ (pyridoxine) | Meat, liver, yeast, whole grains, fish, vegetables | Stable except to light | Functions in amino-acid metabolism | Dermatitis |
| Vitamin B₁₂ (cyanocobalamin) | Meat, liver, eggs, milk, yeast | Unstable to acid, alkali, light | Necessary for production of red blood cells and growth | Pernicious anemia |
| Vitamin C (ascorbic acid) | Citrus fruits, tomatoes, potatoes, cabbage, green peppers, broccoli | Least stable of the vitamins; destroyed by heat, alkali, air; dissolves in cooking water | Essential for cellular metabolism necessary for teeth, gums, bones, blood vessels and tissue repair | Scurvy; poor teeth, weak bones, sore and bleeding gums, easy bruising, poor wound healing |

NOTE: Several other water-soluble vitamins are believed to be essential to human nutrition, but are not as well understood as the above vitamins and their deficiency is less common.

metabolic breakdown of stored food. Since there are variables both in water needed and water available from different sources, it is not possible to state the specific amount of water a person should drink each day. In general, a person should drink a little more water than is sufficient to satisfy his thirst. The slight excess beyond thirst provides for good kidney health.

# FOOD PRESERVATION AND ENRICHMENT

One of the greatest problems with food is its relatively short storage life. In the past, man has used many methods to try and preserve perishable foods—the most common being drying and salting, or adding salt, sugar, or spices.

### Additives

Chemicals added to food as a result of our food technology are known as food *additives* and *residues.* Some compounds are added directly; others are produced as the result of processing. Some occur accidently such as residues from seed, soil, or crop treatment; from chemicals fed to animals; or from packaging materials surrounding food. By conservative estimates, there are at least ten thousand such compounds.

*Antioxidants.* Some foods, particularly unsaturated fatty acids, tend to oxidize. Frozen peaches become brown and unattractive. Some cake mixes become useless unless the shortening in them is kept fresh. Antioxidants are used to minimize these problems.

*Acids.* Baking powder or cream of tartar (tartaric acid) reacts with baking soda and produces carbon dioxide to leaven bread and cake, making it light. Certain other acids (phosphoric, citric, malic) are used to counteract the excessive sweetness of many soft drinks.

*Emulsifiers.* Emulsifiers break up fats and oils into very small particles. They are used in bakery goods to improve uniformity of texture, fineness, and softness; in ice cream to control particle size (smoother ice cream); in salad dressing to prevent the oil and vinegar from separating.

*Artificial Sweeteners.* Substitute sweeteners (sweet-tasting compounds with no food value) have a long history. Two of the most important are saccharin and cyclamates. These have long been used by diabetics. Saccharin is over 300 times as sweet as table sugar (sucrose), while cyclamates are only about 30 times as sweet as table sugar. Although safe within recommended doses and as used by diabetics, their use is restricted or prohibited in some countries because they are nonfoods (contain no food value) and are possibly dangerous when consumed in large quantities.

*Vitamins and minerals.* Vitamins and minerals are added to certain food products to replace those that have been lost during processing or to make up for an inherent deficiency in the food. For example, white flour has several vitamins and minerals added to replace those lost in milling, and most milk has vitamin D added because it is normally present in only trace quantities.

*Enrichment Chemicals.* Some chemicals are added to white flour in order to "enrich." The food industry insists these chemicals are identical to the vitamins and minerals which have been removed in processing. The problem is that the "enriching" may restore only 25 to 60 percent the original amount (a net loss).

*Others. Pectin* is a thickening agent which is added to certain fruits in order to give a consistent and desirable thickness to jams and jellies. Wieners, like other sausages, require *flavoring agents.* Canned shredded coconut requires a *humectant* to keep it moist. Table salt, powdered sugar, and malted milk powder all require *anticaking* agents. Salt and sugar are still used as preservative and flavoring agents.

### Hazards Posed by Additives

Official policy governing the use of additives varies widely. While strict in some countries, the United States has allowed wide proliferation of new additives (preventing adequate evaluation of each new one). Many are loosely accorded "generally recognized as safe" (GRAS) status, on the basis of long-established use without "evidence of harm." Relatively few food additives have been accepted for specific and limited uses on the basis of sound investigation.

It is acceptable for food processors to give food a reasonable shelf life, but not to "embalm" food that can no longer be considered fresh.

Some additives are now under suspicion. The antioxidant butylated hydroxytoluene (BHT) is suspected of inhibiting the uptake of oxygen by hemoglobin in the red blood cells. One emulsifier, polyoxyethylene (no longer used in the United States), was found to greatly increase the rate of iron absorption in some animals—leading to too great an absorption of vitamin A.

The most disturbing element with the use of additives is that they are not always fully investigated *before* being used in foods. This is particularly true of substances in use prior to the Food Additives Amendment to the Federal Food, Drug, and Cosmetic Act, as well as with those included in GRAS. In some cases, the disuse of a particular additive, with great food industry resistance, has come *only* after the fact—after possible physical damage to unwary and trusting consumers.

Before purchasing processed foods, read the ingredients list on the label. The ingredients are listed in descending order of abundance—the first item listed is the most abundant. If there seem to be more chemicals than food, you might consider buying another product. Remember that some of the ingredients with chemical-sounding names, such as ascorbic acid, are actually important vitamins or other nutrients. Some foods, such as ice cream, can still be sold with no ingredients listing, although a multitude of chemicals may be included.

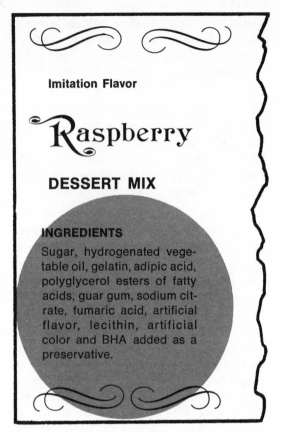

**Imitation Flavor**

# Raspberry

## DESSERT MIX

### INGREDIENTS
Sugar, hydrogenated vegetable oil, gelatin, adipic acid, polyglycerol esters of fatty acids, guar gum, sodium citrate, fumaric acid, artificial flavor, lecithin, artificial color and BHA added as a preservative.

Be aware of what you eat. Notice from the ingredients panel above that this dessert has very little actual food in it. It is important to note that ingredients must be listed in order of their proportion.

## NUTRITION AND HEALTH

Good health is much more than the absence of disease; it is also physical and intellectual vigor, vitality, and freedom from emotional and functional illnesses of all kinds. The level of general public health in the United States has been improving through the years, but consistent health problems do trouble certain segments of our population. Diet, the customary amounts and types of food and drink taken by a person from day to day, and nutrition, the relationship between the needs of our body and the food we consume, are important factors in good health. In fact, to a certain extent, food is the basis of good

health. How adequate our diet and nutrition are in contributing to good health may be measured in the following ways.

### Nutritional Levels

Adequate nutrition is attained when an individual is eating a diet that enables him to grow, mature, reproduce, and function in a healthy and normal manner. Insufficient nutrition occurs when the nutritional level and diet are inadequate for an individual to maintain adequate health. It may result from one of two things—undernutrition or malnutrition. The effects of these two may appear separately or together.

*Undernutrition.* This is an insufficiency of calories in the diet, and is usually caused by an insufficient supply of food. When famine strikes, those most severely hit are the very young, the old, and those in the lower socioeconomic groups. It is estimated by the United Nations Food and Agricultural Organization (FAO) that 10 to 15 percent of the world's population is undernourished.

The most obvious symptoms of continued calorie deficiency are the conditions of underweight and starvation. The undernourished body begins to utilize its own fat, protein, and other tissues, causing first a loss of weight and then a stunted growth and development. In serious cases of starvation, the metabolic rate is reduced, the pulse is slowed and weakened, the blood pressure is reduced, muscle tone is decreased, the skin becomes less elastic, and there is mental dullness and easy fatigue. In cases of extreme starvation the body becomes severely waterlogged, and death commonly occurs from heart failure.

Pregnant women suffering from severe undernourishment may have longer periods of labor at childbirth, creating hazards to both child and mother. Since the mother's production of milk is often affected, infant mortality increases sharply. The famines in certain European countries occupied by the Germans during the 1940s caused a reduction in the size of children at birth. There is even some evidence that poor nutrition during pregnancy may increase the incidence of congenital handicaps.

During a temporary famine, the growth of a child slows down, but then catches up with that of normal children when food is available. There is no permanent effect on eventual size and weight. During periods of chronic undernutrition, however, children show reduced resistance to diseases such as tuberculosis. Their muscular development is weakened, their skeletal development delayed, and permanent bone abnormalities may be produced.

*Malnutrition.* Malnutrition is a type of "selective starvation." It is the absence of some of the needed nutrients in the diet and is responsible for the deficiency diseases that affect human beings.

Protein deficiency may result from severe hemorrhaging, extensive burns, severe injuries, or loss of the body fluids. This can cause shock and circulatory collapse. More commonly, protein deficiency occurs when there is an inadequate protein intake or excessive body breakdown of proteins.

Kwashiorkor, a severe protein-disease, is the world's most widespread and most serious deficiency disease in the world today. It affects children from the time of their weaning to their sixth year of life. Kwashiorkor is common in southern Mexico, northern South America, tropical Africa, India, and much of China—all countries with low agricultural productivity. It also occurs among the very poor in the United States.

Toward the end of the child's first year of life, if his mother's milk fails to supply enough protein and supplementary foods given to him are largely carbohydrates, he has a greatly reduced protein intake, causing serious symptoms. The syndrome usually includes severely retarded physical and mental growth, apathy, loss of appetite, tissue swelling, loss of pigmentation, diarrhea, and anemia, as shown in the photograph. The word kwashiorkor, of Ghanaian origin, means either "red boy" in reference to the change in skin and hair pigmentation among afflicted African blacks, or "displaced child" in reference to the onset of the disease in the elder child when a younger child is nursed by the mother. Before modern medical facilities were available in Africa, the mortality rate there from this disease ranged from 30 to 100 percent. Treatment consists of a diet largely of dry skim milk.

In the United States, the symptoms of kwashiorkor include the inability to combat such diseases as pneumonia, measles, whooping cough, diarrhea, and tuberculosis.

Vitamin A is necessary for normal bone growth, normal vision, and normal skin. In victims of xerophthalmia, a vitamin A deficiency disease, there is impaired night vision, a breakdown of the layers of the skin, and a tendency for secondary infection to readily occur. Conditions such as these can be avoided by including vitamin A or carotene in the diet.

Because of increased cloud cover, the northern latitudes tend to receive less winter sunshine than do more southerly ones. Within the United States, for example, the percentage of winter sunshine varies from 20 to 40 percent around the Great Lakes area to 70 to 90 percent in the Southwest. The amount of sunshine a person receives relates directly to the amount of ultraviolet radiation he absorbs and, in turn, determines the amount of vitamin D in his body. Ultraviolet light hitting the skin causes the body to produce vitamin D, which is essential to the proper utilization of calcium and phosphorus in the formation of bones and teeth. Fish liver oils (liquid extracts of the vitamin-rich storage tissues of the liver) are useful sources of vitamin D and are frequently given to children, especially in regions and at times when sunshine is insufficient.

Rickets and osteomalacia are vitamin D deficiency diseases typical of cold climates where foods are unavailable that are rich in vitamin D or have it added (such as whole milk). The bones of a child with rickets enlarge at the extremities (the arms and legs) and become so soft that they bend under the weight of the body. The disease has its most serious effects during the first two years of life, when growth of the long bones is most rapid. Osteomalacia, a softening of the bones due to vitamin D deficiency, occurs chiefly in adults. Although not killers, these two diseases retard and deform, thus reducing one's work capacity and resistance to disease.

Thiamin deficiency (deficiency of vitamin $B_1$) is associated with diets based primarily on milled rice, which causes the disease beriberi. This deficiency disease is largely restricted to the rice-eating areas of the world, such as Southeast Asia, Venezuela, and Madagascar. In dry beriberi, the lower extremities become weak and unresponsive, seriously restricting walking. In wet beriberi, edema (accumulation of large amounts of fluids in the intercellular tissue spaces of the body) occurs, causing swelling. Cardiac beriberi is associated with heart failure. Infantile beriberi may occur in nursing infants when the mother is thiamin deficient. All forms of beriberi may be fatal. Infantile beriberi is the leading cause of infant mortality in many developing areas of the world.

Niacin deficiency can cause the nutritional disease called pellagra. Prevalent in the temperate zones of the world, it is more severe during the warmer months. It appears to occur where corn is the principal food crop. During the last century it was epidemic among Europeans until their diets were corrected. It is important to realize that the cause of the disease is not the eating of corn, but rather the niacin deficiency patterns which are epidemic in those regions where corn and other starches might be relied upon in place of niacin-rich foods—such as whole grains, organ meats, and eggs.

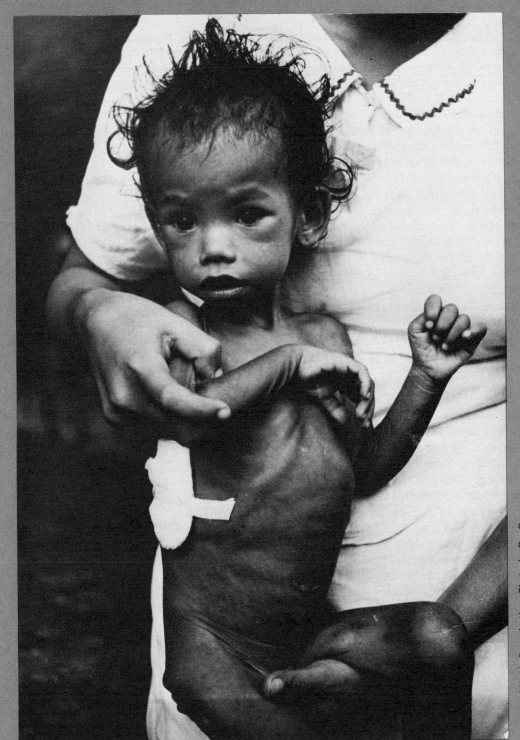

World Health Organization, Photo by Dr. Oomen

# WHO GOES HUNGRY?

The history of the discovery of causes of deficiency diseases consistently shows this same type of pattern. A particular food is consumed to the exclusion of another food; any change in diets occurring within that population permits the observation of a comparison between the two. For example, in China, beriberi was most common among the upper classes, the only portion of the population which could afford the expensive process of hulling and husking its rice. The vitamin $B_1$, held onto the rice grain by the thin hull of the grain, was removed in the rice going to those who could afford the more attractive white rice. The poorer population ate the hull and the grain and so its incidence of the disease was much lower.

This is also true in the case of scurvy. Scurvy is a deficiency disease caused by lack of ascorbic acid (vitamin C). Its incidence was consistently higher among those people who were unable to consume fresh fruits and vegetables—sailors on long voyages, and rural populations during the inactive winter. It was so common during English winters that it took on the name "London's disease." Scurvy can cause pain in the joints, hemorrhaging, gum softening, and tooth loss. Inadequate amounts of vitamin C can occur in a person of any age or sex, regardless of his general level of health. In fact, during the 1950s, a slight outbreak of scurvy's milder symptoms was observed in a wealthy Michigan suburb, probably as a result of the American tradition of skipping breakfast—the one time of the day when most people try to get some vitamin C in their diet.

Iodine deficiency can be due to an insufficient supply in the diet or the inability of the body to use the iodine available. Insufficient amounts of iodine in the body mean inadequate amounts of thyroxin, a hormone responsible for the rate of metabolism in the body. Thyroxin is manufactured by the thyroid gland in the neck. An iodine deficiency can cause the thyroid to enlarge in an attempt to produce sufficient thyroxin. This enlargement of the thyroid gland is called goiter, a condition more unsightly than serious in its early stages.

Iodine is most commonly found in sea water and in the plants and animals in the ocean. A useful way of assuring a sufficient supply of iodine is to include some fish in one's diet. In inland regions of the United States, the inavailability of fish used to be a serious problem, because of the iodine shortage, but iodized salt has successfully reduced the prevalence of this deficiency in the United States.

Reduction in the number of red blood cells or the amount of hemoglobin in red blood cells is called anemia. Since hemoglobin contains iron, an iron deficiency may reduce the hemoglobin concentration and cause an iron-deficiency type of anemia. Eating food rich in iron, such as liver, meat, shellfish, egg yolk, legumes, and dried fruits, can prevent this type of anemia.

### Other Nutritional Disorders

Many kinds of human disorders arise from faulty nutrition. For example, certain types of high blood pressure (hypertension) can be related to too much salt in the diet; thus the use of low-salt diets is commonly recommended for those with high blood pressure. The depositing of cholesterol in the inner layer of the arteries relates to the formation of blood clots and blood vessel diseases. An excessive cholesterol level in the blood may be related to the amount and kinds of fats or carbohydrates in the diet. Nutrition plays an important role in such metabolic diseases as gout, diabetes, and obesity. Acne, eczema, dermatitis, and other skin diseases often have nutritional origins. The skin is affected by many nutritional problems—the lack of vitamins A and C, and protein. Also, well-nourished skin appears better able to resist skin infections. High-quality nutrition helps to counteract both physical and emotional stresses.

Inadequate amounts of protein in the diets of children have a direct bearing on their intellectual development. Lysine, one of the amino acids, plays an important part in supplying adequate protein which, according to some authorities, may play a significant role in how the memory operates.

## TOTAL PROTEIN AND ESSENTIAL AMINO ACID CONTENT OF SELECTED FOODS (IN GRAMS)

| | | ESSENTIAL AMINO ACIDS | | | | | | | |
|---|---|---|---|---|---|---|---|---|---|
| | TOTAL PROTEIN[a] | TRYPTO-PHAN | THREO-NINE | ISO-LEUCINE | LEUCINE | LYSINE | METH-IONINE | PHENYL-ALANINE | VALINE |
| RECOMMENDED DAILY ADULT INTAKE | | 0.5 | 1.0 | 1.4 | 2.2 | 1.6 | 2.2 | 2.2 | 1.6 |
| FOOD, QUANTITY: | | | | | | | | | |
| *Animal sources:* | | | | | | | | | |
| Cow's milk, whole or skim, 1 cup | 8.5 | 0.12 | 0.39 | 0.54 | 0.84 | 0.66 | 0.21 | 0.41 | 0.59 |
| Egg, 1 large | 6.4 | 0.11 | 0.32 | 0.42 | 0.56 | 0.41 | 0.20 | 0.37 | 0.48 |
| Beef, 4 oz | 20.6 | 0.24 | 0.91 | 1.08 | 1.69 | 1.80 | 0.51 | 0.85 | 1.15 |
| Chicken, 4 oz | 23.4 | 0.28 | 0.99 | 1.23 | 1.69 | 2.05 | 0.61 | 0.92 | 1.15 |
| Fish, 4 oz | 20.6 | 0.21 | 0.89 | 1.05 | 1.56 | 1.81 | 0.60 | 0.77 | 1.10 |
| Pork, 4 oz | 18.6 | 0.24 | 0.86 | 0.95 | 1.37 | 1.53 | 0.46 | 0.73 | 0.97 |
| Gelatin, 1 tbsp | 8.6 | 0.00 | 0.19 | 0.14 | 0.29 | 0.42 | 0.08 | 0.20 | 0.24 |
| *Plant sources:* | | | | | | | | | |
| Beans, common, 1 oz | 6.1 | 0.06 | 0.26 | 0.34 | 0.52 | 0.45 | 0.06 | 0.33 | 0.37 |
| Soybeans, 1 oz | 9.9 | 0.15 | 0.43 | 0.58 | 0.84 | 0.68 | 0.15 | 0.54 | 0.57 |
| Peanuts, 1 oz | 7.6 | 0.10 | 0.23 | 0.36 | 0.53 | 0.31 | 0.08 | 0.44 | 0.43 |
| Corn, meal, 1 cup (4 oz) | 10.9 | 0.07 | 0.43 | 0.50 | 0.41 | 0.31 | 0.20 | 0.49 | 0.55 |
| Rice, 1 cup (6.7 oz) | 14.5 | 0.16 | 0.57 | 0.68 | 1.25 | 0.57 | 0.26 | 0.73 | 1.01 |
| Wheat flour, whole grain, 1 cup (4 oz) | 16.0 | 0.20 | 0.46 | 0.69 | 1.07 | 0.44 | 0.24 | 0.79 | 0.74 |
| Potatoes, 4 oz | 2.2 | 0.02 | 0.08 | 0.10 | 0.12 | 0.12 | 0.02 | 0.10 | 0.12 |

[a]Total protein need varies with size, age, sex, pregnancy, lactation, and quality of protein.

NOTE: The quantities of foods listed vary.

SOURCES: M. G. Wohl and R. S. Goodhart, *Modern Nutrition in Health and Disease*, 3rd edition, Philadelphia, Lea and Febiger, 1964; and U.S. Department of Agriculture, *Food, The Yearbook of Agriculture*, Washington, D.C., 1959.

*193*

# 10
# Input
# and Output

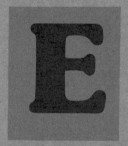

**E**very cell of the human body requires certain chemical nutrients in the fluids that surround it. In order to supply these nutrients, the body must break down complex foods into molecules small enough to pass through tissues, enter the bloodstream or lymphatic systems, and be delivered in a soluble form to the various body cells. This breaking down of insoluble forms is known as digestion; the passage of such substances into the blood or lymph is known as absorption.

## THE DIGESTIVE SYSTEM

The human digestive tract is a long, muscular tube (up to 25 feet in length) that begins at the mouth and ends at the anus. This tube consists of the oral cavity, pharynx, esophagus, stomach, small intestine, and large intestine.

Several glands, located outside the digestive tract, are also important in the digestive process. These glands, known as accessory glands, are connected by ducts to the digestive tube. These accessory glands include the salivary glands, liver, gallbladder, and pancreas. Each gland produces secretions that function in the digestive process, and each is therefore part of the digestive system (see illustration on the next page).

### The Process of Digestion

Digestion involves many enzymes, chemicals, and physical processes within the digestive tract. According to the area in which digestion is carried on, these digestive processes may be classified as salivary digestion, when occurring in the mouth; gastric digestion, in the stomach; and intestinal digestion, in the small intestine. In the large intestine (the last section of the digestive tube) no digestion takes place. Here water is absorbed, bacteria grow, and the unabsorbed solid-residue wastes of digestion collect and are excreted as feces.

# GASTROINTESTINAL DISORDERS

The digestive system is one of the largest systems in the body, and its disorders are serious to the body's health. Many significant diseased conditions are directly related to the structures and functions of this system.

## Indigestion

Common causes of digestion are eating too much, eating too rapidly, inadequate chewing (often due to teeth lost prematurely and not replaced, malocclusion, and neglected dental caries that may make teeth painful to chew upon), eating during emotional upsets, and swallowing large amounts of air with the food. Other factors that may cause prolonged and frequently serious forms of indigestion are excessive smoking, constipation (infrequent or difficult evacuation of the feces), eating poorly cooked foods or foods high in fat content, eating highly spiced foods, and disease.

The major symptoms of indigestion are nausea, heartburn, and flatulence (an excessive accumulation of gas in the stomach or intestine). Nausea may be produced by any condition that increases the tension on the walls of the lower end of the esophagus, stomach, or intestine. Distension of any part of the esophagus may result in what is usually called "heartburn." Flatulence may be produced by any of the conditions just mentioned.

A physician should be consulted whenever indigestion is severe enough to produce excessive discomfort. Common indigestion may be relieved by eating a balanced diet, allowing adequate time for eating a meal (preferably an hour), slowly and thoroughly chewing food, and, whenever possible, eating the meal in a pleasant, quiet, relaxed environment. After a meal the person should avoid excite-

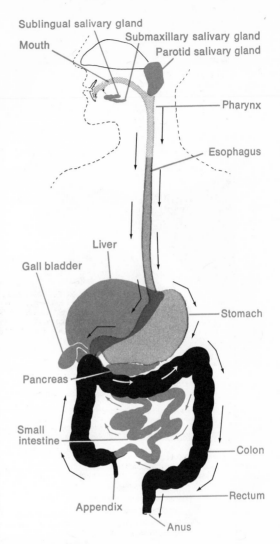

Structure of the human digestive system. The functions of this system are shown on the facing page.

ment. Smoking immediately after a meal frequently causes indigestion.

## Peptic Ulcer

A peptic ulcer is an open sore in the lining of the digestive tube in one of four places—the

195

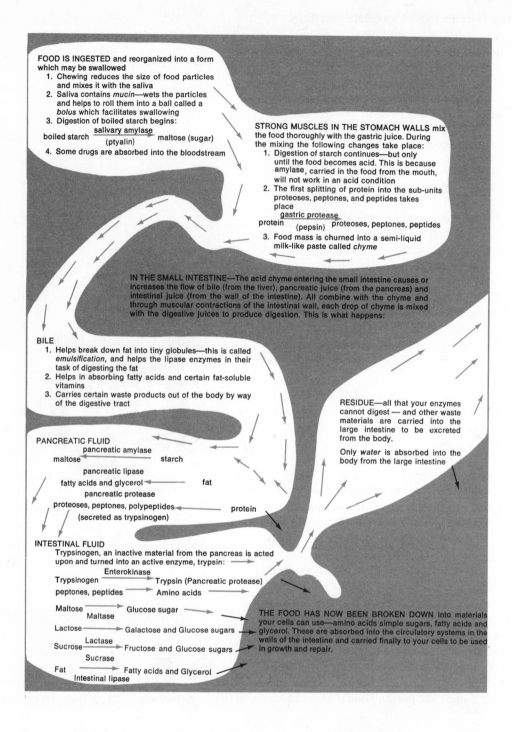

**FOOD IS INGESTED and reorganized into a form which may be swallowed**
1. Chewing reduces the size of food particles and mixes it with the saliva
2. Saliva contains *mucin*—wets the particles and helps to roll them into a ball called a *bolus* which facilitates swallowing
3. Digestion of boiled starch begins:

boiled starch $\xrightarrow[\text{(ptyalin)}]{\text{salivary amylase}}$ maltose (sugar)

4. Some drugs are absorbed into the bloodstream

**STRONG MUSCLES IN THE STOMACH WALLS mix** the food thoroughly with the gastric juice. During the mixing the following changes take place:
1. Digestion of starch continues—but only until the food becomes acid. This is because amylase, carried in the food from the mouth, will not work in an acid condition
2. The first splitting of protein into the sub-units proteoses, peptones, and peptides takes place

protein $\xrightarrow[\text{(pepsin)}]{\text{gastric protease}}$ proteoses, peptones, peptides

3. Food mass is churned into a semi-liquid milk-like paste called *chyme*

**IN THE SMALL INTESTINE**—The acid chyme entering the small intestine causes or increases the flow of bile (from the liver), pancreatic juice (from the pancreas) and intestinal juice (from the wall of the intestine). All combine with the chyme and through muscular contractions of the intestinal wall, each drop of chyme is mixed with the digestive juices to produce digestion. This is what happens:

**BILE**
1. Helps break down fat into tiny globules—this is called *emulsification,* and helps the lipase enzymes in their task of digesting the fat
2. Helps in absorbing fatty acids and certain fat-soluble vitamins
3. Carries certain waste products out of the body by way of the digestive tract

**RESIDUE**—all that your enzymes cannot digest — and other waste materials are carried into the large intestine to be excreted from the body.

Only *water* is absorbed into the body from the large intestine

**PANCREATIC FLUID**

maltose $\xleftarrow{\text{pancreatic amylase}}$ starch

fatty acids and glycerol $\xleftarrow{\text{pancreatic lipase}}$ fat

proteoses, peptones, polypeptides $\xleftarrow{\text{pancreatic protease}}$ protein
(secreted as trypsinogen)

**INTESTINAL FLUID**
Trypsinogen, an inactive material from the pancreas is acted upon and turned into an active enzyme, trypsin:

Trypsinogen $\xrightarrow{\text{Enterokinase}}$ Trypsin (Pancreatic protease)

peptones, peptides $\xrightarrow{}$ Amino acids

Maltose $\xrightarrow[\text{Maltase}]{}$ Glucose sugar

Lactose $\xrightarrow[\text{Lactase}]{}$ Galactose and Glucose sugars

Sucrose $\xrightarrow[\text{Sucrase}]{}$ Fructose and Glucose sugars

Fat $\xrightarrow[\text{Intestinal lipase}]{}$ Fatty acids and Glycerol

**THE FOOD HAS NOW BEEN BROKEN DOWN** into materials your cells can use—amino acids simple sugars, fatty acids and glycerol. These are absorbed into the circulatory systems in the walls of the intestine and carried finally to your cells to be used in growth and repair.

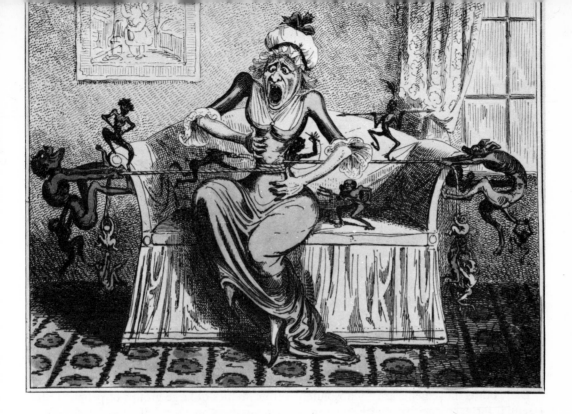

Along with mechanical stomachs, balloons, faucets, and the other "explanations" given by the Television Age is this view of indigestion, first published in 1819. *From Mary Evans Picture Library.*

lower end of the esophagus, the stomach (gastric ulcer), the duodenum (duodenal ulcer), or at the junction of the duodenum and jejunum.

The exact causes of peptic ulcers are unknown. Emotional tensions seem to play an important part in the formation of ulcers by producing an oversecretion of the acid in the stomach and upsetting the overall digestive processes.

If not promptly and properly treated by a physician, an ulcer can become an extremely dangerous condition. All treatment of an ulcer should always be under the immediate supervision of a physician.

### *Appendicitis*

Appendicitis is an inflammation of the vermiform appendix. The inflammation results from an obstruction and from the infection of the wall of the appendix by the numerous bacteria always present in the large intestine.

Typically, appendicitis is characterized by a pain in the umbilical region, which may be accompanied by nausea or vomiting. After several hours, the pain often shifts to the lower right portion of the abdomen, becomes continuous, dull or severe, and may be accompanied by coughing or sneezing.

Early diagnosis and treatment are necessary to save the life of an appendicitis victim. Use of antibiotics and surgery are common treatments. If treated early by surgery, deaths from appendicitis are extremely low—in many hospitals, less than 1 percent.

The use of a laxative or purgative, or application of heat to the abdominal area can cause the appendix to rupture into the abdominal cavity, which may cause death.

### Constipation

This is the difficult or infrequent passage of feces caused by large quantities of very dry, hard feces accumulating in the descending lower colon.

People who are tense, nervous, anxious, and hurried may suffer periodically from constipation. Individuals with long-standing poor eating or bowel habits, who have food allergies, or who overuse laxatives may frequently become constipated.

Daily bowel movements are not absolutely essential for everyone. No real harm comes from not having a bowel movement for a period of up to four days. But the use of laxatives, suppositories, and enemas can, over a period of time, cause the colon to lose its elasticity and muscular strength.

## RECOMMENDATIONS FOR A HEALTHY DIET

A healthy diet must meet certain basic requirements. It should provide sufficient amounts of all the nutrients known to be required by good health; it should provide these substances in amounts that are compatible with the needs of the individual; and it should not provide any nutrient in dangerous excess. (Some nutrients can be stored in the body if excess occurs; other nutrients can be eliminated if more than the basal amount is provided; other nutrients might be toxic

in high concentrations in the body.) A diet should include a variety of textures to maintain good intestinal tone and should provide a sufficient amount of water. There are several guidelines—some developed by research agencies in government and private industry, some provided by educational institutions to help in the teaching of sound nutrition—which can help you select a good diet.

### Recommended Dietary Allowances

The Food and Nutrition Board of the National Research Council has developed formulas of daily food intake considered adequate for maintaining good nutrition for people living in the United States. These formulations are called the *recommended dietary allowances* (RDA). As new information becomes available, recommendations are changed and revisions are made.

The RDA's are based on statistics gained from studies of large groups of people. Individuals vary in terms of physical structure and biochemical makeup. Since some people need more, some less, than the recommended amounts of certain nutrients, it must not be automatically assumed that certain food practices are poor or that people are malnourished simply because the recommendations are not being completely met. Also, the RDA's are ample enough to provide some margin of safety for each nutrient above the bare requirements in order to take care of variations between different individuals. For most people in this country, the recommended allowances can be considered adequate for maintaining good health and preventing nutritional diseases.

In addition, it is important to remember that the RDA's are not specific for all people in the population. The RDA's are directed toward a "reference" man and woman. The reference man for the RDA's is 22-years-old, weighs 154 pounds, and is 5 feet, 8 inches

## DESIRABLE WEIGHTS FOR ADULTS

| HEIGHT[a] (IN.) | WEIGHT (LB) MEN | WOMEN |
|---|---|---|
| 60 | | 109 ± 9[b] |
| 62 | | 115 ± 9 |
| 64 | 133 ± 11 | 122 ± 10 |
| 66 | 142 ± 12 | 129 ± 10 |
| 68 | 151 ± 14 | 136 ± 10 |
| 70 | 159 ± 14 | 144 ± 11 |
| 72 | 167 ± 15 | 152 ± 12 |
| 74 | 175 ± 15 | |
| 76 | 182 ± 16 | |

[a]Heights and weights are without shoes and other clothing. Weights are based on those of college men and women.
[b]Desirable weight for a small-framed woman at this height would be approximately 109 lb minus 9 lb, or a total of 100 lb; for an average-framed woman, 109 lb; for a large-framed woman, 109 lb plus 9 lb, or a total of 118 lb.

SOURCE: National Academy of Sciences Food and Nutrition Board, *Recommended Dietary Allowances*, 7th ed., National Research Council, Washington, D.C., 1968.

tall. The reference woman is 22-years-old, weighs 128 pounds, and is 5 feet, 4 inches tall. They are presumed to live in a climate with a mean temperature of 68° F and to be moderately active physically. (See table of recommended dietary allowances on pp. 202 and 203.)

### Calculating Calorie Allowances

Calorie needs are actually the simplest to determine. By examining the activity patterns, body-frame size, height, age, and the possible presence of other complicating conditions (such as pregnancy), nutritionists can determine the amount of food energy, as expressed in calories, an individual should receive each day from his diet in order to maintain a desirable weight. (See the table.)

The major reasons for the distinction (shown in the figure on recommended calorie allowances) between men and women is that women generally have smaller body frames and are less physically active, and therefore have a smaller proportion of muscle in their body weight.

The table (p. 204) on the adjustment of calorie allowances shows the shift in caloric needs that occurs during one's lifetime. The steady decline in caloric requirements after the age of about 18 years is due to a reduction of the basal metabolism rate and the typical decline in daily activity after late adolescence.

### Sources of Calories

As explained previously, the energy available from the various foods is measured in units of calories. Calories are available from fats, proteins, and carbohydrates. Carbohydrates are the primary source of calories for most of the world's people, because they are the cheapest calorie source in most countries. In the United States, the average person derives about 45 percent of his energy from carbohydrates, 40 percent from fats, and 15 percent from proteins. These are not necessarily the optimum proportions. In fact, authorities differ on just what the optimum ratios really are. Apparently the human body is adaptable enough so that it can function well in a wide range of dietary mixtures. Some general guidelines are: a *maximum* of 66 percent of caloric intake as carbohydrates; between 20 and 40 percent of calories as fats, and *at least* 10 percent of calories in the form of proteins. What is certain is that each of the three food types *must* be present in the daily diet and that it is unwise to totally eliminate any of them for reducing or other purposes.

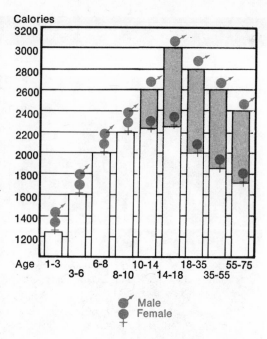

Recommended daily caloric allowances for average individuals within a given age group.

## DIET AND WEIGHT CONTROL

Among the many paradoxes in this world, not the least is that while much of the world's population is fighting starvation, more than 25 percent of the people in the United States are overweight due to excessive eating. The preoccupation which captivates many people in this country is that of weight control. The magnitude of the problem is shown by the one-quarter to one-half billion dollars a year that Americans pay "fat doctors" to help in overcoming this problem. Such concern is not only a reflection of the importance we attach to proper weight, but also a frank commentary on the failure many people encounter in their attempts to maintain a satisfactory weight.

Appetite and hunger control relate to the ability to control weight. Appetite and hunger are known to be controlled by a small area in the brain called the "appetite center" or appestat. It is composed of two sets of nuclei.

One determines your perception of hunger and one determines your perception of a satisfied feeling; your willingness to eat is regulated by the comparison between the two. Thus, the appestat works something like a thermostat controlling the temperature of a room.

As to what activates the appestat, there is still some question. It may be the glucose level (blood-sugar level) in the blood, body temperature changes, or the level of amino acids in the blood. But it is known that the appetite center has nerve connections with the cortex of the brain and may also be consciously controlled. This would mean that emotional factors, as well as chemical ones, appear to control appetite. Worry, tension, frustration, and conflicts in interpersonal relations can influence a person's appetite. Other research has shown that appestats vary in different individuals. Thus a person may inherit a "higher setting" in his appestat than another person and require more food before he feels satisfied. Consequently, we can say that appetite is regulated by emotions, body chemistry, and inheritance. All of these factors influence the ability to control weight.

The Food and Nutrition Board of the National Research Council believes that a desirable weight is normally achieved by age 22. The age 22 weight is the focus of determinations of desirable weight and is the standard by which one should judge one's weight in later years.

Most of us succeed in accomplishing things we want to accomplish; we do things that interest or motivate us. If we are to maintain a desirable weight we must want to. Reasons for losing weight or maintaining a desirable weight that appeal to or motivate people include the following.

1. A desire to look attractive. Whether a person likes it or not, he must admit that clothing styles are directed toward slender figures. Of course, larger sizes are provided for those who need them, but these are not the fashion ideal. Few people are not influenced by the fashion market. Then again, it's always pleasant to "fit" into a standard-size theater or lecture-hall seat, or to take no more than our third of the car seat. The overweight person faces such dilemmas daily.

2. Longer life. According to studies, a man 45 years of age, of medium height and frame, and weighing 170 pounds, can expect to live 2 to 4 fewer years than a similar man weighing 150 pounds. A man 45 years of age, of medium height and frame, weighing 200 pounds, can expect to live 4 to 6 years less than a similar man weighing 150 pounds.

3. Fewer diseases. Cardiovascular disease, diabetes, gallbladder disease, cirrhosis of the liver, certain forms of cancer, and arthritis occur more often or can be more serious in overweight people than in those of desirable weight.

4. Fewer painful conditions. Overweight is a factor in such common conditions as varicose veins, high blood pressure, gout, pulmonary emphysema, nephritis, and toxemia in pregnancy. It is estimated that for every pound of added fat an additional two-thirds of a mile of blood vessels are required to keep this pound of fat alive.

Excess fat complicates all surgery and increases surgical risks. The same is true in the delivery of a child. It takes extra body effort to carry body weight that is not needed; thus, the overweight person is more often tired. Fat accumulates around internal vital organs (such as the heart and lungs) and tends to crowd them. The overweight person is less agile, has more balancing problems, moves more slowly, and has more physical accidents than a person of normal weight.

### Patterns of Obesity

Obesity is the medical condition of overweight caused by excess fat on the body frame. It is thought to be due to one of two basic causes. It may be due to a difference in the ability of the body to utilize food in the same manner as the majority of people (known as metabolic obesity). Or obesity can be due to an inability to regulate food intake, called regulatory obesity.

Metabolic obesity depends on the rate at which food is being built up for storage and broken down for use (the rate of metabolism) which varies from person to person. These differences occur in response to specific hormone and enzyme activities in the body. Rate differences may be the result of inherited or developmental differences, or they may be the result of disease in the pituitary gland

| | | AGE (years) From—To | WEIGHT (lb) | HEIGHT (in.) | kcal | PROTEIN (gm) | FAT-SOLUBLE VITAMINS | | |
|---|---|---|---|---|---|---|---|---|---|
| (lb) | (in.) | | | | | | VITAMIN A ACTIVITY (IU) | VITAMIN D (IU) | VITAMIN E ACTIVITY (IU) |
| Infants | | 0–1/6 | 9 | 22 | kg × 120 | kg × 2.2 | 1,500 | 400 | 5 |
| | | 1/6–1/2 | 15 | 25 | kg × 110 | kg × 2.0 | 1,500 | 400 | 5 |
| | | 1/2–1 | 20 | 28 | kg × 100 | kg × 1.8 | 1,500 | 400 | 5 |
| Children | | 1–2 | 26 | 32 | 1,100 | 25 | 2,000 | 400 | 10 |
| | | 2–3 | 31 | 36 | 1,250 | 25 | 2,000 | 400 | 10 |
| | | 3–4 | 35 | 39 | 1,400 | 30 | 2,500 | 400 | 10 |
| | | 4–6 | 42 | 43 | 1,600 | 30 | 2,500 | 400 | 10 |
| | | 6–8 | 51 | 48 | 2,000 | 35 | 3,500 | 400 | 15 |
| | | 8–10 | 62 | 52 | 2,200 | 40 | 3,500 | 400 | 15 |
| Males | | 10–12 | 77 | 55 | 2,500 | 45 | 4,500 | 400 | 20 |
| | | 12–14 | 95 | 59 | 2,700 | 50 | 5,000 | 400 | 20 |
| | | 14–18 | 130 | 67 | 3,000 | 60 | 5,000 | 400 | 25 |
| | | 18–22 | 147 | 69 | 2,800 | 60 | 5,000 | 400 | 30 |
| | | 22–35 | 154 | 69 | 2,800 | 65 | 5,000 | — | 30 |
| | | 35–55 | 154 | 68 | 2,600 | 65 | 5,000 | — | 30 |
| | | 55–75+ | 154 | 67 | 2,400 | 65 | 5,000 | — | 30 |
| Females | | 10–12 | 77 | 56 | 2,250 | 50 | 4,500 | 400 | 20 |
| | | 12–14 | 97 | 61 | 2,300 | 50 | 5,000 | 400 | 20 |
| | | 14–16 | 114 | 62 | 2,400 | 55 | 5,000 | 400 | 25 |
| | | 16–18 | 119 | 63 | 2,300 | 55 | 5,000 | 400 | 25 |
| | | 18–22 | 128 | 64 | 2,000 | 55 | 5,000 | 400 | 25 |
| | | 22–35 | 128 | 64 | 2,000 | 55 | 5,000 | — | 25 |
| | | 35–55 | 128 | 63 | 1,850 | 55 | 5,000 | — | 25 |
| | | 55–75+ | 128 | 62 | 1,700 | 55 | 5,000 | — | 25 |
| Pregnancy | | | | | +200 | 65 | 6,000 | 400 | 30 |
| Lactation | | | | | +1,000 | 75 | 8,000 | 400 | 30 |

or the thyroid gland. Such conditions can cause overweight or underweight, but less than 5 percent of all cases can be blamed on the glands.

Regulatory obesity occurs far more often; this is the result of failure on the part of a person to voluntarily control his food intake. If such overeating is continued long enough, it may cause basic metabolic changes. Some factors that can affect a person's eating habits and his weight include the following.

1. Family eating and exercise habits. According to U.S. Department of Health, Education, and Welfare (HEW) statistics, over two-thirds of the parents of obese children are themselves obese. It has not been determined to what extent hereditary factors are responsible for this relationship, but it does seem that nonhereditary factors are also im-

| WATER-SOLUBLE VITAMINS | | | | | | | MINERALS | | | | |
|---|---|---|---|---|---|---|---|---|---|---|---|
| ASCORBIC ACID (mg) | FOLACIN (mg) | NIACIN (mg equiv) | RIBOFLAVIN (mg) | THIAMIN (mg) | VITAMIN $B_6$ (mg) | VITAMIN $B_{12}$ ($\mu$g) | CALCIUM (g) | PHOSPHORUS (g) | IODINE ($\mu$g) | IRON (mg) | MAGNESIUM (mg) |
| 35 | 0.05 | 5 | 0.4 | 0.2 | 0.2 | 1.0 | 0.4 | 0.2 | 25 | 6 | 40 |
| 35 | 0.05 | 7 | 0.5 | 0.4 | 0.3 | 1.5 | 0.5 | 0.4 | 40 | 10 | 60 |
| 35 | 0.1 | 8 | 0.6 | 0.5 | 0.4 | 2.0 | 0.6 | 0.5 | 45 | 15 | 70 |
| 40 | 0.1 | 8 | 0.6 | 0.6 | 0.5 | 2.0 | 0.7 | 0.7 | 55 | 15 | 100 |
| 40 | 0.2 | 8 | 0.7 | 0.6 | 0.6 | 2.5 | 0.8 | 0.8 | 60 | 15 | 150 |
| 40 | 0.2 | 9 | 0.8 | 0.7 | 0.7 | 3 | 0.8 | 0.8 | 70 | 10 | 200 |
| 40 | 0.2 | 11 | 0.9 | 0.8 | 0.9 | 4 | 0.8 | 0.8 | 80 | 10 | 200 |
| 40 | 0.2 | 13 | 1.1 | 1.0 | 1.0 | 4 | 0.9 | 0.9 | 100 | 10 | 250 |
| 40 | 0.3 | 15 | 1.2 | 1.1 | 1.2 | 5 | 1.0 | 1.0 | 110 | 10 | 250 |
| 40 | 0.4 | 17 | 1.3 | 1.3 | 1.4 | 5 | 1.2 | 1.2 | 125 | 10 | 300 |
| 45 | 0.4 | 18 | 1.4 | 1.4 | 1.6 | 5 | 1.4 | 1.4 | 135 | 18 | 350 |
| 55 | 0.4 | 20 | 1.5 | 1.5 | 1.8 | 5 | 1.4 | 1.4 | 150 | 18 | 400 |
| 60 | 0.4 | 18 | 1.6 | 1.4 | 2.0 | 5 | 0.8 | 0.8 | 140 | 10 | 400 |
| 60 | 0.4 | 18 | 1.7 | 1.4 | 2.0 | 5 | 0.8 | 0.8 | 140 | 10 | 350 |
| 60 | 0.4 | 17 | 1.7 | 1.3 | 2.0 | 5 | 0.8 | 0.8 | 125 | 10 | 350 |
| 60 | 0.4 | 14 | 1.7 | 1.2 | 2.0 | 6 | 0.8 | 0.8 | 110 | 10 | 350 |
| 40 | 0.4 | 15 | 1.3 | 1.1 | 1.4 | 5 | 1.2 | 1.2 | 110 | 18 | 300 |
| 45 | 0.4 | 15 | 1.4 | 1.2 | 1.6 | 5 | 1.3 | 1.3 | 115 | 18 | 350 |
| 50 | 0.4 | 16 | 1.4 | 1.2 | 1.8 | 5 | 1.3 | 1.3 | 120 | 18 | 350 |
| 50 | 0.4 | 15 | 1.5 | 1.2 | 2.0 | 5 | 1.3 | 1.3 | 115 | 18 | 350 |
| 55 | 0.4 | 13 | 1.5 | 1.0 | 2.0 | 5 | 0.8 | 0.8 | 100 | 18 | 350 |
| 55 | 0.4 | 13 | 1.5 | 1.0 | 2.0 | 5 | 0.8 | 0.8 | 100 | 18 | 300 |
| 55 | 0.4 | 13 | 1.5 | 1.0 | 2.0 | 5 | 0.8 | 0.8 | 90 | 18 | 300 |
| 55 | 0.4 | 13 | 1.5 | 1.0 | 2.0 | 6 | 0.8 | 0.8 | 80 | 10 | 300 |
| 60 | 0.8 | 15 | 1.8 | +0.1 | 2.5 | 8 | +0.4 | +0.4 | 125 | 18 | 450 |
| 60 | 0.5 | 20 | 2.0 | +0.5 | 2.5 | 6 | +0.5 | +0.5 | 150 | 18 | 450 |

SOURCE: National Academy of Sciences Food and Nutrition Board, *Recommended Dietary Allowances*, 7th ed. National Research Council, Washington, D.C., 1968.

portant. The role of the parent as model for eating and exercise habits seems particularly significant. Some individuals come from homes in which parents provide meals that are excessive in calories. Others are accustomed to heavy between-meal eating of soft drinks, candy, ice cream, and pastries. Still others have been accustomed to too little exercise as a result of easily available transportation, too few sports, modern conveniences, and sheer laziness.

2. Emotional factors. Some people use food as a comfort, crutch, or compensation for feelings of frustration, unhappiness, or

## ADJUSTMENT OF CALORIE (KCAL) ALLOWANCES[a] FOR ADULT INDIVIDUALS OF VARIOUS BODY WEIGHTS AND AGES [AT A MEAN ENVIRONMENTAL TEMPERATURE OF 68°F, ASSUMING LIGHT PHYSICAL ACTIVITY]

| BODY WEIGHT | RMR[b] AT AGE 22 | 22 | 45 | 65 |
|---|---|---|---|---|
| **MEN** | | | | |
| 110 | 1540 | 2,200 | 2,000 | 1,850 |
| 121 | 1620 | 2,350 | 2,150 | 1,950 |
| 132 | 1720 | 2,500 | 2,300 | 2,100 |
| 143 | 1820 | 2,650 | 2,400 | 2,200 |
| 154[d] | 1880 | 2,800 | 2,600 | 2,400 |
| 165 | 1970 | 2,950 | 2,700 | 2,500 |
| 176 | 2020 | 3,050 | 2,800 | 2,600 |
| 187 | 2110 | 3,200 | 2,950 | 2,700 |
| 198 | 2210 | 3,350 | 3,100 | 2,800 |
| 209 | 2290 | 3,500 | 3,200 | 2,900 |
| 220 | 2380 | 3,700 | 3,400 | 3,100 |
| | | | | |
| **WOMEN** | | | | |
| 88 | 1280 | 1,550 | 1,450 | 1,300 |
| 99 | 1380 | 1,700 | 1,550 | 1,450 |
| 110 | 1460 | 1,800 | 1,650 | 1,500 |
| 121 | 1560 | 1,950 | 1,800 | 1,650 |
| 128[d] | 1620 | 2,000 | 1,850 | 1,700 |
| 132 | 1640 | 2,050 | 1,900 | 1,700 |
| 143 | 1740 | 2,200 | 2,000 | 1,850 |
| 154 | 1830 | 2,300 | 2,100 | 1,950 |

[a]Kcal allowance (males) = (RMR + 13w) × (percent adjustment for age); kcal allowance (females) = (RMR + 7w) × (percent adjustment for age); w = wt in kg. Values are rounded to the nearest 50 kcal.

[b]RMR = resting metabolic rate, approximately 10 percent above the metabolic rate measured under basal conditions.

[c]Age adjustments:

| Age | Adjustment (percent of kcal allowance at age 22) |
|---|---|
| 22–35 | 100–95 |
| 35–45 | 95–92 |
| 45–55 | 92–89 |
| 55–65 | 89–84 |
| 65–75 | 84–79 |
| 75–85 | 72 |

[d]Reference man and woman.

SOURCE: National Academy of Sciences Food and Nutrition Board, *Recommended Dietary Allowances*, 7th ed., National Research Council, Washington, D.C., 1968.

worry. They overeat to counteract domestic troubles, financial problems, family illness, or social upsets.

3. Poverty. Some families, because of limited finances, buy cheap foods that tend to be high in carbohydrates or fats, in place of more expensive protein-rich foods.

4. Uncontrolled snacking and nibbling. This habit can lead to the consumption of uncounted calories. When such snacking is added to regular meals, it can mean more calories taken in than the body is using, and thus more stored fat. Controlled nibbling is not damaging as long as the nibbling does not interfere with good nutrition and excesses are avoided.

5. Failure to cut down eating during reduced activity. It has already been pointed out that as a person becomes less active with age or occupation, he requires fewer calories to maintain his weight level. If, on the other hand, his food intake is not decreased but remains about the same, he puts on added weight.

6. Ignorance. Some people are frankly ignorant of caloric values of various foods. They tend to confuse the wide differences in the caloric content of favorite foods and drinks (see table).

Regardless of the underlying causes of obesity, the basic problem is simply one of taking in more calories than are needed for one's total activities—basal metabolism, heat loss, work, and exercise. Unused calories from any source are stored in the body as fat; each pound of stored fat is the equivalent of 3500 calories. All calories taken in are either stored or used, and the more calories that are stored, the greater the degree of obesity.

### Reducing

Reducing calls for unyielding determination. A person must be prepared to face the rigors of ignoring the sight and smell of appealing food within his reach. This calls for high motivation and willpower.

A person must accept a personal responsibility for his weight problem. It cannot be blamed on family problems, spouse, unmanageable children, lack of friends, or troubles in general. Although admittedly these may affect the obese person, in the end it is that person who has been overfeeding himself—he has voluntarily overeaten.

A reducing diet is based on the principal that reducing the calorie intake will permit daily caloric needs to exceed the available amount from the diet. In this way, stored body fat can be used up and weight can be reduced.

*Reducing Diets.* There are many ideas and suggestions about how to lose weight. These range in severity from the "miracle diets" that guarantee to take off 10 pounds in 2 weeks to the oils, tablets, seeds, juices, extracts, and high-fat or protein diets. There are also prepared formulas on the market in the form of canned drinks or cookies. Some of these have value, some are worthless, and some are outright dangerous.

Low-carbohydrate diets have been prominent in recent years. While they are known by many names and variations, the basic premise of all of these diets is that if carbohydrates are restricted enough, other calorie sources, even fats and alcohol, may be consumed in unlimited quantities without interfering with weight loss. While such diets have enabled many people to lose weight, at least temporarily, there are strong warnings from many medical authorities regarding the dangers inherent in an extreme low-calorie diet. The AMA Council on Foods and Nutrition has stated: "The council is deeply concerned about any diet that advocates an unlimited intake of saturated fats and cholesterol-rich foods. Individuals responding to such a diet with a rise in blood fats will have an increased risk of coronary artery disease and atherosclerosis, particularly if the diet is maintained over a prolonged period." Another concern is that when carbohydrate intake is very low, fats are broken down to chemicals called ketones, creating an acidic condition in the blood. Among the known or suspected effects of extreme low-carbohydrate diets are weakness, faintness, depression of the functions of the central nervous system, kidney and liver damage, and the development of gout (a painful accumulation of uric acid crystals in the body).

1. *See a physician.* A doctor should decide whether it is safe for you to lose weight, how much to lose, and how long the reduction should take.

2. *Choose a practical diet.* Under the direction of your physician you should choose a reducing diet that can be followed without undue punishment or undue cost. It should be compatible with eating habits you are accustomed to. It is not necessary to stop eating the foods you cherish, but it will be necessary to regulate the amount of them that you eat. Such regulation is demanded not only for losing pounds, but also for maintaining a desirable weight when it is reached. Once the reducing diet is over and you have lost the unnecessary pounds, you should never return to the old excessive weight. Unless you learn to live on a maintaining diet, all of your agonies of losing weight will have been in vain.

3. *Reduce the calories taken in.* Opinions vary on whether caloric reduction can best be done by limiting carbohydrate intake, fat intake, or protein intake. But whatever the method, there is no doubt that calories do count (even if you refuse to count them). You must watch your foods, particularly the rich ones. Some of these tantalizing and irresistible foods are loaded with calories. Remember that fats have over twice the calories, per unit of weight, of carbohydrates or proteins, so learn what the high-fat foods are and how to cut down on them.

4. *Plan the diet.* One of the most important facts about weight reduction is that the same number of nutrients must be "fitted" into a smaller number of calories. Your reducing plan should include all the basic food groups—meat, milk, vegetables, fruits, mineral, vitamins, and water. Also, your body will still need a daily supply of proteins, minerals, vitamins, and limited calories. A good reducing diet should provide at least 1200–1800 calories a day. Some commercially prepared, canned reducing formulas supply a minimum of 900 calories per day. These are acceptable when they contain carefully measured supplements of essential vitamins and minerals. The 1200 calorie-per-day table shows how many combinations of food are available for a well-planned diet.

5. *Know your reducing goal.* You should know how many pounds you intend to lose and how long the reduction should take. Each pound of body fat represents 3500 calories. To lose 1 pound in 1 week, you must reduce your calorie intake by 3500 calories over that period of time. "Crash" diets that claim to take off 10 pounds in 2 weeks mean a calorie reduction of 2500 calories a day, which is more than some people normally eat altogether.

6. *Graph your progress.* Since you gain weight gradually, you should lose it slowly. But, because gradual reducing plans can be discouraging, you may lose sight of your goal. Therefore, a good psychological aid is to keep track of progress by setting up a simple graph at the beginning of the program. You should plan to lose 1 or 2 pounds a week, and construct a typical reducing graph similar to the

# THE CALORIE CONTENT IN SOME FAVORITE FOODS AND DRINKS

| BREAKFAST | CALORIES | DRINKS | CALORIES |
|---|---|---|---|
| 1 scrambled egg | 110 | Whole milk, 1 cup | 160 |
| 2 slices fried bacon | 100 | Nonfat milk, 1 cup | 90 |
| Ham, slice, lean and fat | 245 | Malted milk, 1 cup | 280 |
| 1 wheat pancake | 60 | Cocoa, 1 cup | 235 |
| 1 waffle | 210 | Orange juice, frozen, | |
| Grapefruit, ½ whole | 55 | 1 cup diluted | 110 |
| Cantaloupe, ½ melon | 60 | Apple juice, 1 cup | 120 |
| Corn flakes, 1 oz | 110 | Grape juice, canned, 1 cup | 165 |
| Oatmeal, 1 cup | 130 | Yoghurt, 1 cup | 120 |
| White bread, 1 slice | 60 | Cola drink, 1 cup | 95 |
| Butter, 1 pat | 50 | Ginger ale, 1 cup | 70 |
| Jam, 1 tablespoon | 55 | Beer, 1 cup | 100 |
| LUNCH OR DINNER | | SNACKS | |
| Tomato soup, 1 cup | 90 | Cheddar cheese, 1-inch cube | 70 |
| Spaghetti, meat balls and | | Bologna, 1 slice | 85 |
| tomato sauce, 1 cup | 335 | Peanut butter, 1 tablespoon | 95 |
| Pork chop, 1 slice lean | 130 | Peanuts, roasted, 1 cup | 840 |
| Roast beef, 1 slice lean | 125 | 10 potato chips | 115 |
| Hamburger, meat only, 3 oz | 245 | Raisins, dried, 1 cup | 460 |
| 1 frankfurter, cooked | 155 | 1 apple | 70 |
| Chicken, ½ breast | 155 | 1 banana | 85 |
| Mashed potatoes, buttered, | | 1 orange, navel | 60 |
| 1 cup | 185 | 1 peach | 35 |
| Pizza, 1 section | 185 | Watermelon, 1 wedge | 115 |
| Cottage cheese, creamed, | | Popcorn, 1 cup | 65 |
| 1 cup | 240 | 2 graham crackers | 55 |
| Custard, 1 cup | 285 | 1 doughnut, cake type | 125 |
| Angelfood cake, 1 section | 110 | Candy, milk chocolate, 1 oz. | 150 |
| Iced chocolate cake, | | Marshmallows, 1 oz | 90 |
| 1 section | 445 | Pretzels, 5 small sticks | 20 |
| Apple pie, 1 section | 345 | 1 fig bar | 55 |
| Ice cream, 1 cup | 285 | 1 cookie, 3-inch | 120 |
| Sherbet, orange, 1 cup | 260 | | |
| Cornstarch pudding, 1 cup | 275 | | |

SOURCE: U.S. Department of Agriculture, *Nutritive Value of Foods*, Home and Garden Bulletin No. 72, rev. ed., Washington, D.C., September 1964.

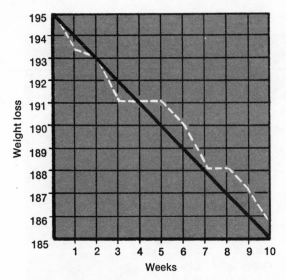

A typical weight-reducing graph. The straight line shows the "ideal" weight change from steady maintenance of a low-calorie diet plan; the dotted line is the more realistic pattern of expected weight change.

one shown here. In constructing the graph, you should allow as many weeks as there are pounds to lose, draw a straight line from where your beginning weight is to where it should be at the end, weigh in each morning on the bathroom scales, and place a dot on the graph at your weight point for that day. The graph can be a reminder of your progress and keep you determined to succeed.

7. *Exercise regularly.* A reasonable program of regular exercise helps to burn up energy, improves muscle tone, and creates a feeling of well-being, both physically and emotionally. Many people, including certain authorities, have tended to underestimate the role of exercise in weight control and of inactivity as a contributing factor in obesity. But now, many authorities are placing added emphasis on the importance of exercise in addition to diet. Some people rationalize their inactivity, stating that exercise would increase their appetite, canceling its beneficial effects. But this is rarely so. In fact, for most people exercise lets the appestat function more effectively, reducing the amount of "nervous" eating that is often the result of inactivity. Thus exercise may actually decrease the appetite of a sedentary person.

### Underweight

Whether or not someone should be called underweight should not be determined by weight alone, but on the presence or absence of associated symptoms of malnutrition. It is possible to eat a balanced diet, in moderation, and remain in excellent health even though slender. But symptoms such as lack of endurance, easy fatigue, frequent infections, intermittent diarrhea, or sores on the skin or mucous membranes might indicate a definite problem of undernutrition—there is not enough food intake for normal body function. In severe cases, the results can include deficiency diseases, injury to vital organs (especially heart and kidneys), and even death. Underweight can be due to emotional state (nervousness, worry, anxiety), diseases, malnutrition (poor selection of foods), hormonal disorders, or unrealistic dieting.

The treatment of underweight is not always just a simple matter of starting to eat more. There should be a physician's consultation to detect the presence of any infectious or glandular disease or other contributing condition. If the problem appears to be purely dietary, emphasis should be on a good balanced diet, adequate in protein and other nutrients. If the problem is an emotional one, as is often the case, efforts should be made to either correct, or learn to cope with, the underlying conditions. Increased exercise may help relieve nervous tension, leading to improved diet.

## A 1200-CALORIE-PER-DAY DIET PATTERN

**BREAKFAST**

Fruit—1 medium serving, fresh, frozen, or canned
Egg—1, poached or boiled
Toast—1 slice with 1 teaspoon butter or margarine

or

Cereal—½ cup with ¼ cup milk, no sugar
Coffee or tea—no cream or sugar

**MIDMORNING SNACK**

Nonfat milk or buttermilk—1 glass

**LUNCHEON**

Meat or cheese—1 3-oz. portion
Vegetable—1 medium serving; may be raw, as a salad such as lettuce and tomato,
    or cooked; use lemon or vinegar for seasoning rather than butter or salad dressings
Fruit—1 medium serving, fresh or unsweetened canned
Bread—1 slice
Butter or margarine—1 teaspoon or 1 pat
Tea or coffee—no cream or sugar

**MIDAFTERNOON**

Iced tea, lemonade, or a soft drink

**DINNER**

Bouillon or consommé or vegetable-juice cocktail—1 serving
Meat—1 3-oz portion
Potato or a substitute for potato—1 small serving of mashed or baked potato, steamed
    rice, corn, lima beans, or macaroni; or 1 slice bread
Vegetable—1 serving, raw, as a salad, or cooked; one vegetable a day should be a
    green, leafy one
Butter or margarine—1 teaspoon, for potato
Fruit—1 medium serving, fresh or unsweetened canned
Tea or coffee—no cream or sugar

**EVENING OR BEDTIME**

Nonfat milk, buttermilk, soft drink, or glass of beer
Crackers or pretzels—2

## TOTAL FITNESS

Fitness, according to Dr. Roger Bannister (the first 4-minute miler), is one of the most misused words in the English language. It can mean anything from "that feeling of pleasure which a person experiences when he stands by an open window early in the morning to—for those with vested interests—some recommendation that we ought to drink more milk or beer."

### The Measure of Total Fitness

Total fitness implies the ability to function at an optimum level of efficiency in all daily living. This encompasses the whole philosophy of the science of health: intellectual, emotional, and social, as well as physical conditioning. A totally fit individual has the strength, speed, agility, endurance, and social and emotional adjustments appropriate to his age.

All body activities require energy. Very simply, energy is produced by breaking down foods (carbohydrates, fats, and proteins) in the presence of oxygen. The body can store food, but it cannot store oxygen. If the body takes in more food than is needed, it uses what it needs and stores the rest for later. Not so with oxygen. We cannot store oxygen, so we breathe in and out every moment of our lives to keep the supply coming in. If the oxygen supply were suddenly cut off, the oxygen stored in the body would not last more than a few minutes. The brain, the heart, all body tissues would cease to function, and we would die. The oxygen in the air is readily available; as we need it we breathe it in. The problem is getting enough oxygen to all parts of the body where food is burned.

Most of us produce enough energy to per-

| ENERGY EXPENDITURE PER HOUR DURING DIFFERENT TYPES OF ACTIVITY FOR A 70 KILOGRAM MAN [154 lbs] | |
| --- | --- |
| FORM OF ACTIVITY | CALORIES PER HOUR |
| Sleeping | 65 |
| Awake lying still | 77 |
| Sitting at rest | 100 |
| Standing relaxed | 105 |
| Dressing and undressing | 118 |
| Tailoring | 135 |
| Typewriting rapidly | 140 |
| "Light" exercise | 170 |
| Walking slowly (2.6 miles per hour) | 200 |
| Carpentry, metal working, industrial painting | 240 |
| "Active" exercise [brisk walking] | 290 |
| "Severe" exercise | 450 |
| Sawing wood | 480 |
| Swimming | 500 |
| Running (5.3 miles per hour) | 570 |
| "Very severe" exercise | 600 |
| Walking very fast (5.3 miles per hour) | 650 |
| Walking up stairs | 1100 |

Extracted from data compiled by Professor M. S. Rose.

SOURCE: A. C. Guyton, *Basic Human Physiology*, 4th ed., Philadelphia, W. B. Saunders, 1971.

form ordinary daily activities, that is, walk, talk, think, or study. However, as the activities become more vigorous, we sooner or later reach our maximum performance or maximum oxygen consumption. A person's maximum oxygen consumption is known as his *aerobic capacity*. The range between our minimum oxygen requirements (amount of oxygen used at rest) and our maximum capacity is one factor in the physiological measure of our total fitness. The most totally fit persons have the greatest range of capacity, the least fit, the narrowest range. In some persons, their minimum energy requirements and maximum physical capacity are almost identical. A totally fit individual should have, among other qualities, adequate aerobic capacity and physical strength to engage in daily physical activities, including such sports as tennis, swimming, bicycling, and handball, without producing undue fatigue.

To achieve this level of fitness an individual must participate in a daily fitness program. Programs must be individually tailored to the goals of the person. For example, the term *weight lifting* applies to the competitive weight lifter whose objective is to see how much weight he can lift. *Body building* involves lifting weights to build up muscles. *Weight training* is done to improve an individual's strength so that he can perform in other physical activities or sports. All three types of lifting might involve the same lifts but each lift would be tailored to the individual's objectives. A shot putter would do an *olympic lift* to improve his putting, while a body builder would do a *power lift* to improve his physique. Fitness programs to achieve adequate total fitness can be intelligently planned to meet the physiological needs and skill-performance goals for any individual.

As early as the preschool years, the growth and maturation of the neuromuscular system and the establishment of locomotor movement patterns lay the foundations for future learning and development of skills and attitudes of the individual toward physical fitness. Strong physical play forms the basis for a person's strength, agility, and coordination. To maintain these skills an individual must maintain a daily activity program throughout life. In school, activities for children can be planned with specific objectives to develop muscular strength, endurance, aerobic capacity, skill, and to perform in sports and physical activities at a *social level* throughout life.

The development to the social level of physical fitness, or the redevelopment of fitness (for the individual who has been inactive for a number of years) requires regular periods of physical activity within individually designed programs. The individual must start with low-energy-use programs (such as walking) and gradually increase the stress placed upon the body in terms of speed, workload, and duration of activity (termed the "overload principle") until the level of performance the individual is striving for is reached. High-energy-use programs such as jogging, running, swimming, bicycling, handball, and rope skipping are what you are working toward—but, it takes hard work and time.

Total fitness implies that a person is "in condition." Such a level of fitness is also called *overall fitness, endurance fitness,* or *working capacity* (the ability to do prolonged work without undue fatigue). If an individual is working toward a level of fitness needed for competitive sports he should do so only under the direction of a professional physical educator. In this section we are restricting our definition of "in condition" to that of the American Medical Association's Committee on Exercise and Physical Fitness. They stated in 1967 that fitness is "the general capacity to adapt and respond favorably to

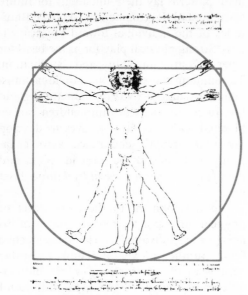

The proportions and symmetry of the totally fit human body attracted the scientific artistry of Leonardo da Vinci.

timum diet and total fitness. An estimation of normal aging becomes an estimate of the decline of the vitality of an individual. Under optimum conditions of energy supply, oxygen supply, waste removal, and periods of functioning and rest, the cells and the body tend to live longer. Body-age estimations based on such factors determine *biological age.* This bears no relationship to one's *chronological (year) age.*

The body shows biological age in terms of changes in structure and functioning of the major body systems. Various physiological functions change within these systems at different rates. Some changes take place rapidly, others appear to be age-resistant. The biological aging process can be speeded up by a deficient food supply, inactivity (the nonexerciser), infection, traumatic injury, and physical irritation. Rapid biological aging leads to deterioration of the body, disease, and *premature death* (death prior to the estimations for the general population).

The struggle for a better life has brought about impressive improvement in the living conditions of humans. Our infant mortality rate has lowered and, over the last hundred years, the average length of life in the United States has increased. This has been due to the control of *communicable diseases,* such as pneumonia and influenza, which caused the majority of deaths in the past. With control of the communicable diseases (over the past 100 years), life expectancy in the United States has been extended from 40 to over 68 years for males and over 75 years for females.

Parallel to the fact of increased life expectancy is that these longer-living individuals often are not able to function normally or adequately in the later years and die of diseases which formerly were uncommon. Today's deaths are more commonly caused by various *degenerative conditions* (the out-

physical effort. The degree of physical fitness depending upon the individual's state of health, constitution, and present and previous activity." This is also our definition of a person's *total fitness.*

### The Meaning of Total Fitness

Many individuals may be classified as "nonexercisers." This individual represents passive fitness; he makes no effort to keep his body fit. He does only what he has to during his daily routine. There is nothing physically wrong with him—not yet—nor is there anything really right with him. If he is lucky, he may remain like that for years. But, without increasing his physical activity, such an individual's body is essentially deteriorating.

The vitality and health of an individual is determined by many factors including op-

come of biological aging). These diseases cause or are the result of bio-changes in the structure and functioning of the body: arteriosclerosis, coronary thrombosis (cardiac infarction), cerebral thrombosis (stroke), as well as cancer of various organs.

Exercise physiologists show that physical exercise, if sufficiently intensive and regular, can override the various phenomena of aging—such as the decrease in muscle mass, diminished oxygen intake, reduced heat production, and the fall in total blood quantity. Physical exercises are also intensive overall cerebral activities. They stimulate the neural controls of metabolism, respiration, blood circulation, digestion, and the activities of the glands of internal secretion. A correct combination of alert mental activity and physical exercise is at present the best method of preserving, for as long as possible, at a high level, the activity of the brain cells.

This control of the phenomena of aging—the desire for longevity—should begin as early as possible, before you have completed your physical development (between 14 and 22 years of age). It is considerably more difficult to control premature biological aging after it has already set in. A regular exercise program contributes to vitality and healthful good looks throughout the middle years. A person who has maintained a successful personal fitness program can enjoy his middle and later years more fully. This is why the habits of physical exercise and total fitness should be formed from earliest childhood.

Total fitness is produced when someone engages in balanced activities, strengthening all body systems; particularly the cardiovascular system, the respiratory system, the nervous system, and the muscular system. But, it is very important to realize that total fitness is produced by *optimum* intensity and duration of physical activity. The amount and duration of physical activity required is different for every person. This is directed toward the female as well as the male. The values of total fitness are the same for both.

Contrary to some common thought, involvement in exercise programs and sports will not develop unfeminine or bulky muscles in women. Such a program that would *over*-develop specific muscles would be unhealthy for males or females. Exercise improves the female figure by "normalizing" it and causing it to become better proportioned. If the arms or legs are too heavy, exercise works toward slimming; if too thin, exercise develops them. Women should engage in regular physical programs and sports. They will help develop the beautiful, womanly figure that is slender and graceful, and has curves in the right places. Many beautiful feminine women are involved in daily (or three times a week) exercise programs and participate in sports.

### Activity Programs

Your likelihood of maintaining a physical fitness program depends on how interesting it is to you. In order for someone to perform within an activity program throughout the years it must maintain their interest. Most of the well-publicized physical fitness programs that stress exercises, machines, or rely on an athletic club need great motivation to be maintained throughout life. The best way for an exercise program to be fun is for you to take part in an individual activity or dual sport. But, you can not receive satisfaction out of a sport that you are not in condition to perform. Consequently, an individual must have a general conditioning program, which is routine (usually 3 days a week) and can be maintained easily to stay in condition for any sport. (See example on p. 214.)

An individual, while he is in school or college, should develop skills in several dif-

## WEIGHT PROGRESSION CARD[a]

| EXERCISES | MAY 1 SET | REP | WGHT | MAY 2 SET | REP | WGHT | MAY 3 SET | REP | WGHT | MAY 4 SET | REP | WGHT | MAY 5 SET | REP | WGHT | MAY 8 SET | REP | WGHT | MAY 9 SET | REP | WGHT | MAY 10 SET | REP | WGHT | MAY 11 SET | REP | WGHT | MAY 12 SET | REP | WGHT | NOTES |
|---|---|---|---|---|---|---|---|---|---|---|---|---|---|---|---|---|---|---|---|---|---|---|---|---|---|---|---|---|---|---|---|
| Two-arm standing press | 3 | 10 | 40 | skip | | | 3 | 10 | 40 | skip | | | 3 | 10 | 40 | 3 | 10 | 45 | skip | | | 3 | 10 | 45 | skip | | | 3 | 10 | 45 | increase weight 10 lbs. |
| Rowing motion | | | | | | | | | | | | | | | | | | | | | | | | | | | | | | | |
| Shrug | | | | | | | | | | | | | | | | | | | | | | | | | | | | | | | |
| Squat | | | | | | | | | | | | | | | | | | | | | | | | | | | | | | | |
| Rise on toes | | | | | | | | | | | | | | | | | | | | | | | | | | | | | | | |
| Lateral bench raise | | | | | | | | | | | | | | | | | | | | | | | | | | | | | | | |
| Barbell curl | | | | | | | | | | | | | | | | | | | | | | | | | | | | | | | |
| Lateral raise | | | | | | | | | | | | | | | | | | | | | | | | | | | | | | | |
| Side bend | | | | | | | | | | | | | | | | | | | | | | | | | | | | | | | |

[a]You may want to add the following to a weight progression card:
1. Dimensions of wrist, waist, thighs, and neck.
2. Holes so that the card can be put into a ring binder for future reference.
3. Space for notes on progress.
4. Charts should be for two-week periods.

ferent activities to participate in throughout life. Five major factors should be considered as one plans his physical fitness activities for later life. He should develop his (1) muscular strength, (2) muscular endurance, (3) circulatory endurance, (4) flexibility, and (5) skill (coordination). Physical education courses should help the individual to gain knowledge in activities and sports that develop and maintain these factors.

The concepts of exercise, but not the principles, have changed drastically in recent years. Modern total fitness programs are the result of laboratory studies that have added greatly to our knowledge. Exercise is accepted today as being essential to counterbalance our oversedentary life style. Now, the question becomes, "how much and what kind of exercise?" Dr. Kenneth H. Cooper, in his book *The New Aerobics,* points out that the body needs oxygen and the rhythmic physical activity that supplies the body with oxygen. During exercise, the blood is richer in oxygen and nutrients and more effectively eliminates wastes from the muscles and other organs. Activities that promote such efficient body functioning include walking, running, swimming, cycling, dancing, skiing, and tennis. Also, for exercise to be effective, it must be routine and done at one's capacity. But what is your capacity?

If your current total fitness status is adequate and you are satisfied with your ability to function, then all you need is to maintain this level. But, if you are dissatisfied with your physical condition and capacity and want to improve it there are several steps to take prior to starting a total fitness program.

1. Have a complete medical examination, especially if you are 30 years of age. (No one over 30 should ever start on any total fitness program without first consulting a physician.)

2. A major part of your medical examination should be an *exercise capacity test* (bicycle ergometer or treadmill test), as shown in the following photograph. It may be necessary to ask your physician for this test.

3. Recondition yourself before starting any regular exercise program. If you have not exercised regularly for a number of years, you must "recondition," as explained later in this chapter, on a warm-up basis to keep from injuring yourself.

4. Have an individual program worked out for you by a competent exercise physiologist or physical education specialist. It is important that you have a *balanced* activity program which improves the condition of your lungs, cardiovascular system, muscular system, and total fitness of your body.

Too often sedentary persons start an exercise program without considering these four points. Many individuals who die while exercising (jogging, running, or swimming) have rushed into a daily exercise program without consulting a physician or a physical educator. The least that can happen to such individuals is that they will become sore or injured because their muscles and joints are not ready for such activity or to carry their body weight while exercising. A warm-up program, of from 15 to 20 minutes at a very slow pace, starts with light, rhythmical calisthenics, accompanied by stretching and deep breathing. This helps to stretch and loosen the muscles and raise the heartbeat and body temperature enough to promote sweating. Following this with slow jogging and walking will help prevent soreness and muscle injury. Such a program should be followed until the body is reconditioned enough to withstand more vigorous exercise. An individual should allow a minimum of six weeks or one month of such reconditioning for each year he has been out of condition.

*Exercise tolerance* is the level at which the body responds favorably to exercise. An individual's exercise tolerance is his ability to perform a series of exercises, participate in a sport, or enjoy a walk without undue fatigue. All exercises should be adapted to an individual's tolerance level. Activities which are too easy or are impossible should not be attempted.

The body has great ability to adapt to stress and increase one's exercise tolerance. Therefore, people who wish to improve their performance and physical condition should continually increase the duration and intensity of their exercises. Extending oneself beyond usual physical effort is called *overloading,* or, more recently, *interval training.* This involves increasing physical stress by:

1. Gradually and progressively increasing the speed of performing an exercise.
2. Gradually increasing the total *resistance,* amount of weight to be lifted.
3. Progressively increasing the total time that a given position, contraction, or resistance can be held or sustained.
4. Maintaining a constant resistance and progressively increasing the total number of *repetitions,* the total number of. times a weight is lifted at one time or exercises are performed.

Fatigue may be delayed by reducing the work load (resistance), by slowing the rhythm, and by breathing regularly and deeply. In using interval training, a person may alternately run and walk to give himself periods to recover from fatigue. The principles of overloading should help increase efficiency and performance. As you master an exercise program, progress to more strenuous exercises. All fitness programs should provide for progression. Generally, increasing the intensity or the tempo of a program is much more important than just increasing the time spent in your daily exercise program.

The intensity of an activity should be as high as possible, based upon the individual's tolerance level. A fitness activity should last from 30 to 60 minutes every other day. Heart rate should be increased to 60 percent of the way from rest to maximal capacity and maintained at this level for 15 minutes at a time for improvement to occur. A pulse rate of 151 beats per minute for a person under 30 years of age and 131 beats per minute for a person over 30 years of age may be taken as showing that the heart is working at 60 percent of capacity. After 30 years of age a person should not let his pulse rate go too much over 131 beats per minute, because of the greater chance of a heart attack or stroke with increasing age. A rule of thumb for maximum heart rate is never let your heartbeat increase above your age (after 30 years of age) subtracted from 200. (For example, $200 - 50 = 150$ beats per minute *maximum.*)

Prior to any total fitness program an individual must be able to possess sufficient muscular strength to support his body weight easily and have muscular endurance needed to complete the activities. Two types of muscular contractions, *isometric contractions* and *isotonic contractions,* have been used to develop muscular strength and endurance.

Isometric contractions are produced by pushing or pulling against an immovable object. The best results appear to be obtained by using maximal contraction of the muscles, held for 5 to 8 seconds and repeated 5 to 10 times daily.

Isotonic contractions are produced when an individual continues to raise, lower, or "move" a moderate load. Within isotonic exercise programs there are many combinations of *repetitions, resistance,* and *sets* (the number of groups of repetitions of a specific exercise, to be done without resting). Muscular strength is best developed when the resistance is relatively high and the number of repetitions is low—such as in a weight training program. Muscular endurance, flexibility, and coordination, or the ability to control muscular movement, are best developed when the resistance is relatively low and the number of repetitions is high. Body weight is considered low resistance and calisthenic-type exercises best serve to produce these isotonic contractions.

Circulatory endurance exercises are activities that stimulate an increase in cardio-respiratory functioning, thus producing results known as "conditioning," "training effect," or "aerobic capacity." Essentially, isotonic activities that are strenuous enough to increase the pulse rate to 151 beats per minute (for anyone under 30 years of age) or 131 beats per minute (for those over 30 years of age) and continued over a period of time (a minimum of 15 minutes) will improve circulatory endurance.

During such periods of sustained activity, heavy demands are made upon the heart, lungs, and circulatory system. Several months of such activity results in:

1. Increased oxygen-carrying ability of the blood due to an increase in the number of red cells and total blood volume.
2. Increase in the number or involvement of more capillaries.
3. Greater cardiac efficiency and output which results in a lower pulse rate and a more rapid return to a normal pulse rate after physical activity.
4. Reduction of body fat by about 8 percent (overall weight loss of about 2 percent).

A woman should take special care to select exercise programs which provide *balance*— ones which develop muscular strength, muscular endurance, and circulatory endurance. Programs should also emphasize exercises which strengthen abdominal and back muscles, improve posture and balance (such as tennis, volleyball). A pregnant woman should consult her obstetrician about any exercise program. If she has been participating in a regular daily exercise program, which includes activities to strengthen abdominal and back muscles, she should be able to carry her child easily, deliver easily and swiftly, and rapidly regain her figure after delivery. Normally, such a woman should be able to continue her regular exercise program, if it isn't too strenuous, up to the sixth month of pregnancy. During the last three months, she may engage only in a simple walking program.

Each time one exercises or participates in a sport, the body should be warmed up by light conditioning and stretching exercises, such as those shown, before heavier, more strenuous activities are attempted. Proper warm-up increases body temperature, stretches ligaments, and slightly increases cardiovascular activity in preparation for exercise. The amount of warm-up necessary will vary between individuals and generally will increase with age.

Just as the body needs warming up it also needs easing off after exercise. This helps return the blood to the heart and get the body temperature back to normal. One should keep moving for several minutes after vigorous activity until the breathing has returned to normal, the stress of the activity has subsided, and the body has cooled.

*Calisthenics.* They provide an opportunity to exercise specific groups of muscles or the whole body. These figures are a series of test exercises which can provide a foundation from which a calisthenic program may be developed. You should not, however, go on to more vigorous calisthenics (progression) until you can complete these tests. There are many basic calisthenic programs designed for the whole body. In the early 1960s the Royal Canadian Air Force originated two programs which have proved to be very successful. The

## Some Sample Exercises

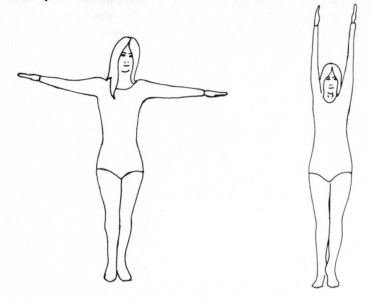

Deep breathing exercise. Stand tall; rise on your tiptoes, and inhale deeply. As you inhale and rise, raise your arms until your hands come together over your head. Hold this extended position for 1 or 2 minutes. Then lower your arms and drop back to the standing position as you exhale.

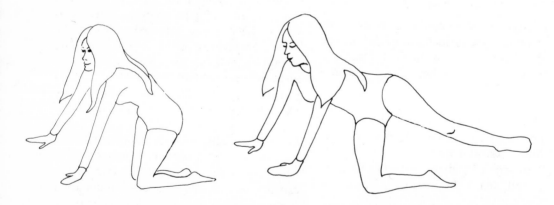

Hydrant exercise. Start on your hands and knees on a soft surface. Keeping your left knee bent, raise it to the side until it is level with your hips. Extend the leg straight out to the side, keeping it at hip level. Then bend the knee back and return it to the floor in the starting position. Repeat with right leg.

## Some Sample Exercises (Continued)

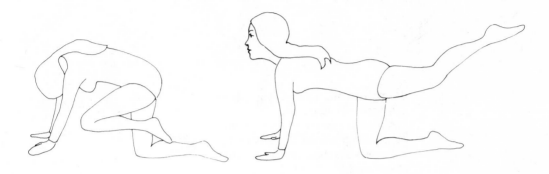

Knee-to-nose kick. Get down on your hands and knees on a soft surface. Bend your head down and bring your left knee as close to your nose as possible. Hold for 2 seconds. Next, extend the left leg back and up, at the same time bringing your head up. Hold for 2 seconds. Repeat action with right leg.

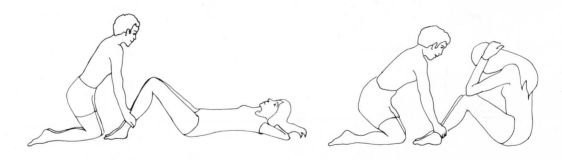

Bent-knee sit-ups. Lie on your back with your hands clasped behind your head, your knees bent, and your feet held down. Keeping your chin on your chest and your back rounded, roll up into a sitting position. When you are in a sitting position, straighten your back, lift your head, and press your elbows back. Hold for 2 seconds, then drop your head, round your back, and roll slowly down to the starting position.

# Some Sample Exercises (Continued)

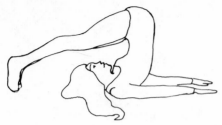

Yoga plow. Lie on your back with your arms beside your body. Lift both legs at once and slowly swing them up and over until your toes touch the floor behind your head. Your shoulders and arms should remain on the floor. Hold, then return to original position.

Arm rotation. Extend your arms straight out from the shoulders, and rotate them so that your hands are tracing circles about 1 foot in diameter. Rotate arms foward, then backward.

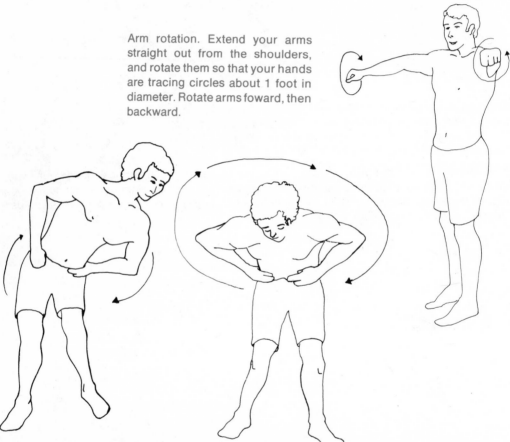

Body rotation. With your legs wide apart and hands on hips, lean forward and bend at the waist. Now rotate your body from the waist in great, slow circles. Lean far enough to the right, rear, left and front so you feel the muscles stretch. Now rotate to the left, rear, right and front.

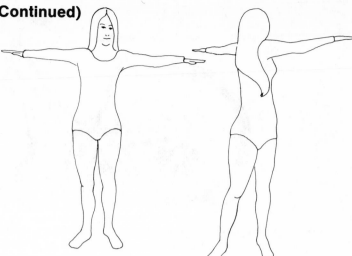

Standing body rotation. Stand with your feet well apart, and extend your arms at shoulder level. Twist your upper body all the way around to the right following it with your eyes; hold for 1 second. Twist back to the left as far as possible; hold for 1 second.

Windmill. Stand with your feet well apart and arms extended at shoulder level. Bending at the waist, touch right hand to left foot, keeping your left arm extended. Return to an upright position and repeat action, this time touching left hand to right foot.

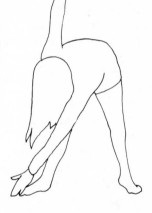

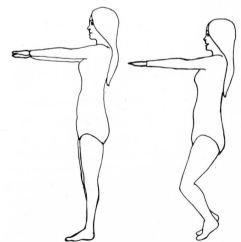

Half knee bends. Stand with your legs together and feet parallel. Rise to the toes for a count of 1 and bring your arms forward for balance. Tighten the muscles of the seat, abdominal area, thighs, and knees. Keeping your back very straight, lower yourself until your knees are only half-way bent. Do not go into a deep knee bend. Rise again to your toes and then lower yourself to your heels.

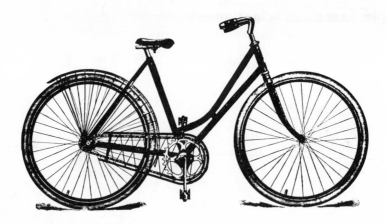

Now more popular than ever, the bicycle provides an enjoyable and healthful form of exercise. It is also an effective and inexpensive means of transportation for the ecology minded.

*5BX* (Five Basic Exercises) *Plan for Physical Fitness* for men and *XBX* (a series to ten exercises) *Plan* for women are simple calisthenic exercises which can be completed in 11 minutes each day. You should either follow an organized program such as this one or have a physical educator design a program especially for you.

*Weight training.* Lifting weights does not develop circulatory endurance. It does increase muscular strength and endurance through application of the principle of *progressive resistance exercises.* In other words, as strength increases, resistance is increased. Progressive resistance occurs when a person moves a given resistance (barbells or weights) a definite number of times (repetitions). Resistance exercise programs may be as extensive or as simple as the individual desires (competitive weight lifting, body building, or weight training); but no program should ever deviate from the principle of resistance progression. A person who simply wants to see how much weight he can lift may injure muscles and joints. Weights should be increased only as strength increases.

For an individual interested in increasing his strength in order to participate socially in medium- and high-energy sports, weight training will help him produce the strength needed for participation. Weight training combines weight lifting with calisthenics. Weight training takes time; a person may not reach the strength needed by some sports for months or years of continuous progression.

If you are interested in weight training, you may want to follow a trial program like one presented in this section. You should remain in it for three months to determine whether there is an improvement in strength. Work out three times a week on alternate days. Start with a weight, such as those recommended in the suggested poundage table, that is light enough to do ten repetitions comfortably. Often, individuals starting their second workout find themselves stiff, sore, and tired, and the weights feel heavier than they did during the first workout. If this happens, reduce the weights by 5 pounds for one week or by 10 pounds for two weeks, or until the weights feel comfortable. Then return to the point at which you began, grad-

| EXERCISE | AVERAGE POUNDS TO START WITH | RANGE OF CHOICE OF STARTING WEIGHT |
|---|---|---|
| Two-arm standing press | 40 | 30–50 |
| Rowing motion | 35 | 25–45 |
| Shrug | 45 | 35–60 |
| Squat | 45 | 35–55 |
| Rise on toes | 45 | 35–60 |
| Lateral bench raise | 7½ each | 5–10 each |
| Barbell curl | 35 | 25–45 |
| Lateral raise (standing) | 7½ each | 5–10 each |
| Side bend | 35 | 30–40 |

ually increasing the weights once a week. Perform the exercises in numbered order, doing one set of ten repetitions at each workout. Rest 2 to 3 minutes between exercises. Increase the poundage whenever the weight in any one exercise feels light. Plan your program in writing; make out a "program card" such as the one shown on p. 214 listing your exercises, poundages, and number of repetitions. Do not engage in any other regularly scheduled exercise program.

1. *Two-arm standing press.* Stand with weight at your shoulder. Now, using the strength of the arm, shoulder, and upper back only, push the weight above your head. Lower to your shoulder and repeat.

2. *Rowing motion.* Stand with your legs apart and your body in front bending position; keep your arms straight down. Without any body motion, pull the weights up until the bar touches your chest. Lower and repeat.

3. *Shrug.* Hold weight while standing with arms straight out. Keeping your elbows straight, pull your shoulders up toward your ears; do not move your whole body. Relax and repeat.

4. *Squat.* Stand erect with weight held across your shoulder. Keeping your heels on floor, bend your knees until your thighs are parallel to the floor. Keep your back as straight as possible. Rise to the standing position and repeat.

5. *Rise on toes.* After performing the squat, do not remove the weight from your shoulders. Rise up on your toes and lower your heels back to the ground. Repeat.

6. *Lateral bench raise.* Lie on your back on a bench. Start with a pair of dumbbells held straight up at arm's length. Breathe in deeply, and slowly lower the weights to your side. Return to starting position and repeat.

7. *Barbell curl.* Hold weight at your thighs with both your hands. Without moving your body except to bend your elbows, raise the weight to the shoulders. Lower and repeat.

8. *Standing lateral raise.* Hold a pair of dumbbells down the sides at arm's length. Keeping your elbows stiff, raise the dumbbells straight out from your shoulders. Bring the pairs together above your head. Lower and repeat.

9. *Neck exercise.* Take a light dumbbell and wrap a towel around the handle. Place it on your forehead, and raise and lower your head up and down.

10. *Side Bend.* Hold a weight in one hand and place the other hand behind your head.

As you hold the weight, bend as far as you can to the side. Return to a standing position and repeat. Do this exercise for both sides.

11. *Sit-up.* Lie on the ground and hook your feet under a barbell. Raise your body to a sitting position. Lower and repeat.

Remember that hard work is required to obtain results and results occur very slowly. The trial program outlined here should begin to increase your strength within three months. If you enjoy this program, ask a physical educator to design a weight training program for you. Weight programs are often part of a college or university curriculum, a men's club, the YMCA, or a gym.

*Walking.* This is the most natural of all forms of exercise. A person may walk at any time with almost no medical risk. Brisk walking for a period of time or distance sufficient to accelerate the pulse strengthens heart, lungs, and leg muscles. Extremely inactive people may obtain endurance effects and begin a regular exercise program by walking; later, however, they must increase their rate of speed to obtain further benefits. Inactive, sedentary men (more than women) over fifty years of age should walk for exercise. They should not try jogging or running because of the increased chance of heart attack after fifty.

*Jogging.* The next step up from walking, jogging is steady, slow running. Jogging may be alternated with breath-catching periods of walking. Jogging became popular in the late 1960s with the publication of *Jogging* by William J. Bowerman, track coach at the University of Oregon, and W. E. Harris, M.D., a heart specialist. This book presents a detailed, complete program for anyone interested in jogging as part of his exercise program. Jogging is pleasant, free, easy, relaxing, and fun. It can be done alone or in groups. Jogging is especially good for main-

taining circulatory endurance. To achieve this purpose, however, college age students must alternate jogging with intervals of hard running after the first month or two of progression.

A jogging program begins with a short period of trotting and walking. As jogging progresses, the jogger covers greater and greater distances. You may want to attempt the following trial program for one month. If you enjoy it, obtain the book *Jogging* or ask a physical educator to design a program for you.

Schedules are planned for Monday, Wednesday, and Friday. You may rearrange them (Tuesday, Thursday, and Saturday) to fit your own schedule if you will remember

## SCHEDULE I AND II

### WEEK 1 (TOTAL DISTANCE: ½ MILE)

| | |
|---|---|
| Monday | Warm up (always do warm-up exercises). Jog 55 yards in 25–30 seconds; then walk 55 yards.ª Repeat four times. |
| Tuesday | Walk for 5–10 minutes after warming up. |
| Wednesday | Jog 110 yards in 55–60 seconds; then walk 110 yards. |
| Thursday | Walk for 5–10 minutes after warming up. |
| Friday | Jog 55 yards in 25–30 seconds; then walk 55 yards. Repeat two times. |
| Saturday and Sunday | Walk for 5–10 minutes after warming up. |

ªYou need only estimate distances; they do not have to be accurate. A track is usually 440 yards in length with each straightaway and turn 110 yards. Using a car odometer or a pedometer, lay out a course beforehand. City blocks are about 220 feet by 500 feet. Telephone poles are about 100 yards apart. Any watch with a second hand is adequate for timing.

| WEEK 2 (TOTAL DISTANCE: ¾ MILE) | WEEK 2 (TOTAL DISTANCE: 1 MILE) |
|---|---|
| **Monday** Jog 55 yards in 25–30 seconds; then walk 55 yards. Repeat four times. Jog 110 yards in 55–60 seconds; then walk 110 yards. Repeat four times. Jog 55 yards in 25–30 seconds; then walk 55 yards. Repeat four times. | **Monday** Jog 55 yards in 25–30 seconds; then walk 55 yards. Repeat four times. Jog 110 yards in 55–60 seconds; then walk 110 yards. Repeat four times. Jog 55 yards in 25–30 seconds; then walk 55 yards. Repeat four times. |
| **Wednesday** Jog 55 yards in 25–30 seconds; then walk 55 yards. Repeat three times. Jog 110 yards in 55–60 seconds; then walk 110 yards. Repeat three times. Jog 55 yards in 25–30 seconds; then walk 55 yards. Repeat three times. | **Wednesday** Jog 55 yards in 25–30 seconds; then walk 55 yards. Repeat three times. Jog 110 yards in 55–60 seconds; then walk 110 yards. Repeat five times. Jog 55 yards in 25–30 seconds; then walk 55 yards. Repeat three times. |
| **Friday** Jog 55 yards in 25–30 seconds; then walk 55 yards. Repeat four times. Jog 110 yards in 55–60 seconds; then walk 110 yards. Repeat two times. Jog 55 yards in 25–30 seconds; then walk 55 yards. Repeat four times. | **Friday** Jog 55 yards in 25–30 seconds; then walk 55 yards. Repeat two times. Jog 110 yards in 55–60 seconds; then walk 110 yards. Repeat six times. Jog 55 yards in 25–30 seconds; then walk 55 yards. Repeat four times. |

the "hard-easy" principle of all exercise programs—exercise one day, rest the next. No exercise program should be followed every day. If you jog for 55 yards and it leaves you gasping and too breathless to talk with your fellow joggers, you are running too fast or you have not worked yourself into the condition to perform in this program. If the 110-yard jogs were not too much for you, try Schedule II in the second week. If the first week's schedule seemed comfortable and you were pleased with your performance, continue on Scheduled I for the second week.

By the fourth week you should know whether jogging is an exercise program that you enjoy. Also, you will know enough about it to use it for change of pace in other exercise programs. Exercise must be fun if an indi-

vidual is to continue on with it. Therefore, expose yourself to a number of different exercise programs. You may maintain your interest in fitness activities by alternating exercises if one set of exercises begins to bore you.

If you decide to continue jogging, refer to William J. Bowerman's book, *Jogging.* It provides schedules for reaching 4 or 5 miles a day. It also contains complete programs and many suggestions for varying your program to maintain interest.

Jogging may be satisfactory to an individual during the initial phase of conditioning. After the goal of 1 mile is achieved, however, running often replaces jogging. Running can provide a challenge as well as good circulatory endurance. The progression of jogging

| Monday | Jog 55 yards in 22–25 seconds, then walk 55 yards. Repeat four times. Jog 220 yards in 90–100 seconds, then walk 220 yards. Repeat one time. Jog 110 yards in 45–50 seconds, then walk 110 yards. Repeat two times. Jog 55 yards in 22–25 seconds, then walk 55 yards. Repeat four times. |
|---|---|
| Wednesday | Jog 55 yards in 22–25 seconds, then walk 55 yards. Repeat two times. Start a slow, steady jog for 2 or 3 minutes. The pace is 55 to 75 seconds for 110 yards. Walk whenever you need to; walk at the end of the 3 minutes. Jog again steadily for 2 or 3 minutes. Jog 55 yards in 22–25 seconds, then walk 55 yards. Repeat two times. |
| Friday | Jog 55 yards in 22–55 seconds, then walk 55 yards. Repeat two times. Jog 110 yards in 45–50 seconds, then walk 110 yards. Repeat one time. Jog your slow, steady pace for 2 or 3 minutes. Then walk until wind is back to normal. Jog 55 yards in 22–25 seconds, then walk 55 yards. Repeat two times. |

and walking outlined previously may be used to progress toward the goal of running 1 mile. Some people, however, may want to increase the time period in the schedule to two months. Before you try to run a mile, be sure that you can jog comfortably for this distance. Don't worry about your time at first. When you can jog for a mile, start pacing yourself and reducing your time. You should pace yourself so that you are running at a constant rate. Avoid any bursts of speed because they greatly reduce your efficiency and cause fatigue. Reduce your time by 10 seconds a week until you can run a mile in 6 minutes. This is considered excellent time for maintenance of circulatory endurance.

When space or weather restricts your ability to run, *running in place* can be a very effective means of maintaining circulatory endurance. The important factors in running in place are the cadence of the step and the duration of the activity. The most comfortable time length seems to be 5 minutes. To

| Monday | Jog 55 yards in 22–30 seconds, then walk 55 yards. Repeat four times. Jog 110 yards in 45–60 seconds, then walk 110 yards. Repeat two times. Jog 220 yards in 90–100 seconds, then walk 220 yards. Repeat two times. Jog 110 yards in 45–60 seconds, then walk 110 yards. Repeat two times. |
|---|---|
| Wednesday | Start to establish a steady, comfortable jogging pace for the required distance. Start at about 110 yards in 56 seconds. This is 4 miles per hour. See how long you can continuously jog with comfort. Walk when too winded to talk with companions. Jog and walk for 1¼ miles. |
| Friday | Jog 110 yards in 45–50 seconds, then walk 110 yards. Repeat four times. Jog steadily 330 yards in 2 minutes 48 seconds. Walk until wind is back to normal. Jog 110 yards in 45–50 seconds, then walk 110 yards. Repeat four times. |

## RUNNING IN PLACE

| NUMBER OF SESSIONS | RUNNING TIME |
|---|---|
| 1–5 | 1 minute |
| 6–10 | 1½ minutes |
| 11–15 | 2 minutes |
| 16–20 | 2½ minutes |
| 21–25 | 3 minutes |
| 26–30 | 3½ minutes |
| 31–35 | 4 minutes |
| 36–40 | 4½ minutes |
| 41–45 | 5 minutes |

reach a 5-minute goal, begin by running in place for 1 minute. Then increase your time by 30-second intervals. Run for five sessions at each time level before progressing to the next interval.

When you can run in place for 5 minutes, you may begin to increase your step cadence.

*Aerobics* is a total fitness program first published in 1968. The originator of the program was Major Kenneth H. Cooper, M.D., of the U.S. Air Force Medical Corps. The key concept in this program is oxygen consumption. Because oxygen cannot be stored in the body, it must be continually replenished. Consequently, the fatigue level of an individual is controlled by the ability of his respiratory and circulatory systems to supply oxygen to the muscles.

Dr. Cooper's aerobics system consists of a point count assigned to different physical activities that increase circulatory endurance. In his physical activities an individual progresses to the point where he can perform activities worth thirty points each week. The number of points represents the amount of the physical activity necessary for maintenance of the cardiorespiratory system.

Points are obtained by performing specific circulatory endurance activities in a specific amount of time. Such activities include run-ning, swimming, bicycling, walking, running in place, and participating in strenuous games of squash, handball, and basketball. Dr. Cooper's book *The New Aerobics* (a revised version of the program published in 1968) provides standards against which a person may gauge his aerobic fitness. For beginners to the program the test of aerobic fitness is the distance that can be covered by running in 12 minutes.

After you have determined your fitness category, refer to *The New Aerobics* and choose the schedule you should follow to obtain thirty aerobic points per week.

*Circuit training.* A *circuit* refers to a number of carefully selected exercises which are arranged and numbered consecutively; the exercises range over a given area. Each numbered exercise within the circuit is called a *station*. An individual moves at his own speed from one station to another until he completes the entire circuit. In most cases he repeats the total circuit more than once (usually three times) and records the total time of performance. This is a convenient and different approach to exercising—one that is physically, physiologically, and psychologically sound.

Circuit training involves two valuable activities; weight training and running. The best physical activity for development of muscular strength and muscular endurance is weight training. One of the most effective methods of developing and maintaining circulatory and respiratory endurance involves running (others are swimming, bicycling, and rope skipping). A well-planned circuit involves both weight training and running. Thus, circuit training increases muscular strength, muscular endurance, and cardiovascular endurance.

The value of circuit training lies in its extreme adaptability to a great variety of situations. A circuit can be designed to fit

227

## DISTANCES COVERED IN 12 MINUTES BY RUNNING

| AGE GROUPS | FITNESS CATEGORIES | AGE GROUPS |
|---|---|---|
| Under 30 years | | 30 to 39 years |
| Less than 1.0 mile | Very poor | Less than 0.95 mile |
| 1.0 to 1.24 miles | Poor | 0.95 to 1.14 miles |
| 1.25 to 1.49 miles | Fair | 1.15 to 1.39 miles |
| 1.50 to 1.74 miles | Good | 1.40 to 1.64 miles |
| 1.75 miles and over | Excellent | 1.65 miles and over |
| 40 to 49 years | | Over 50 years |
| Less than 0.85 mile | Very poor | Less than 0.80 mile |
| 0.85 to 1.04 miles | Poor | 0.80 to 0.99 miles |
| 1.05 to 1.29 miles | Fair | 1.00 to 1.24 miles |
| 1.30 to 1.54 miles | Good | 1.25 to 1.49 miles |
| 1.55 miles and over | Excellent | 1.50 miles and over |

any individual, group, area, or condition (it is even adaptable to medical rehabilitation). Circuit training enables an individual or a group of people to progress through a series of exercises and check the progress against a clock.

Circuit training utilizes three variables: load, repetitions, and time. Weight training exercises provide the load, and sets provide the repetitions. Interval running, engaged in between stations, provides repetitions and time.

On a circuit, progression is produced by decreasing the time required to complete one circuit, increasing the work load (weight or sets), or a combination of both. Progression is assured because an individual works at his present capacity and can progress as his capacity increases. Circuit training provides a series of progressive time goals which are achieved step by step. This time factor provides built-in motivation; it encourages a person to push himself to do better. The circuit layout in which a person moves from one station to another offers variety; this is appealing to most people.

The progressions used in weight training may be used in circuit training. Loads can be increased by progressively increasing the size of the weights to be lifted. In circuit training it is not necessary to change weights as frequently as it is in weight training because weight training is only one of the variables involved in the program.

Calisthenic exercises may be used in a circuit. When this is done, the load is a person's own body weight. The load is increased by modifying the exercise. For example, the following changes will increase the work load in a push-up: standard push-up; push-up, pushing hands off the floor; push-up, pushing off the floor and clapping hands; pushing up, pushing off the floor and slapping the chest. Such modifications make calisthenic exercises very useful in circuit training. Load can also be increased by increasing the number of repetitions, or sets, at each station or by increasing the number of times the circuit is run. Laps may be added; in that case, a person runs the length of the circuit without performing at the stations. Another way to increase the load is to decrease the time needed to perform a circuit. In maintaining good progression the most important factor is to increase the work load gradually and at a rate that can be handled with ease and safety.

An individual should know his goals before beginning any exercise program. You should be able to say what purpose you want the program to serve. In planning a circuit, remember that your circuit must be based on your personal goals. Choose exercises that are strenuous. Each exercise should contribute toward progression by increasing both work load and work rate. This automatically eliminates the very light warm-up exercises which should be performed before the circuit is run. Also, do not include "duck waddle," deep knee bends, or any other exercise which can cause joint, ligament, or muscle damage if done too fast. Perform each exercise the same way every time so that you are able to observe and evaluate your improvement.

Select exercises that balance other exercises so that all groups of muscles receive proper exercise. Improper balance of strength between antagonistic muscle groups can produce permanent body damage. To avoid improper balance, classify the muscle groups into three categories: the arm, neck, and shoulder group; the abdomen, back and chest group; and the buttock, hip, and leg group. When arranging your stations, avoid consecutive placement of exercises that involve similar muscle groups. For example, both arm curls and chin-ups involve the arm, neck, and shoulder muscle group. If you include both these exercises in a circuit, separate them. A circuit designed for general body conditioning should include exercises which involve all three of the muscle groups.

The amount of time you have available for performing a circuit is a factor in determining both the difficulty of exercises and the number of stations to be included in the circuit. The spacing and the arrangement of the stations are determined by the amount of space you have available and by the kinds of exercises you want to emphasize. If your basic purpose is general body conditioning (an emphasis on cardiovascular endurance), you should choose a large area for your circuit, allowing for distances between stations for running and movement. There should always be enough room for exercise which is strenuous, yet free-flowing and uninterrupted. Where there is available space and facilities, several circuits (or variations of one circuit) may be organized, utilizing the same area or equipment.

The *recommended circuit* is useful for general body conditioning. However, a person with a little experience, skill, and understanding may design circuits to meet the fitness needs of nearly any vigorous sport or activity.

*Rope skipping.* This is an excellent cardiovascular exercise. A person who jumps steadily for 5 minutes is getting a good workout. A 10-minute daily program of rope skipping improves and maintains cardiovascular endurance as well as a 30-minute program of jogging. Rope skipping may be either a program in itself or a bad-weather substitute for a jogging, running program.

Obtain a piece of rope which is anywhere from 6 to 9 feet long. An easy way to determine the correct length for you is to make the length of the rope two times the distance from your arm pit to the ground, or a length which is comfortable. Tape the ends so they will not fray.

Variations within a rope skipping program can add interest and incentive. They may also provide progression. (Progression may also be achieved by performing a specific number of jumps in a certain amount of time.) The normal skipping style may be modified by jumping on one foot, alternating feet, or jumping with both feet together. Running

## RECOMMENDED CIRCUIT

| EXERCISES (IN THE ORDER TO BE DONE) | REPETITIONS | | | WEIGHT IN POUNDS |
|---|---|---|---|---|
| | 1 | 2 | 3 | |
| Bench press | 8 | 10 | 12 | 60 |
| Side bends | 7 | 9 | 11 | |
| Chins | 1 | 3 | 5 | |
| Back extension | 7 | 9 | 12 | 10 |
| Two-arm curl | 8 | 10 | 12 | 25 |
| Squat | 10 | 13 | 16 | |
| Bent-leg sit-ups | 15 | 20 | 25 | |
| Three-quarter squat | 9 | 12 | 15 | 25 |
| Lateral raise | 8 | 10 | 12 | 7½ |
| Shuttle run | (5–10 yards) | | | |

NOTE: This is a short 10-minute circuit which utilizes some of the exercises discussed in the *calisthenics* section. Follow the recommendations listed with each exercise for progression. Determine your own time limit by judging how well you perform the circuit when you first try it.

with skipping increases timing and coordination. Jumping backward is a simple maneuver in which various foot styles can be used. Make some forward-to-backward changes and then some backward-to-forward changes. This is difficult because you must jump an extra time as the turn is completed.

A double jump is challenging. This is done by spinning the rope faster and jumping a little higher. When you have increased your skill, shorten the rope slightly by winding it within the hand, and stay in the air longer by bending the knees and keeping them high. You may achieve a triple jump. Double and triple jumps have an effect similar to that caused by sprints in running; they rapidly increase the heart rate.

A front cross may be achieved by crossing the arms when the rope starts downward. This makes a loop through which you may jump. On completion of the jump, the arms are uncrossed and the next jump is made in the normal manner. If you have difficulty performing a front cross, lengthen the rope slightly and either lower the hands as the arms cross or cross the arms far enough to bring the elbows together. These changes will give you a wider loop to jump through. A back cross may be done by performing a regular back jump with arms crossed in front of the body (cross your arms so your elbows touch each other).

Make your own modifications. Try jumps such as a double jump with a front cross, or try to run while you change jumping forms. Again, make some forward-to-backward changes and then some backward-to-forward changes.

### Sports

Sports and other recreational activities may serve as conditioning programs. However, some individual and dual sports require such small amounts of physical activity that they are not adequate for a fitness program. Golf is such a sport. It has many psychological and social values but little physical value. The main energy expenditure in golf comes from walking. This walking is usually not vigorous enough to elevate the pulse significantly.

If a sport is to supply the requirements

of a physical fitness program, it must be vigorous. Also, a person should participate in it for at least three sessions a week. Each session should last for a minimum of 30 minutes. Ideally, a person who is using a sport as the basis of a fitness program should participate in the sport for 60 minutes every day.

When you participate in a sport, you should remember that your expenditure of energy depends on several factors:

1. *The number of participants.* In calisthenics, weight training, and running, you control the expenditure of energy. In dual sports, however, you must consider the number of participants. Handball may be least demanding in a game of doubles, more demanding in a game of singles, and most demanding in a game involving three people ("cutthroat").
2. *The skill of the participants.* Generally, a high level of skill is reflected in greater efficiency. Thus a skilled person can participate at a lower energy cost. As your skill develops, you should either increase the amount of time you devote to a sport or pit yourself against people who are more skillful than you are.
3. *The duration.* The longer the duration of an activity, the greater is the energy expenditure. Each participant should be vigorously active for 30 to 40 minutes; in a 60-minute game, then, you should be moving one-half to two-thirds of the time.
4. *The speed of the necessary physical movements.* Sports which require occasional bursts of speed are more demanding and require a greater expenditure of energy than are sports in which the participants can establish a steady pace. You should participate in such sports only after you feel your physical condition is adequate.

In choosing sports, remember the value of developing and maintaining circulatory endurance. Sports which improve circulatory endurance include individual activities such as swimming, scuba diving, snorkeling, hiking, running, and bicycling; dual activities such as wrestling, and judo; and court games such as badminton, handball, squash, tennis, and volleyball.

Dual sports and court games require at least two participants. Court games further require a court. These requirements may limit your opportunities to engage in exercise. Individual activities usually offer more opportunities for participation.

Some sports are much more beneficial to fitness than are others. Golf is the least beneficial. It is followed, in increasing benefit, by court games, dual sports, individual sports, weight training, jogging, and running.

### Use of Leisure Time

The automobile, television, and liquor are unfortunate distractions we turn to as we leave our hectic work pace and go to leisure activities. Abolition of these, however, would not cause us to become more involved in programs of physical conditioning. Whether one exercises regularly or changes his life style to be compatible with the environment depends on motivation. People must understand how to condition themselves and what certain activities do for total fitness to produce the motivation needed to exercise.

Psychological as well as physiological limits increase with exercise, making one feel better, be more decisive, and have a more positive and confident outlook on life. It enables one to actively participate in many activities that are part of a natural life-style.

Leisure time is well spent pursuing nonpowered, nonspectator activites that reacquaint one with the environment. One should seek out activities that provide healthful exercise, are pleasurable, and cost much less than any form of motorized recreational vehicles, or seats at a spectator sport.

# 11
# Your Investment in Good Health

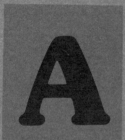special report by *Business Week* (January 1970) stated that "a lot of Americans would rather die than get seriously sick. For millions, going to the hospital means going broke or close to it. For many more, good medical care is nonexistent." Underlying the cost of disease to this country is the fact that the total health bill for America now stands at over 75 billion dollars a year. This represents 7.4 percent of our gross national product (a greater proportion than in any other country). It amounts to almost 300 dollars per person per year for medical goods. The Consumer Price Index shows that, over the years, health-care costs increase faster than any other major personal expense. From the base period of 1957–59 to 1971, medical costs rose over 65 percent.

Unfortunately, even with this great expenditure of money, the United States has been falling behind other nations in the major standards of health care. For example, in infant mortality we ranked fourteenth at the end of the 1960s, by 1972 we had dropped to fifteenth. As the infant mortality table shows, Sweden ranks first and spends only 5 percent of her gross national product on health services. They are also first in life expectancy.

According to the National Health Survey by the United States Department of Health, Education, and Welfare in 1971, Americans experience about 3 billion days of restricted activity annually. This amounts to about 16 days per year of restricted activity per every man, woman, and child in the country. This total includes over 424 million lost workdays and over 220 million days of school absenteeism per year.

Americans suffer over 250 million cases of acute illnesses each year. Included in these statistics are only those conditions for which a doctor was consulted or conditions which caused a person to restrict his normal activities for at least one day. Nearly 220 million of these cases are respiratory infections (such as the common cold); 48 million of all acute illnesses are nonrespiratory or parasitic diseases (measles, hepatitis, mumps, etc.); 23 million are acute digestive conditions; 59 million are due to injuries; and over 23 million are due to chronic diseases or impairments that limit activity.

## MAJOR CAUSES OF DEATH
## IN THE UNITED STATES

The effects of disease have changed significantly during the past 70 years, as the table on the major causes of death shows.

The causes of death differ for different age groups. Accidents top the list from childhood through age 45. Below we list the five leading causes of death in order of frequency for different age groups.

1. *Infant mortality (under 1 year of age).* (1) premature birth, (2) postnatal asphyxia, (3) congenital malformations, (4) other diseases of early infancy, and (5) pneumonia and influenza.

2. *Preschool children (ages 1 through 4).* (1) accidents, (2) influenza and pneumonia, (3) congenital malformations, (4) cancers, and (5) meningitis.

3. *Elementary and junior high school students (ages 5 through 14).* (1) accidents, (2) cancers, (3) congenital deformities, (4) influenza and pneumonia, and (5) heart diseases.

4. *Senior high school and college-age persons (ages 15 through 24).* (1) accidents, (2) cancers, (3) homicide, (4) suicide, and (5) heart diseases.

5. *Young adults and parents (ages 25 through 44).* (1) accidents, (2) heart diseases, (3) cancers, (4) suicide, and (5) homicide.

## INFANT MORTALITY PER COUNTRY

| RANK | COUNTRY | INFANT MORTALITY PER 1000 BIRTHS[a] |
|------|---------|------------------------------------|
| 1 | Sweden | 11.1 |
| 2 | Finland | 11.3 |
| 3 | Netherlands | 11.4 |
| 4 | Norway | 12.7 |
| 5 | Japan | 13.0 |
| 6 | Iceland | 13.2 |
| 7 | France | 13.3 |
| 8 | Denmark | 14.2 |
| 9 | Switzerland | 14.4 |
| 10 | New Zealand | 16.5 |
| 11 | Australia | 17.3 |
| 12 | Canada | 17.6 |
| 13 | Germany (East) | 17.7 |
| 14 | United Kingdom | 18.0 |
| 15 | United States | 18.5 |
| 16 | Hong Kong | 19.0 |
| 17 | Ireland | 19.6 |
| 18 | Belgium | 19.8 |
| 19 | Singapore | 21.0 |
| 20 | China (People's Republic of) | Not available |

SOURCE: *1973 World Population Data Sheet,* Population Reference Bureau, Washington, D.C., 1973.
[a]Annual deaths to infants under one year of age per 1000 live births.

## LIFE EXPECTANCY PER COUNTRY

| RANK | COUNTRY | LIFE EXPECTANCY AT BIRTH (IN YEARS) | |
|------|---------|:---:|:---:|
| | | F | M |
| 1 | Sweden | 77 | 72 |
| 2 | Netherlands | 77 | 71 |
| 3 | Norway | 77 | 71 |
| 4 | Iceland | 76 | 71 |
| 5 | Denmark | 76 | 71 |
| 6 | France | 76 | 69 |
| 7 | Canada | 75 | 69 |
| 8 | United States | 75 | 67 |
| 9 | Germany (East) | 74 | 69 |
| 10 | Japan | 74 | 69 |
| 11 | Germany (West) | 74 | 68 |
| 12 | Switzerland | 74 | 69 |
| 13 | Australia | 74 | 68 |
| 14 | Belgium | 74 | 68 |
| 15 | New Zealand | 74 | 68 |
| 16 | United Kingdom | 74 | 68 |
| 17 | Austria | 74 | 67 |
| 18 | Czechoslovakia | 74 | 67 |
| 19 | USSR | 74 | 65 |
| 20 | Israel | 73 | 70 |
| 21 | Bulgaria | 73 | 69 |
| 22 | Italy | 73 | 68 |
| 23 | Ireland | 72 | 68 |
| 24 | Spain | 72 | 67 |
| 25 | Hungary | 72 | 62 |

SOURCE: *1973 World Population Data Sheet*, Population Reference Bureau, Washington, D.C., 1973.

6. *Middle-aged persons (ages 45 through 64).* (1) heart diseases, (2) cancers, (3) stroke, (4) accidents, and (5) cirrhosis of the liver.

7. *The elderly (ages 65 and over).* (1) heart diseases, (2) cancers, (3) stroke, (4) influenza and pneumonia, and (5) hardening of the arteries.

Leading the major disease killers are heart diseases and cancers. Over 50 percent of all deaths in the United States are due to the effects of the cardiovascular diseases (heart, cerebral hemorrhage, and other vascular lesions); 16 percent are due to cancers and other malignant growths; and 6 percent are due to accidents. (In 1900, these causes were responsible for all deaths in the United States in this proportion: cardiovascular diseases, 14 percent; cancers and other malignant growths, 4 percent; and accidents, 4 percent.) It is further estimated that one adult in four can anticipate developing a fatal heart ailment during his life. Likewise, one in every four adults can expect to suffer from cancer. Among these victims, two out of every three (67 percent) will die from the effects of the disease.

## THE HIGH COST
## OF MEDICAL CARE

The American public spends an average of 128 percent more in health care now than 10 years ago. In terms of kinds of care, the total percentage increase breaks down this way: hospital care, up 160 percent; physician's services, up 129 percent; medicines and appliances, up 104 percent; and all other medical care, up 143 percent. For the same period, the amount spent for all personal items (including health care) increased 65 percent.

There is no question but that much of this higher cost represents proportionately better care. A study from Massachusetts General Hospital is a case in point. It is a comparison of patients coming into the hospital with heart attacks in terms of cost per patient and fatalities for years 1920, 1940, and 1970:

| YEAR | PATIENTS | FATALITIES | COST PER PATIENT |
|------|----------|------------|------------------|
| 1920 | 100 | 40 | $200 |
| 1940 | 100 | 30 | $400–600 |
| 1970 | 100 | 16 | $3500 |

In spite of past increases in medical costs, all indications are that if medical services are to be improved to any extent, the costs will go higher. Medical authorities predict that medical advances can be measured in terms of more expense, and that by the end of the 1970s, personal medical expenses will take no less than 8 percent of the gross national product. Some are even suggesting that by 1980 hospital costs may rise to at least 1000 dollars per day per bed. Already costs of 100 dollars per day per bed are common, with intensive care beds now averaging about 300 to 500 dollars per day.

Why the great increase in medical costs? Answers are multiple. Costs per square foot on new construction have soared; hospital employee salaries and benefits are up (63 percent of the hospital budget goes into salaries and benefits); new equipment becomes obsolete before it is worn out. It is estimated that every year about half of the major equipment in a hospital becomes obsolete. Hospitals are expected to be open and available 24 hours a day, 365 days a year, emergencies or not. A high-quality acute-care hospital hires an average of six employees for every patient.

There is public apathy about hospital costs; people are confident that, unreasonable cost or not, their health insurance will bail them out (often unaware their insurance will pay only one-fourth to one-third of most hospital bills). Welfare payments are rarely enough to pay the true cost of public care. To make ends meet, hospitals overcharge private patients (and their insurance companies). Some private insurance policies provide coverage only if the patient is admitted to the hospital overnight (although overnight admission may not be required for the emergency). People abuse their health insurance—figuring the care is coming to them, forgetting that each such unnecessary use helps boost the cost of health insurance. People go to the hospital when the same care might be provided just as well and with much less cost in a physician's office or clinic.

Although disturbing, there is evidence that the medical profession (at least the AMA) has been opposed to both better and cheaper medical care. Many physicians are guilty of greater concern over maintaining their high income than providing medical service their patients can afford. Medical care costs everyone. It should be used discreetly and only at those times it is required.

## PAYING MEDICAL BILLS

The traditional method of financing medical costs has been for each family to pay off their medical bills as they arise, always hoping that there is sufficient money available in the bank to cover major episodes. For some families this amounted to a "pay-as-you-go" method, hoping the money for the week held out; for others it was a matter of budgeting, reserving money each month for medical costs. Were all medical expenses "average," it wouldn't be too difficult for a family to budget money each month for such a purpose, just like a budget for other household expenses. But medical expenses are often erratic, with times of great expense separated by times of lesser expense, so budgeting becomes almost impossible. All of us know of some families that seem to be hit repeatedly by heavy medical expenses which go way beyond the average. As a result of the erratic unpredictable nature of medical costs for a family, there has been a greatly increasing trend toward collective financing of medical expenses.

It is the boast of the health insurance field that over 89 percent of our population holds some form of health insurance. Studies show that in the long run medical care tends to be a little cheaper in the form of a prepaid plan. In this manner people are protected somewhat against sudden large medical expenses by being forced systematically to lay away funds.

The current methods of collective financing of medical costs fall into one of two basic categories—public (tax-supported) and private (voluntary) health insurance.

### Public Medical Care

*Care of the Poor.* Most of the first organized medical programs were those for the poor.

In the mid-1930s, Congress passed the Federal Social Security Act. Among other things, this act provided medical services for several categories of poor people: the elderly, the blind, and dependent children. In January 1966 *Medicaid* (Title 19 of the Social Security Act) gave funds to states to expand their public assistance programs to persons, regardless of age, whose incomes are insufficient to pay for health care. *Medicaid* greatly increased medical care for the poor.

According to the Bureau of the Census, over 13.7 percent of all Americans live *below* the poverty line. By federal definition, the "poor are those who are not now maintaining a decent standard of living—those whose basic needs exceed their means to satisfy them."

While 68 percent of the poor are white, 32 percent are nonwhite. But the number of poor whites and nonwhites to their total populations is another picture. Over 9 percent of *all* whites are poor, but over 32 percent of *all* nonwhites are poor.

A part of the basic needs of people is adequate medical care. Those poor living in urban areas generally have greater access to such services than rural poor. Significantly, slightly over one-half of all poor families live in metropolitan areas, and slightly less than one-half in nonmetropolitan areas. Of all poor families in the country, almost one-half live in the South.

Although pressures on health facilities exist everywhere, they tend to be greater for the rural poor. They include the presence of a hospital or clinic, the lack of physicians in the rural places, transportation—general accessibility. Also important is the difference in level of welfare provisions in the various states. Southern states tend to be lower in their state health care provisions than other regions of the United States.

*Medicare.* Medicare is a program of health

insurance under Social Security which helps the elderly pay for medical care. It includes hospital insurance, which covers most inpatient care, and medical insurance, which is designed to cover most physicians' fees. The plan is voluntary and people must sign up for it in order to be eligible. The monthly premiums are shared equally by those who sign and by the federal government.

*Military Coverage.* A military veteran may receive care for any condition inflicted or activated during his service. The veteran will be taken care of at government expense through the Veterans' Administration hospitals. Wives and children of military personnel who are on active duty or who are retired from the service are eligible for the Aid to Military Dependents Program. Children are covered until they are 18 years of age.

*Special Diseases.* There are tax-supported medical programs for certain noncommunicable diseases that are of particular social concern. State hospitals for the mentally ill and neurologically disabled have been provided for almost 100 years. Clinics and hospitals for drug problems are on the increase both by the federal government and within individual states.

*Communicable Diseases.* Communicable diseases are of high public concern. Venereal diseases (syphilis and gonorrhea) are of epidemic proportions in this country. Public medical care centers, often city or county, provide both public education, diagnosis, and treatment. There is a public hospital for lepers at Carville, Louisiana. In some of the larger cities there are special hospitals for other infectious diseases.

*General Hospital Care.* Most counties and larger cities in the country provide a county or general hospital for their citizens. Although these hospitals usually provide gen-

eral medical care, they tend to be strongly oriented to the care of poor persons or those with chronic illnesses.

*County or Local Health Departments.* Virtually every county government in the United States supports some kind of county health department. Services provided vary from county to county, but usually include some or all of the following: (1) communicable disease control, (2) tuberculosis control, (3) venereal disease control, (4) local community health offices, (5) public health nursing services, (6) public health social services, (7) public health nutrition services, (8) child and maternal health consultations, (9) public health dentistry, (10) sanitation inspection and supervision, (11) maintenance of vital records, (12) public health education, (13) air pollution control, and (14) school and industrial health services.

Eligibility for services from county health departments and general hospitals varies from place to place and depends on the restrictions thought necessary by the local agency.

### Private Health Insurance Programs

Private health plans, like public facilities, operate on the basis of the advantages of collective cost and risk sharing. Unlike the public insurance plans, the costs of private health coverage are maintained solely by the beneficiaries. The major advantage of private health insurance at the present time is that it does permit the insured to select specific provisions and types of coverage that might be unavailable through public plans. Another advantage of private health insurance coverage is that it encourages the insured to take better care of himself—to see a physician or have necessary diagnostic work done, knowing that he is already allotted a specific amount of money for this purpose. With Medicare in

237

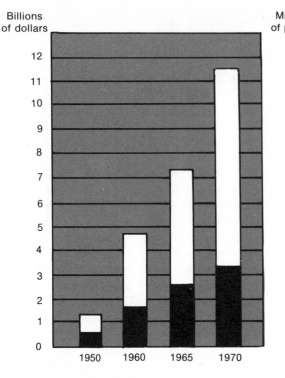

Billions of dollars

Health insurance premiums of insurance companies by type of policy. Group policies, white; individual policies, shaded. Source: *1971–72 Source Book of Health Insurance Data,* Health Insurance Institute, New York, 1973.

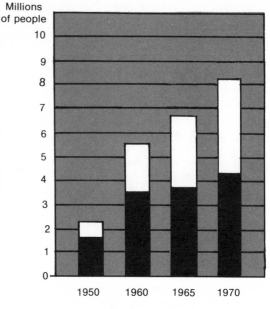

Millions of people

Number of persons with health insurance by type of insurer. Group policies, white; individual policies, shaded. Source: *1971–72 Source Book of Health Insurance Data,* Health Insurance Institute, New York, 1973.

effect, most health care policies now terminate at age 65, or when the insured individuals become eligible for Medicare.

### Kinds of Subscriptions

The most favorable premium rates (the cost of insurance) have been gained through the formation of groups of subscribers. A group is composed of a number of individuals or families who subscribe to a similar insurance plan. Group plans are generally available only through an employer, educational institution, or fraternal organization. Typically, only one type of plan is available to the group, with a similar premium charge to each

subscriber within the group who holds a similar contract. (There may be some small differences in premium rate depending on the size of the family.) It generally costs more for an unaffiliated individual to buy insurance of the same type and coverage, or else his policy might provide fewer benefits. The graph on health insurance premiums demonstrates the differences in cost. As shown in the second graph, the majority of people covered by health insurance today belong to group plans.

### Types of Benefits

In terms of benefits (the services upon which

the insurance plan makes payment), there are two general plans: *service* and *cash indemnity* plans. Service plans are generally in the form of contracts between the policyholder and the hospital or physician. The hospital agrees to provide certain services to anyone who is a policyholder under such a plan and who can present a policy identification card. The hospital or physician then agrees to accept the fees allowed under the plan as full or near-full payment for the care that is given. After the hospital (or physician) has completed its service, its office fills out a claim form and sends it to the insurance company. Reimbursement is then made directly to the hospital or physician according to the provisions of the policy.

Cash indemnity plans pay benefits in the form of cash to the policyholder. He is reimbursed directly for the medical costs he has incurred or paid. The patient is generally required to present either a physician's or hospital's statement showing the exact amount due or a receipt confirming payment already made.

### Types of Insurers

There are no two health insurance plans that are exactly alike. There are several hundred different health insurance companies in the country today. Their plans, however, tend to fall into several main categories.

*Blue Cross.* Blue Cross is a nonprofit operation with over 68 million members. This represents about 34 percent of the population, and 68 percent of all Blue Cross members belong to a group plan. Through seventy-five plans in the United States, Blue Cross insures members against costs of hospital care, physicians' services, drugs, and laboratory costs. Even though all plans bear the name Blue Cross, each is sold exclusively within a given geographical area, and is gov-

erned independently by a local board made up of community, hospital, and medical leaders.

Types of coverage range from several weeks to a full year of hospital service. The most widely sold policies cover the partial or complete cost of 30 days of hospital care. Other plans also cover services of physicians, anesthetists, x-ray diagnosis and therapy, drugs, and laboratory tests. Most plans also now include extended coverage—benefits payable in the event of a long period of illness. Claims may be paid directly to the contracting hospital or physician or may be mailed to the subscriber who, in turn, endorses the check and mails it to the hospital or physician.

*Blue Shield.* Set up along the same general lines as Blue Cross, Blue Shield plans claim over 60 million subscribers through seventy-two different plans. Organized in 1946 and endorsed by the American Hospital Association, Blue Shield plans are designed to provide prepaid coverage for physicians' services and at the same time help to assure the collection of physicians' fees. In some areas, such as Southern California, Blue Shield prepays both physician and hospital costs. Blue Shield is available in most states.

*Commercial.* Most of the health insurance plans available are being written by commercial insurance companies. Although their coverage is similar to Blue Cross and Blue Shield, the approach of the commercial companies is often quite different. Their plans tend to be of the cash indemnity type or are a combination of service-cash indemnity. The commercial health insurance companies in no way engage in setting up contracts with hospitals or physicians and thus do not seek to control the quality of medical services rendered to their policyholders. A wide variety of plans are available, even from one given company, thus a family can select a policy which is tailor-made to its needs.

Commercial companies have helped in the development of certain other forms of health insurance such as the following:

1. *Major medical.* Just as the name implies, these plans are set up to give large amounts of coverage for major expenses. They are not designed or intended to pay for smaller medical expenses which the insured individual can easily pay out of his own pocket or which can be covered by the regular type of health insurance plan. Accordingly, major medical plans usually contain a deductible clause, excluding payments on medical expenses under 100 dollars for a given period; this figure can range as high as 500 dollars. The policyholder is expected to pay this amount himself. Beyond this, some policies provide coverage for 75 to 80 percent of the costs above the deductible amount; the policyholder agrees to pay the remainder.

2. *Comprehensive plans.* Contracts of this type are designed to provide regular (basic) medical care *plus* major medical coverage. They are designed to combine the best features of the other types of policies. They can be purchased either on a group or individual basis. Some Blue Cross plans now offer comprehensive coverage.

3. *Income (disability) insurance.* A person may not realize his need for income protection until his income ceases. Many people look upon accident and serious illness as things that happen to "other people."

Most income contracts are written on a scheduled basis. The insured elects to take such coverages as he believes will benefit him. He can tailor his contract to his particular needs and his ability to pay. His total premium will be determined by the kinds and amounts of coverages he takes, his occupation, age, and sex. Accident coverage may include total disability, loss of life, limb, or sight, and blanket medical expense. Sickness coverage may include total disability, hospital room and board, surgical operation, in-hospital physician, and nurse expense.

The most important part of the contract is the provision for total or partial disability. Most companies use a 30-, 60-, or 90-day clause requiring that disability commence within this time period following the accident.

It is important that a person look carefully at the insuring clause in accident policies, because they are not uniform. Income benefits for sicknesses are not sold separately from accident income protection. It is likely that both will be issued in the same contract; a separate contract covering accidents usually is drawn up only for those who specifically request such a policy.

4. Health insurance companies continue to develop new types of insurance to meet the changing needs of the American public. Health insurance explorations have begun in such areas as vision insurance, group travel insurance, and special risk insurance. Also, experiments are underway in developing new ways to control health costs, delivery of services, and use of facilities to decrease health costs to the individual.

*Independents.* There are, in addition, several hundred smaller local plans. They have been organized by labor unions, corporate managements, physicians, and laymen. They tend to be unique in that most of them provide their own salaried physicians, their own clinics, and sometimes their own hospitals. They go under such names as the Health Insurance Plan of Greater New York, the Kaiser Foundation Health Plan, and the Community Health Association of Detroit. Patients are expected to use the staff physician who is provided, and not bring a nonstaff physician into the clinic or hospital. Plans lacking their own hospitals have agreements with specific hospitals to provide services.

Although the independents are generally local, it does not mean they are small. Many are large organizations. New York, California and other states have a number of such plans.

### Purchasing Health Insurance

The novice can easily be totally confused by his first attempt at purchasing health, hospital, surgical, or accident insurance. It is literally a concern of life and death and should not become a battle of wits between the buyer and seller. In purchasing health insurance the buyer must be careful not to end up with a policy that does not give him the coverage he needs, or makes him pay for additional provisions he does not need.

Generally, a person should begin the purchase of health insurance by first determining (1) the type of health care expenses he desires to be protected against, and (2) the extent (proportion) to which he desires these expenses insured. One should have a clear picture of the regular, periodic payments he is obligated to pay—such as auto loans, rent or loan payments on a house, educational fees, furniture payments, and so on. A family must be sure that the expected health insurance premiums can be added to the budget and be paid. It is also wise to remember that the family with more financial obligations has as much, if not more, need for health insurance than the family with fewer financial obligations. If a financially obligated person were to encounter huge unexpected medical bills and not be able to keep up payments on his car, refrigerator, or house, these could be taken away from him through repossession or foreclosure. Therefore, the financially obligated person particularly needs adequate health insurance. It must not be something a person plans to buy when all the rest of his bills have been paid.

Observing these points should enable a person to make a wise selection of health insurance. In certain types of employment the health insurance is automatically provided as a fringe benefit, and an employee does not have the problem of selection.

Here are some questions that should be asked of the insuring company:

1. Is the company or prepayment plan licensed to do business in your state?
2. What is the organization's reputation for fulfilling its obligations to its policyholders?
3. Is there a claims payment office located either in the state or otherwise reasonably near?
4. Does the company's agent have a good reputation in the community?

There are three classes of medical expenses—hospital costs, physicians' fees, and paramedical costs (laboratory, x-ray, nursing, physical therapy, and pharmaceuticals). The first two lend themselves more readily to the provisions of health insurance. A prospective buyer of health insurance should be aware of the prevailing costs for these services in his community and measure these costs against the benefits offered by specific policies.

There is a wide range of contract provisions which limit the insuring companies' liability and which frequently are discovered only too late by the subscriber. Among these are:

1. *Insuring clause.* Be sure the coverage includes the types of benefits you require.

2. *Exclusions or conditions not covered.* Most policies exclude certain types of costs including (1) cosmetic or plastic surgery; (2) elective surgery (operations performed at the patient's convenience); (3) occupational illnesses and accidents covered by public insurance programs, such as Workmen's Compensation; (4) conditions resulting

from acts of war and riot; (5) pre-existing illnesses; and (6) dental work.

3. *Waiting periods.* There is usually a time interval between the issuing of a contract and the date certain benefits are payable. Examples of such benefits might be maternity, elective surgery, or pre-existing illness.

4. *Benefit reductions.* Benefits might be reduced if services are performed in a nonparticipating hospital or by a nonparticipating physician.

5. *Persons covered.* Usually policies include coverage for spouses and unmarried dependent children. These names must be specified in the policy.

6. *Age limits.* Some policies specify maximum and minimum age limits; most policies will cover a dependent child only up to a stated age.

7. *Cancellation and renewal provisions.* Many policies are cancelable by the insuring company; some policies state that the company can elect not to renew the policy at any premium-due date.

8. *Limited choice of a physician or hospital.* All limits should be explicitly understood, such as the restrictions on selection of a physician and the coverage of a nonparticipating physician's costs.

Your own physician's advice in the selection of a health insurance plan can be very useful. He can advise you of the record of the specific company in honoring its commitments.

It is wise to periodically review your health insurance policy. Changes in income, marital status, obligation to dependent children, and employment might substantially affect your policy and your needs for certain types of coverage. It is particularly important to be aware of employee plans which are carried by the employer; a change of job might terminate your coverage.

Regardless of how a family provides for its medical care, it is obvious that some form of payment planning is essential. Most people are directly dependent on a continual income, and financial protection against physical disability is a most important asset. Not only must a family protect its ability to earn money, it must also protect its savings and investments against large unanticipated medical and hospital costs. A well-planned, well-balanced health insurance program can do just this.

# 12
# Selecting Health Services

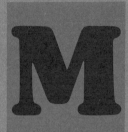

odern medicine has made unbelievable advancements within the past century. Rather than slowing down, the tempo of discovery in medicine has been picking up in recent years. During the past 15 years, vaccines have been developed for poliomyelitis, measles, and rubella (German measles). Research is making a massive assault on the causes of and cures for cancer. Mental retardation, once considered to be an unpreventable malady, is now known to have several causes, some of which are preventable. Many diseases are so well controlled today we give little or no thought to them; the causes and cures of others will, without doubt, be uncovered within the immediate future. The importance of all this is that a child born today can anticipate a life expectancy half again as long as his grandparents could anticipate 50 years ago.

Such medical advancements come to us not only through work in the research laboratory, but through the availability of quality medical counsel and patient care. But wanting the best in medical care and getting it can be two different matters. It becomes essential for a person to know how to choose medical care.

## THE PEOPLE WHO PRACTICE MEDICINE

A major problem facing the medical profession today is the increasing shortage of physicians. It is estimated that the current shortage of physicians in the United States is about 50,000. Rather than improving, the situation is getting worse. Just 60 years ago, there was one physician for every 568 persons in the United States; by a recent census, there is now one for every 616 persons. Such ratios are mild compared to some of the underdeveloped countries, but they do present a serious threat to the maintenance of a high level of general health care in this country.

In addition to the need for more physicians, the ones available are not always evenly distributed throughout the population. The physician-patient ratio is more favorable in urban areas and less favorable in rural areas. Many physicians prefer to practice in urban locations close to modern medical facilities. Here they can render the highest type of medical care, the income is higher, and there are more cultural advantages both for themselves and their families. The upshot of such concentration, of course, is that scattered rural populations are often deprived of adequate medical personnel. A further problem is that not all physicians are available for general health care. Actually, at present, there is only one general practitioner available for every 3000 persons, and only one internist available for every 4000 persons.

Although the number of physicians per 100,000 population has increased in recent years, more and more physicians have restricted their practice to specialized fields of study because of the flood of new medical information. Specialists outnumber general practitioners by almost four to one. This results in reduced numbers of general practitioners per 100,000 population, depriving many of adequate medical care. Consequently, a change is taking place from reliance on a family physician (who was usually a general practitioner) to reliance upon group practice or clinic medicine, composed of a group of specialists. This has caused some confusion as to what kind of physician to consult. Compounding the problem is the increasing demand the American public is making on the physician's services. Today the average American sees a physician five times a year, twice as often as he did in 1930.

### The Specialties

The more a physician concentrates his attention on a given system of the body, the less time he has for the whole person and the less proficient he is in general practice. To thoroughly know one area of medicine, he must confine himself to it to the exclusion of other areas. Such concentration has been necessary for medicine to make its great strides in heart surgery, cancer treatment and prevention, psychiatry, orthopedics, surgery, and other areas. A recognized specialist must have completed a full program of medical training and passed the written examination required of his particular specialty. Brief descriptions of several fields of specialization follow:

*Family Practice.* Family practice is a newly recognized specialty (1969). It has been created to give specialist status to the general practitioner in hopes of encouraging more doctors to remain in general practice. In recent years only about 12 percent of medical school graduates have entered general practice; the rest elect to specialize. This has resulted in a serious shortage of general practitioners in many parts of the United States.

*Internal Medicine.* The internist specializes in diagnosis and is particularly suited for both preventive medicine and coordinating the work of specialists needed to treat the specific problems the patient faces. Generally, internists do not deliver babies, practice surgery, deal with eye diseases or refractory corrections, or treat children. The internist often serves as a family doctor.

*Obstetrics and Gynecology.* Obstetrics is the care of the woman in pregnancy and child birth. It is frequently combined with gynecology, the care of women's diseases. Stressing preventive medicine, the obstetrician sees the mother early in pregnancy, supervises her health, and handles the delivery. Such attention has reduced infant mortality in this country and assures the best possible health for both the child and the mother.

*Pediatrics.* Pediatricians specialize in the care of infants and children. They advise parents, give checkups, diagnose congenital deformities, administer immunizations, and treat childhood diseases. Some pediatricians con-

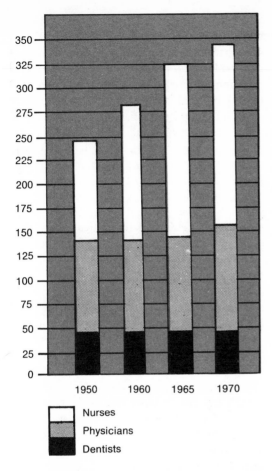

350 —
325 —
300 —
275 —
250 —
225 —
200 —
175 —
150 —
125 —
100 —
75 —
50 —
25 —
0 —

1950    1960    1965    1970

☐ Nurses
▨ Physicians
■ Dentists

Health Professionals per 100,000 population. Physicians refer to all physicians, active and inactive. Dentists refer to dentists in private practice. Source: *1971–1972 Source Book of Health Insurance Data,* Health Insurance Institute, 1973.

fine themselves to certain types of children's diseases, such as cardiovascular disorders or pediatric allergies.

*Surgery.* The work of the surgeon involves surgically operating on a patient to correct some physical condition. It may involve removing a cancer, repairing a defective heart, setting a broken bone, or attempting to correct a damaged brain. Since the body is so intricate, this specialty is subdivided into specific areas, such as neurosurgery, thoracic surgery, orthopedic surgery, and abdominal surgery.

*Psychiatry.* Dealing with emotional illnesses and disturbances is the work of the psychiatrist. Rather than using the scalpel, as does the surgeon, he treats his patients through psychotherapy, shock therapy, drugs, or combinations of these methods. Some psychiatrists are also specialists in neurology (the study of disorders of the nervous system). As with all other medical specialties, a psychiatrist must first earn an M.D. (Doctor of Medicine) degree, then study toward his specialty.

Some other fields of medical specialty are:

1. *Anesthesiology,* the science of administering general and local anesthetics.
2. *Dermatology,* the science of treating diseases of the skin.
3. *Neurology,* the science dealing with physical diseases of the brain and nervous system.
4. *Ophthalmology,* the medical branch treating the eye and its diseases.
5. *Otorhinolaryngology,* the medical branch treating diseases of the ear, nose, and throat.
6. *Pathology,* the study of the disease process, includes the examination of tissues for the diagnosis of cancer and other diseases. The pathologist may serve as a coroner and perform autopsies. His office is often located in a hospital.
7. *Proctology,* the medical branch treating diseases of the rectum and anus.
8. *Radiology,* the science of using x-rays, radium, and other radioactive sources for the diagnosis and treatment of disease.
9. *Urology,* the science of treating diseases

and abnormalities of the urinary tract in the female and the urogenital tract in the male.

In all, there are thirty-four recognized fields of medical specialization today. Each is governed by its respective board for purposes of examination and certification.

### The General Practitioner

In the past, many Americans looked almost solely to a single physician to diagnose and treat all the family's illnesses. The physician practiced general medicine and attempted to handle the full range of health conditions. Twenty-five years ago general practitioners (GP's) outnumbered specialists three to one. Today, specialists outnumber general practitioners about three to one. They are more commonly found practicing in rural, semi-rural, and suburban areas.

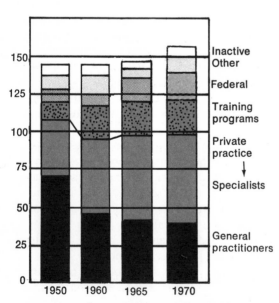

Physicians per 100,000 population. Source: *1970 Health Resource Statistics,* Public Health Service Publication No. 1509.

A physician is entitled to practice general medicine after he has completed his medical school training, has served his internship in general hospital practice, and has passed the examinations required to practice medicine in his particular state. Although not required, more and more physicians are taking additional training of some kind. Today, many physicians have completed at least 2 years of residency training and are members of the American Academy of General Practice. Some physicians direct their postgraduate study to a given area of medicine and may more or less confine their practice to this one area. Many of them conduct a general practice which includes most areas of medicine, except the most specialized ones.

Some unique problems face the general practitioner today. In order to maintain a high-quality practice, he must keep abreast of the mass of new scientific information and changes in medical techniques. He faces a demanding work load. The average GP puts in a 10-hour workday and might see as many as 135 patients a week. He is called upon to treat most of his patient's illnesses, since he is in the best position, medically, to minister to the whole person. During times of infectious outbreaks, the GP must be prepared to be on call for as long as his patients require him. For many physicians, this includes being available for night or home visits.

### Requirements for the M.D.

Before a man is licensed to practice medicine, he must meet certain professional and ethical requirements. Although training standards vary somewhat from state to state, he must take 3 to 4 years of premedical college work. He must then complete a 4-year training program in a medical school approved by the Association of the American Medical Colleges and the Council on Medical Education of the American Medical Association. In addition, most states require that he serve a 1-year internship to gain hospital experience. Before a physician is allowed to practice in a given state, he must be licensed by a board of medical examiners. This license is granted only after the physician has passed either a state or a national board examination. In addition to these basic requirements, if a physician desires to take a residency in a hospital to receive advanced training, or to meet the requirements of a given specialty in medicine, he must spend additional years (2 to 5) in training.

Some standards for the training of physicians as well as the ethics of medical practice are set by the medical profession itself. The medical profession also assumes the responsibility for regulating the professional conduct and ethics of its members. Much of this regulation is handled through local and county medical societies. Most of these societies have adopted standards for their members, such as prohibiting advertising, refraining from guaranteeing cures, adhering to all legalities regarding the taking of human life and the administration of drugs, cooperating with legal authorities, and giving evidence, through all public and private contacts, of their trustworthiness. Not all physicians meet such standards. In this respect, physicians as a whole are no different from other professional groups. In choosing a physician, we should have the privilege and the right of being satisfied both with his reputation, private and public, and his professional qualifications. To him we entrust our lives.

### Osteopathy

Osteopathy is considered another field of medicine, and those trained in it are referred to as physicians. This practice of medicine was started around 1870 by a physician named Dr. Andrew Still. He held that disease could be based on disturbed nerve functions which resulted from a pinching of the nerves as they leave the spinal column. According to this theory, a disease or condition in any particular organ of the body could be traced to a malcondition in the nerve supplying that organ.

The medical profession considers this theory unfounded and contradictory to its knowledge of human anatomy and pathology. Over the course of years, however, osteopathic physicians have been quietly abandoning many of the peculiar tenets originally held in osteopathy and have increasingly emphasized the place of drugs in the practice of sound medicine. This change has progressed to the point where, today, their training and practice is similar to that of traditional medicine. Nonetheless, osteopaths are usually barred from practicing in medical hospitals.

Depending on the state in which a person resides, he will have greater or lesser interest in osteopathy. Moves have been initiated in various state medical societies to unite the medical and osteopathic professions, but only one has been accomplished so far. California, in 1962, recognizing that the quality of osteopathic training was closely similar to that of medicine, passed legislation enabling osteopaths in the state to be considered M.D. s. All former osteopathic colleges in California now bestow the M.D. degree upon their graduates. Significantly, this move came about as the result of a joint effort between osteopathic and medical societies within that state.

Some families prefer the services of an osteopathic physician. A qualified osteopath can satisfactorily serve as a family physician.

### Selecting the Right Physician

In selecting medical care, a person must determine what he or his family needs and then must find out what is available. Some people prefer a general practitioner, while others select several specialists in selected branches of medicine. Since some general practitioners restrict themselves to a narrow branch of practice, it is necessary to know the nature of a physician's practice. If the family includes young children, the same point should be applied to elderly people. A person who cannot find one ideal physician for the entire family may prefer settling for several specialists, such as a pediatrician for the children and an internist for the adults.

In selecting a physician, either for general practice or to deal with a specific problem, there are certain procedures worth following that can help guarantee you will find a physician well suited to your needs and temperament.

1. Consider the reputation of various physicians in your community. Contact a local *accredited* hospital for the names and addresses of the physicians who practice through that hospital. There is usually a relationship between the quality of a hospital and the quality of the physician who practices there.

If considering physicians who have been recommended by friends and relatives, you should be prepared to do some independent investigating. Other people's attitudes toward their doctors and their illnesses might not be useful to you. It is wise, however, to stay away from doctors who consistently cause dissatisfaction among people whose judgment you respect.

2. Visit the office of the physician you are considering. His office should be within easy commuting distance. Find out if the physician is accepting new patients; if his office is neat, clean, and orderly. Discuss with the physician such general questions as whether he can furnish you or your family general medical care, whether he makes house calls, if he is usually available for emergencies, what other physician provides these services in the event he is out of town, his fee schedule and how it compares to that of other physicians in town.

He should be a person you can confide in and who appears interested in your family's health and well-being. If you are satisfied regarding these points, you have found your physician.

### The Patient-Physician Relationship

The patient is entitled to receive careful, professional service from his physician including laboratory test results and consultations with any medical specialists necessary for adequate medical treatment. It may not always be possible for the physician to cure, but the patient should always have reason to feel that the physician is doing his best.

A physician should be as concerned with preventing disease as curing it. He should keep his patients well informed as to when inoculations and periodic examinations should be given. In the practice of preventive medicine, it may be difficult for patients to understand the full benefit of medical care and justify the cost of it. Prevention of illness is not only easier, but less painful, cheaper, and less time consuming. A careful physician would much rather keep a patient from getting ill than attempt to bring him back to health once he is ailing.

The patient should understand his physician's fee schedule. If the cost of medical care is imposing a genuine hardship on the patient or his family, the physician will want to know about it. The physician may be willing to adjust his fees in the case of hardship. The patient should feel no embarrassment about raising such a discussion.

In return, the physician may expect certain courtesies and cooperation from his patient. In nonemergencies, the patient should make

248

appointments and then keep them. He should be punctual. He should be prepared to pay his medical bills promptly or make arrangement to pay them as soon as possible. The patient should follow the physician's instructions exactly. If medication is prescribed he should get it immediately and take it as directed. The physician has a right to expect the confidence of his patient.

A physician is not necessarily under obligation to answer emergency calls from unknown individuals late at night. The physician will have no medical history of the patient, may be subjecting himself to physical hazard, or may be greatly fatigued. Some individuals moving into a new community may fail to contact a new physician until they need him in emergencies or late at night. Then, if difficulty in obtaining care is encountered, they make complaints against the medical profession. In such emergencies, the nearest general hospital should have physicians on duty who can provide care.

A physician can give the best service when he feels his patients appreciate his efforts. As much as he would enjoy being able to cure every physical ailment, medical research has not provided him with all the necessary answers to accomplish that aim. But a good physician will go just as far in diagnosis and treatment as his ability, training, available facilities, and patients allow.

## Chiropractic

It is necessary to make some mention and clarification of chiropractic. This profession is a system of treatment based on the belief that the nervous system largely determines a person's state of health and that any interference with this system impairs normal functions and lowers the body's resistance to disease. Patients are treated primarily by specific adjustment of parts of the body, especially the spinal column. X-ray is used extensively to aid in locating the source of the difficulty. Supplementary treatment measures such as diet, exercise, rest, water, light, and heat are used. Chiropractic treatment by law may not include the use of drugs or surgery. The training of chiropractors, although ranging from 2 to 4 years, consists in most states of 4 years of training in a chiropractic school following graduation from high school. Graduation does not qualify a chiropractor to practice in all states, since not all states license the practice of chiropractic.

Since many of the body's ailments are due to infections or degenerative diseases, any field of the healing arts that does not qualify a practioner in the diagnosis and treatment of these kinds of maladies restricts his usefulness. Accordingly, a chiropractor should not be chosen as a family physician. It is the official position of the American Medical Association that "chiropractic is an unscientific cult whose practitioners lack the necessary training and background to diagnose and treat human disease."

## Dentist

Dental training consists of four years of professional training following two to four years of required college work. A dental specialty usually requires two or three years of additional professional training. The majority of dentists are general practitioners who provide many types of dental care. If an individual is in need of a dental specialist his regular dentist will be more than glad to recommend one who will provide the required treatment.

Although there has been an actual increase in the number of dentists in the United States, the number has not kept pace with the increasing population. Since 1950 there has been a 23 percent increase in dentists, but this has resulted in an 8 percent actual *decrease* compared to the population.

### Nurse

The nursing team is led by the professional or *registered nurse* (R.N.) but also includes the vocational nurses, nursing aides, medical technologists, orderlies, and attendants. Registered nursing training requires two to four years of professional training beyond high school. Additional training can be taken to qualify a nurse in a nursing specialty (such as obstetrics, pediatrics, psychiatry, or surgical nursing).

Since 1950 the number of nurses has increased 87 percent. About 29 percent of all professional nurses work on a part-time basis. Also, the number of male nurses is increasing, and today account for a full 1 percent of all professional nurses.

## FACILITIES FOR PATIENT CARE

As medical techniques have improved, so have facilities for patient care. Today's physician makes few home visits, particularly in urban areas. The home no longer needs to serve as a hospital for delivery of babies, treatment of tuberculosis and pneumonia, and nursing home for elderly people suffering from chronic diseases. Today, only minor illnesses are cared for at home. Improved standards of diagnosis and treatment require facilities that are only available in physicians' offices, clinics, nursing homes, and hospitals.

### Clinics and Nursing Homes

Clinics are often set up in conjunction with a hospital to provide various types of specialized services for patients with venereal diseases, tuberculosis, cancer, and communicable diseases, and for patients needing maternal and child care. These clinics service patients whose cases are not severe enough to require hospitalization, and yet need medical care. Although dealing in diagnosis and treatment, the clinic's efforts go largely toward instructing expectant mothers, providing social services, and giving advice on nutrition and other health problems. In public clinics, patients who can afford the service may be charged; many pay little or nothing.

Some clinics are formed by a group of private physicians and are set up to provide more services than that of the single-physician office. They often provide more complete diagnostic and laboratory services. They may be operated by physicians within a given specialty or include physicians from various specialties. Private clinics generally do not provide surgical or bed services.

Nursing homes provide services, on a more limited scale than a hospital, for convalescing patients or for those with chronic illnesses. Many nursing homes are privately owned and, though smaller, the quality of their care should be no different from that of a hospital.

### Hospitals

Population increases, along with greater physician use of hospitals, have substantially increased the demand for available hospital facilities. Hospitals are usually constructed with funds from community sources, private philanthropists, local or state tax dollars, and grants of federal funds. Due to the increased demand for hospital services and the greatly increased costs of new hospital construction, many hospitals are being built with the aid of public funds. Providing up-to-date hospital equipment and paying new increases in salaries have greatly raised the operating costs of existing hospitals. For these reasons some parts of the country either lack hospital facilities or have substandard ones. Before an older hospital is enlarged or a new one built, it is important that the community consider its needs and the ability of the area to support modern hospital facilities, both financially and professionally.

The three basic types of hospitals in the United States are the government hospital, the voluntary hospital, and the proprietary hospital.

The federal government has established hospitals for military personnel and their dependents, American Indians, merchant seamen, veterans, lepers, and narcotics addicts. Individual states have built specialized hospitals for emotionally and neurologically ill patients and for those with tuberculosis, as well as general hospitals, which are usually associated with a state-supported medical school. City and county hospitals are commonly general hospitals providing general medical care, although some give special attention to communicable-disease control and the care of indigents.

Voluntary hospitals are public facilities set up on a nonprofit basis. They are established by churches, philanthropic individuals, charitable organizations, or the local community. They are run by governing boards, usually selected from the community, which are responsible for their operation, financing, and construction. Such hospitals provide for more than two-thirds of all hospital admissions in this country. Although such hospitals are meant to be self-supporting, their operations sometimes need to be underwritten financially by local organizations. Some federal funds are now available for new construction of voluntary hospitals.

Proprietary hospitals are owned and administrated by individuals or corporations,

and are set up to make a profit. Some are even established by real estate promoters and then leased to physicians at no construction cost to the community. Proprietary hospitals often have a questionable reputation. They tend to prefer the most profitable types of hospital cases, while taking few, if any, charity cases. The majority of these hospitals are small and only about one-third of them are accredited.

*The Accreditation of Hospitals.* In 1952 a Joint Commission on Accreditation of Hospitals (JCAH) came into being to judge the operations of hospitals. It is sponsored by the American Hospital Association, the American Medical Association, the American College of Surgeons, and the American College of Physicians. It has set up national standards for hospital care, it accredits hospitals meeting these standards, and it periodically reviews accredited hospitals. Upon application, a hospital is thoroughly examined for cleanliness, laboratory operations, food handling, records, and the practice of its staff physicians. To be accredited, a hospital must have at least twenty-five beds, belong to the American Hospital Association, and pass its examination. An accreditation is good for 3 years.

It is increasingly important for a hospital to have JCAH accreditation. A nonaccredited hospital may not train interns, residents, or nurses. There may be no doctor's review committee overseeing the treatment which takes place as a guard against unnecessary or inappropriate surgery or other treatments. In some nonaccredited hospitals much needless surgery takes place merely to increase the income of the surgeon. Some medical insurance companies have refused to make payments to nonaccredited hospitals. Today, hospitals representing over 89 percent of the country's total hospital bed space are accredited. Most of these hospitals are voluntary ones.

When choosing between these forms of patient care, it is important to carefully examine the patient's need. Some conditions require hospital care, and in most cases the patient is admitted to a hospital upon application by the physician. In fact, some hospitals will not admit a nonaccident patient unless recommended by his physician.

Those conditions, especially those of the elderly, which require medical attention but not necessarily hospitalization can frequently be accommodated in a nursing home or clinic. Some elderly people have a strong aversion to entering hospitals. Cost is a consideration, and because the level of treatment is usually less intense in a nursing home, and less expensive, most medical insurance plans provide payment for more days in a nursing home than in a hospital.

# 13
# "How Do You Feel?"

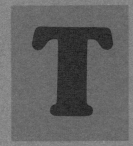

The proper selection of health-related products is more important than that of any other type of consumer goods. Not only can much money be wasted on ineffective products, but a person's health, or even his life, may depend on his getting proper treatment for diseased conditions and avoiding the use of dangerous products. It is essential that self-treatment not be attempted when the services of a physician are needed.

## THE DANGERS OF SELF-DIAGNOSIS AND SELF-TREATMENT

Attempts at self-diagnosis and self-treatment of all types of health problems seem to be a great American tradition. There are several possible explanations for the tendency to "play doctor." As the country was being settled, doctors were scarce and transportation was very poor, so self-treatment was a necessity. Even today, most physicians are very busy, appointments are difficult to get, and, for many people, the cost of proper medical care is discouraging. For many residents of rural areas and ethnic ghetto areas of large cities, transportation to medical facilities is still a problem. In addition to these factors, there is the continuing barrage of advertisements for self-treatment products for ailments of every description. Is it any surprise then that so many people still attempt self-treatment?

There are very real dangers in attempting self-diagnosis and self-treatment of any kind of symptom. The most serious risk is that a major (even life-threatening) disorder can easily be misdiagnosed as some common, minor problem and be treated as such. For example, a person trying self-treatment might take cough drops when he actually had tuberculosis or lung cancer. Not only would the self-treatment be ineffective and possibly harmful, but proper medical treatment would be delayed, perhaps even too late.

Another danger in self-treatment is that not all home remedies and nonprescription drugstore products are completely safe to use.

Some—such as aspirin, laxatives, and antihistamines—are dangerous when used in excessive amounts, in the presence of certain physical disorders, or in combination with other medicines.

It should be apparent by now that in addition to the question of which products to select, there is always the question of whether any product should be selected without the consultation of a physician.

Obviously, people should not run to a physician for every little scrape, bruise, ache, or pain. If they did, our entire system of medical care would be swamped overnight and the doctors would be unable to take care of the more serious problems. How can we know, then, which of the hundreds of different symptoms that can develop require the services of a physician? There are several circumstances under which a physician should always be consulted:

1. *Severe symptoms.* Any type of attack in which the symptoms are severe or alarming —such as severe abdominal or chest pain, or bleeding—should obviously receive prompt medical attention.

2. *Prolonged symptoms.* Any symptoms —such as cough, headache, constipation, or fatigue—that persist day after day should be checked by a physician, even though the symptoms are minor. Serious chronic disorders are often revealed through persistent minor symptoms.

3. *Repeated symptoms.* Symptoms, even though minor, that recur time after time should be reported to a physician because, like prolonged symptoms, they may indicate a serious problem.

4. *Unusual symptoms.* Any symptoms which seem to be unusual, such as unusual bleeding, mental changes, weight gains or losses, digestive changes, or fatigue, call for a visit to a physician.

5. *If in doubt.* If in doubt, the safest action is to see a physician. If there is a serious problem, it can be corrected in its early stages; if there is no problem, then you have paid a very small price for your peace of mind.

## HEALTH PRODUCTS—GOOD AND BAD

### Aspirin

Aspirin is probably the most effective medical substance that can be bought without a prescription. Aspirin, occasionally sold under its chemical name of acetylsalicylic acid, is the principal active ingredient of literally hundreds of nonprescriptive remedies. In many of these preparations, aspirin is the only effective ingredient, but their cost may be many times that of plain aspirin tablets. When advertisements refer to the "pain reliever that doctors recommend most," they mean aspirin. Although certain brands of aspirin have been highly advertised as being more effective than other brands, there is really no significant difference between brands of aspirin.

Aspirin has several beneficial properties. Its most common use is as a pain reliever, especially for headaches and muscular pains. It also has the ability to reduce fever and inflammation. For some people, aspirin may act as a mild sedative.

The "glorified aspirin" products often contain aspirin, phenacetin (another pain reliever), and caffeine (a mild stimulant), or just aspirin and caffeine, or aspirin with a buffering agent. These products have been shown to be no more effective for most persons than plain aspirin, though some people feel that buffers may reduce stomach irritation. Several products which originally contained phenacetin no longer contain this substance, since in large doses it has been shown to occasionally cause permanent damage to the kidneys.

Although the moderate use of aspirin is generally safe, there are certain precautions to follow with it. A few people suffer allergic reactions to aspirin (such as hives); other people find that aspirin causes stomach irritation. The stomach irritation can often be prevented by the presence of food in the stomach. The dosage recommended on the label should not be exceeded. Dosages above this level are not more effective and may be harmful.

Finally, aspirin should be used over long periods of time only on the recommendation of a physician, since it might otherwise be used to relieve the symptoms of a serious disorder which needed medical attention.

Aspirin is among the most common causes of poisoning of young children. It is important that aspirin, like any medication, be kept where children cannot get to it, preferably in a locked cabinet. Specially flavored children's aspirin is a particular problem, since children will eat it as candy. Manufacturers have attempted to devise lids that prevent children from opening the bottles, but this product should still be carefully kept out of the reach of children. Some authorities even recommend splitting adult aspirin tables for use with children rather than keeping the flavored aspirin in the house.

A compound that is similar in its actions to aspirin is acetaminophen. It is contained in over 60 over-the-counter and prescription products, such as Excedrin and Tylenol. It is said to be safer for people with aspirin allergy or bleeding disturbances. When acetaminophen is combined with aspirin, as in Excedrin, these advantages, of course, are lost.

### Remedies for Coughs and Colds

Every year new "miracle" cold remedies are offered to the public in massive advertising

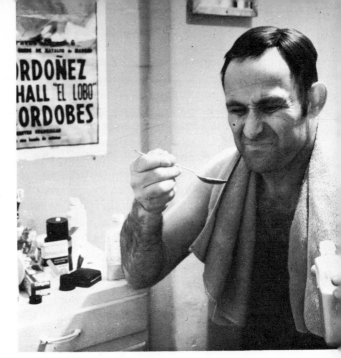

Potions, nostrums, elixirs, "wonder drugs," tonics. Man has swallowed all manner of things in the quest for good health. *Photo by F. Habicht.*

campaigns, only to drop quietly out of the market a few years later when their manufacturers release newer "miracles." The fact remains that, despite the many advances in other fields of medicine, there is still no way to prevent or cure the common cold.

A book by nobel prize winner Dr. Linus Pauling, *Vitamin C and the Common Cold,* has aroused much discussion and not a few warnings. Dr. Pauling recommends as prescription to prevent the common cold, the daily taking of 1 to 5 grams (1000 to 5000 milligrams) of vitamin C. This is well above the recommended 60 milligrams per day. Pauling actually did no research of his own. He just surveyed the literature, drawing heavily on uncontrolled experiments, and talked to his friends (again, no controlled experiments) and reached his own conclusions.

According to the F.D.A. and many scientists, Dr. Pauling's evidence fails to prove his point. In fact, the F.D.A. warns that too much vitamin C (ascorbic acid) can cause severe diarrhea (especially dangerous for elderly people and small children). It can conceivably cause pregnant women to miscarry. Excessive vitamin C causes the body to form oxalic acid, an ingredient in some kidney stones, especially those related to gout. The acidifying effect of vitamin C on urine could interfere with the treatment of diabetes.

The medical consensus is that the effects of massive doses of vitamin C on the human system are yet very poorly understood. But since the average layman would like to believe in miracle drugs, it becomes particularly irresistible to ignore claims for a drug that sounds as harmless as vitamin C. A medical axiom bears repeating, "The taking of any drug not prescribed is unwise."

To put cough and cold remedies into their proper perspective, one needs to understand that a cold is caused by a virus and that, to date, only limited progress has been made toward producing drugs that will cure virus infections. In fact, no drug has been developed that will control cold-producing viruses.

A cough is a reflex action caused by the presence of foreign matter or other irritation within the respiratory system. The purpose of coughing is to remove the irritant. Cough and cold remedies may give symptomatic relief by deadening the cough reflex, opening a stuffed nose, or reducing fever, but they do not get at the basic cause of the trouble. By eliminating the symptoms, but not the source, the cough and cold remedies may in the long run prove harmful. For example, by relieving his symptoms, a person with a cold is tempted to go on with his normal activities when he really should go to bed for 24 hours. This rest period, early in the course of a cold, can often hasten recovery and prevent secondary infections and other complications. The result of "fighting" a cold is often secondary bacterial infection of the middle ear, sinus cavities, or lungs. Coughs can be the result of many serious conditions which need medical treatment rather than just a deadening of the cough reflex. For example, a cough could indicate tuberculosis, pneumonia, other infections of the lungs, or lung cancer.

The reputations of many products for "curing" colds come from the fact that most colds are gone in less than a week. If a cold lasts beyond a week, it is probably due to a secondary bacterial infection, and should be treated by a physician. Antibiotics have no effect on the virus phase of a cold, but may be useful in clearing up the secondary infections. The cold sufferer should not pressure his doctor to prescribe antibiotics unless there is definite evidence of bacterial infection.

Many cold remedies contain antihistamines. These drugs may be effective against certain types of allergies, but not against true colds. If they do seem to cure a cold, there is a possibility that the actual problem was an allergy and not a cold at all. Antihistamines very commonly produce side effects such as dizziness and drowsiness, so they should not be taken when driving a car or operating machinery.

### Products for the Eyes

*Eye Washes.* Many physicians warn against the self-treatment of the eyes with any kind of commercial eye wash or eye drops. The natural flow of tears through the eye is the best means of cleaning the eye of dust, dirt, and other irritating material. As is true with many kinds of self-treatment, eye washes may be used to try to relieve the symptoms of serious eye disorders which really need prompt treatment by a physician. If any of the symptoms for which eye washes are advertised (red eyes, sore eyes) last for more than a day or two, the eyes should be immediately examined by a physician.

*Eyeglasses.* Eyeglasses should not be purchased from variety stores or by mail order. Anyone having difficulty with his vision should have a thorough eye examination by an eye specialist. The optometrist (O.D.) is a nonmedical eye doctor, having attended a college of optometry. He can test the eye and prescribe lenses to correct focusing problems, but he may not administer medications or perform surgery. Thus the optometrist cannot treat diseases of the eye. The ophthalmologist (M.D.) is a specialized medical doctor who can take care of any type of eye problem. The problem may need treatment other than glasses, and in any event glasses should be carefully fitted to the specific eyes of the individual and not purchased at random.

*Contact Lenses.* Contact lenses are small discs that ride on a thin layer of tears directly over the cornea and under the eyelids (see illustration). Recent improvements in their construction have increased their popularity. More often than not, regular vision is improved with "contacts" because there is no distance between the eye and the lens. Another advantage is that they allow greater peripheral vision, which is a great asset in sports and driving. In addition they are practically invisible when worn.

Contact lenses cannot be used by everyone, however, because certain visual defects cannot be corrected satisfactorily by this method. Some disadvantages of contact lenses are that they are more expensive than glasses, they can be easily lost, and they can cause great discomfort when a foreign body enters the eye.

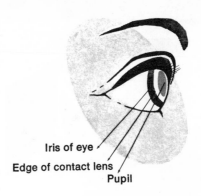

Iris of eye
Edge of contact lens
Pupil

Plastic contact lens, floating on a layer of tears over the cornea of the eye.

Contact lenses must be properly fitted to the eye by a qualified optometrist or ophthalmologist, and it often takes adjustments before they can be worn comfortably. Poorly fitted lenses are very uncomfortable and may even damage the cornea.

*Sunglasses.* Bright sunlight or glare can cause squinting, eyestrain, and headache, and may contain harmful amounts of ultraviolet rays that can gradually damage the lens and retina of the eyes. Sunglasses can reduce the discomfort of bright sun and screen out much of the ultraviolet. Another reason for wearing sunglasses is that vision during the early evening hours is considerably reduced if the eyes have been exposed to bright sunlight during the day. This is hazardous if one is driving.

The prices of sunglasses range from very inexpensive to very expensive. It is wise to pay a little more and get a good pair of sunglasses. There are several requirements for a good pair of sunglasses. First, they should be fairly dark. Second, they should be properly ground, as optical flaws will create eyestrain and headaches just as severe

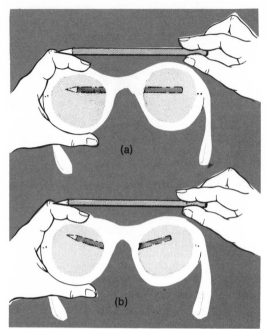

A simple test for optical quality of sunglasses. (a) Properly ground lenses reflect without distortion. (b) Poorly ground lenses reflect a distorted image and transmit it to the eye.

as those produced by the bright sun. The figure illustrating a simple way of determining the optical quality of a pair of sunglasses before buying them shows how to test for distortion. A person who normally wears prescription lenses should have sunglasses ground to his prescription or get the type that clip over his glasses.

Sunglasses should never be worn for night driving, and should never be relied on to protect the eyes during a solar eclipse. There is no safe way of looking directly at the bright sun.

### Pills for Sleeping, Waking, and Relaxing

Since most drugs that really affect the mind are under strict government control and are legally available by prescription only, you might wonder just what is in the nonprescription pills so openly advertised as being useful for going to sleep, staying awake, or relaxing, and relieving nervous tension.

*Pills for Sleeping or Relaxing.* Nonprescription pills for sleeping or relieving nervous tension are entirely different from the pills a doctor might prescribe for the same conditions. These advertised pills generally take advantage of one of the side effects of the antihistamine drugs. Antihistamines, which can be sold without a prescription, are useful in relieving the symptoms of certain types of allergies and are commonly contained in remedies for colds.

Certain of the antihistamines have the side effects of producing drowsiness, which may be rather severe in some people. For this reason, these antihistamines are sold as nonprescription sleeping pills. For many persons, these pills will really produce drowsiness; for some, they may be a psychological aid to sleep (since most sleeplessness is psychologically based); and for some others, there will be no effect at all. For a few people, antihistamines act as stimulants, producing nervousness and sleeplessness, thus contributing to the original problem. The nonprescription sleeping and relaxing pills often contain small amounts of other mild sedatives, such as scopolamine, but not enough to have any real effect.

*Pills for Staying Awake.* The pills that are advertised as helping you stay awake usually contain caffeine. Caffeine, of course, is contained in coffee, tea, and cola drinks. Though not everyone reacts in the same way, many people do find that caffeine acts as a stimulant which can prevent sleep. Caffeine also makes some people feel nervous ("coffee nerves"). So the sleep-preventing pills will do for a person just what coffee does for him.

258

The effect of one tablet is usually about equal to one cup of strong coffee.

The situations that justify taking these pills are rather limited. They do not serve as a substitute for sleep, but merely relieve the symptom of sleepiness. Their use has been compared to "whipping tired horses." They may help you study for an extra hour or two, but beyond that your ability to learn drops considerably. They should not be used to extend driving for more than an hour or two because driving becomes very dangerous beyond that point. A person who badly needs sleep may have dangerous hallucinations while driving or may just suddenly fall asleep at the wheel.

## QUACKERY

The colorful traveling medicine show may be a thing of the past, but medical quackery is still very much a part of the modern scene. Today's quack is much more sophisticated than was the snake-oil salesman of the past, but his goal is still the same—to separate the suckers from their money. The quack seems to be sincerely interested in a person's health, but his real interest is in making money—lots of money. The cost of medical quackery in the United States today is estimated at between 1 and 2 billion dollars a year. Modern quackery takes several common forms: it may involve a direct "doctor-patient" relationship; it may involve the mail-order or house-to-house sale of worthless products; or it may involve the sale in drug or "health food" stores of products that cannot do what is claimed of them.

### Who Are the Quacks?

A quack may be defined as a boastful pretender to medical skill. He is anyone who promises medical benefits which he cannot deliver. He may attempt to go beyond the limits of medical science or the limits of his own training.

Your own mental image of a quack may be that of an odd- or sinister-looking individual, but by actual appearance it would be impossible to tell a quack from an ethical physician. Any quack might be wearing a conservative business suit or a white medical coat. His personality is likely to be friendly, self-confident, and confidence-inspiring; his office walls are covered with "degrees"—you just "know" he is well qualified.

Quacks have various kinds of training. Once in a great while, a licensed medical physician enters into an area of quackery. A few best-selling books have been written by such doctors. Much more common is the quack who has had more limited training, perhaps in chiropractic or naturopathic methods. Many convicted quacks show no record of any formal higher education. College degrees and transcripts are obtainable from print shops and "diploma mill" colleges. The word "Doctor" in front of a name or the degrees after a name may mean nothing. Sometimes the quack is not an individual at all, but a corporation which makes false claims for its products. And, of course, self-treatment is quackery because most individuals are simply not qualified to diagnose and treat their own illnesses.

### Who Turns to the Quacks?

All kinds of people become the victims of quacks—the old and the young, the rich and the poor, and everyone in-between. But quacks do seem to prey particularly on the extremes—the young, the elderly, the very rich, and the very poor.

The young person often becomes the victim of mail-order quackery. There are many deceptive advertisements in certain of the magazines that appeal to young people. The products offered promise good looks, popularity, and sex appeal. There are products which are claimed to help gain weight, lose weight, build muscles, enlarge the breasts, and cure acne. Seldom are these products of any real value.

Elderly people find appeal in products that promise to renew their lost youth and vigor. They often waste their limited money on useless treatments and products that claim to relieve arthritis, impotency, prostate conditions, gray hair, baldness, and "tired blood." The nutrition quack caters to elderly people who are led to believe that all their aches and pains can disappear through the use of certain food products or food supplements. In addition, the elderly are attracted to so-called "clinics" and "health ranches" that claim cures for various chronic diseases through chiropractic, fad diets, and other limited methods.

Quacks are interested in the rich simply because they have money. The poor are receptive to quackery because good medical services are often scarce in low-income areas, the cost of ethical care may seem prohibitive, and the poorly educated may not realize the difference between quackery and ethical medicine.

Much quackery preys on fear. Anyone who has been told by his physician that he has an incurable disease lives in fear—fear of death, fear of pain, fear of surgery, fear of the unknown. He may grasp at any straw of hope offered by the quack, no matter how unscientific or expensive the treatment may be. Sometimes fear keeps a person from seeking an ethical physician in the first place. Afraid of surgery, he may turn instead to a quack who promises a cure without surgery. Sometimes a quack must create fear where none exists. He may, for example, tell a perfectly healthy person that he has a serious disease and then recommend an expensive series of worthless treatments for the nonexistent disorder.

Ignorance and gullibility are strong allies to the quack. Millions of people are almost unbelievably gullible. These people unquestioningly accept almost anything they hear as truth, and anything they read is accepted as absolute gospel. A quack can make his sales talks and his literature seem entirely believable to such people. Even well-educated people who should know better often fall for quack schemes because no one can be completely knowledgeable in all areas.

### *Major Types of Quackery Today*

*Cancer Quackery.* Despite the intensive efforts of government agencies to control cancer quackery, millions of dollars are still being spent every year on worthless cancer treatments. Cancer quackery is one of the most tragic of all rackets because many persons with early, curable cancers waste vital time waiting for a worthless remedy to cure their cancer. By the time they seek ethical treatment using standard methods, their cancers have already progressed to an incurable stage. Early treatment by a competent ethical physician can often result in complete cure of a cancer.

The cancer quack often claims to use an effective treatment which is exclusively his and unavailable to other physicians. Or, he claims that regular doctors don't want to use effective cures for cancer because it would hurt their business. These claims are, of course, ridiculous. Effective medical treatments cannot be kept exclusive in the United States and the ethical doctors certainly do not need dying cancer patients in order to stay busy. There are very few ethical doctors in this country who are not already busier than they would like to be.

A strong ally of the cancer quack is the fear of surgery felt by many people. The quack always promises a cure without surgery, but in ethical medicine, surgery is one of the most important treatments for most kinds of cancer.

*Arthritis Quackery.* Arthritis, sometimes called rheumatism, is an inflammation of the joints. (Rheumatism, broadly defined, includes some muscular conditions as well.) Millions of people suffer from some degree of arthritis, with great pain and crippling in extreme cases. Ethical medicine can offer a real cure for only a few of the many types of arthritis. About half of all arthritis sufferers are therefore led to try quack remedies, at a cost of about a quarter of a billion dollars a year. Many arthritis remedies are just aspirin with a fancy name and a high price.

Some types of arthritis tend to periodically come and go, even without treatment. Thus, quack remedies are often given credit for curing cases of arthritis that would have gone away even if nothing had been done. In arthritis, as well as any other disease, the ethical physician can still be relied upon to offer the most effective, up-to-date treatment available.

### Food Quackery

Food quackery is a big business. Half the money spent on quackery is spent in the area of nutrition. Over 10 million Americans today are living in the shadow of confusion cast by the food faddists and health food quacks. These unfortunate people are encouraged to follow expensive, complicated, and often unpleasant diets. Rather than being better fed as a result, they are actually more likely to suffer from nutritional deficiency than those who eat ordinary diets, following the simple rules of basic nutrition.

Food quackery products are sold in several ways. They are often featured in health food stores, sold by door-to-door salesmen, advertised for mail-order sale, and promoted in "health" lectures. Regardless of the sales approach used, the food quack makes use of scare tactics, calculated to frighten people into buying his products. Almost all operators in this field make use of certain modern myths. Each of these myths may contain some element of truth, but the conclusions drawn by the quack are not supported by scientific evidence. The following are some of these myths.

1. *All diseases are due to faulty diet.* Of course, such deficiency diseases as scurvy are entirely the result of poor diet, and a person's resistance to many infections is lower when his diet is poor. But no known diet can protect a person from all infectious diseases or from cancer, as is claimed by certain quack nutrition products.

2. *A particular product is indispensable.* Salesmen often represent their products as being the only source of a vital food substance and imply that maximum good health is possible only if their products are used. The truth is that every substance known to be important in nutrition is available from a variety of common grocery-store foods. The salesman will often answer this fact by saying that his product contains some substance not yet known to science. However, he has absolutely no basis for such a claim.

3. *Soil depletion causes malnutrition.* A common story is that repeated cropping of the land has removed some substance, which is therefore lacking from the foods produced. The only substance for which a deficiency in the soil is reflected in the crop produced is iodine. Since people today obtain adequate iodine through diet and the use of iodized salt, iodine deficiency is rare. If any other mineral is lacking from the soil, this deficiency is reflected in a lowered *quantity* of

produce, but the nutritional *quality* is not affected.

4. *"Organic" or "natural" foods.* If there is a key word in the "health food" business, it must be either "organic" or "natural." According to the biological or chemical definitions of the word organic (see a dictionary), all foods are organic. The claim is often made that foods grown with commercial fertilizers are inferior to those grown with "natural" fertilizer (manure). The fallacy of this claim lies in the fact that a plant can absorb from the soil only certain simple inorganic nutrients. If manure is used as fertilizer, the organic compounds present must be broken down by bacteria into the same simple compounds present in commercial fertilizers before any absorption into the roots of the plant can take place.

A related claim is that the synthetically produced vitamins are inferior to naturally occurring vitamins. This statement is usually made by salesmen of high-priced food supplement products to indicate the superiority of their products over lower priced products. Actually, the man-made vitamins are chemically identical to the naturally occurring vitamins, are absorbed in the same manner, and function in the body in exactly the same way.

The very word *chemical* is often used in a derogatory manner by the salesman who apparently does not know or chooses to ignore the fact that all food is nothing but a mixture of chemicals. He deplores the use of chemical food additives such as antioxidants, coloring agents, mold inhibitors, and numerous other additives important to modern food processing. Since the 1958 amendment to the Federal Food and Drug Law, such chemicals have been thoroughly screened by their manufacturers for any possible harmful effect before the Federal Food and Drug Administration permits their use

in foods. Though some are dangerous in large dosages, in the amounts used, today's additives are perfectly safe. The food quack is apt to decry even the use of pasteurization, a process of indisputable value and importance for milk and certain other food products.

5. *Overprocessing.* The food quack exaggerates the loss of food value through modern food-processing methods. Although some loss definitely does occur, the public today is much better fed than at any time in the past as a direct result of modern food technology. Highly nutritious processed fruits, vegetables, and meats are available throughout the year, rather than just during limited seasons. Today's processing methods are often less destructive to vitamins than were those of the past. Of course, it is still preferable to use fresh foods—meats, vegetables, fruits, whole grains, and dairy products—whenever they are available.

6. *Protein supplements.* A standard item in health food stores is the protein pill or powder. While these products are, as claimed, rich sources of essential amino acids, their protein is of no better quality or amino acid content than the protein in meats, eggs, or dairy products. In addition, protein supplements are usually much more expensive and less palatable than other protein sources. It is an interesting contradiction when, at the same time, a health food store promotes both "natural" foods and highly processed protein supplements.

7. *Advantages of "raw" sugar.* Most health food stores feature various types of raw or less processed sugar. There are two fallacies involved here. The first is that the nutritional value of less refined sugar is not significantly higher than that of pure sugar. The second is that the sugar content is not much lower. The basic problem is that many people in the United States eat far too much sugar,

a dietary factor that contributes to dental decay, obesity, malnutrition, blood sugar disorders, and possibly heart disease. It makes no difference whether the sugar is "raw" or refined. In many of the "cereal" products that are highly promoted on children's TV programs, the most abundant ingredient is sugar. Even the more "natural" granola-type cereals often have an extremely high sugar content. It is believed that many of today's children are acquiring such a strong desire for sugar that their lifelong eating habits may be altered.

One of the most serious consequences of food quackery is that it frequently interferes with useful, scientific evaluation of nutrition, food processing, and preserving methods. There is presently a good deal of concern about food additives and their known and unknown effects—but this is a different concern from food quackery. In confusion over all the claims and counterclaims, congressional hearings testimony, industry press releases, and "muck-raking" reports, some people turn off their critical faculties and run straight in the other direction. Unfortunately, they usually do not improve their diet and general health in the process; they just substitute one set of myths for another.

### Organized Quackery

There are several national or local organizations of well-intentioned but misinformed people which help to perpetuate certain kinds of quackery. Some examples are the International Association of Cancer Victims and Friends, which runs a bus service from California to Tijuana, Mexico, so people may secure unproven cancer treatments which are illegal in the United States; and the National Health Federation, which has taken stands against immunizations and fluoridation and which helps perpetuate certain myths about foods.

### Some Specific Examples of Quackery

The following specific examples of quackery have been selected from recent issues of *FDA Consumer,* an official publication of the Food and Drug Administration. They should serve to illustrate the types of fraud and deception to which the public is being subjected. (See also the table listing products seized by FDA.)

*Mail Fraud Cases Reported by the Post Office Department.* "Solicitations of orders and sales through the mails of 'Wonder Belt' represented as enabling wearers to reduce and melt away excess fat from any particular part of the anatomy" (December, 1971).

"Solicitations of orders and sales through the mails of 'Vigor-Vite,' a newly created 'Youth-sex pill' that reportedly 'doubles and even triples' the physio-sexual libido capacity in adult men and women" (December, 1971).

(False Representation of a product) "advertising and sale by mail of a product called 'Desk Sitters Diet,' represented to be an effective diet for losing weight." Same company: "advertising and sale by mail of a product called 'Secret Formula,' represented as enabling user to lose up to four inches in girth in 90 minutes" (April, 1972).

(False Representation of a product) "advertising and sale by mail of a product called 'La Fem Climax Cream,' represented to be an effective sex stimulant for women" (May, 1972).

A potato packer in Oregon was charged with false advertising by the Oregon Department of Agriculture's Consumer Officer because of the labeling he was using to promote the sale of his product. Assuming that a large segment of this country's consumers are weight conscious, he used phrases such as "lower in calories" and "less starch" on his labels. The Consumer Officer wanted to know "less starch than what?" and "lower in calories than what?" This violation of the law is punishable by a fine of up to $500 or imprisonment in the county jail for six months or both (February, 1972).

The FDA seized five medical devices that were shipped to chiropractic clinics by a "Post-Graduate School of Chiropractors" and a "Foundation for the Advancement of Chiropractic Research." "The labeling of the devices lacked adequate directions for use for the purposes for which they were intended, namely, for the diagnosis of disease in man; since they were worthless for such purpose" (March, 1972).

### Protection Against Quackery

Many people naively believe that they do not have to worry about quackery because the government doesn't allow it. In reality there are and always will be some worthless treatments and products offered to the public. Although governmental agencies are active and successful in combating quackery, a quack may escape government detection for a period of time. The government must then gather evidence for a case against him. The burden of proof of the fraud is on the government's shoulders; the case may be tied up in the courts for many years until every possible appeal is exhausted. In the meantime, the fraud often persists.

Another problem is that cosmetics do not have to be effective—just "safe"—while a drug must be both safe and effective. Thus many beauty products escape government action by being cosmetics. For example, many suntan products falsely claim to "admit the tanning rays while screening out the burning rays" when in fact both tanning and burning are the result of the same element in sunlight—the ultraviolet content.

It is therefore important for the individual to be able to recognize quackery and to know how to avoid it. Some of the signs of quackery are given below. Some of the signs discussed apply mainly to clinical quackery, where a "doctor" examines the patients and administers drugs. Other signs apply more to the sale of nonprescription remedies through mail order, drugstores, and health stores. Some of the signs apply to both forms of quackery.

*Boastful Advertising.* The code of ethics of most medical, dental, and similar professional associations prohibits or greatly restricts the advertising of services by members. Generally, a simple announcement of name, address, and type of practice is all that is considered ethical.

*Offer of Free or Low-cost Diagnosis.* Less ethical practitioners often advertise complete physical examinations at very low costs ($10 or $15). The practitioner who gives a free or low-cost diagnosis must make his living from the treatments he renders, so he is naturally inclined to make a diagnosis which is going to lead to some of the treatments he provides. These practitioners often treat perfectly healthy persons or else fail to detect the serious disorders a person might have.

*Location.* The ethical practitioner usually prefers a professional environment for his office. Medical offices, for example, are often near a hospital. The practitioner who rents space in a department store or discount store is not necessarily unethical, but one should be alert for other signs of quackery.

*Claim to Cure Diseases that Others Cannot Cure.* The quack often claims that he has the ability to cure some condition that the ethical physician cannot always cure, such as cancer, arthritis, or old age.

*Guarantee of Cure or Satisfaction.* The ethical physician never guarantees a cure; he does the best he can, but medical science has not progressed to the point where results are that

# PRODUCTS SEIZED BY THE FOOD AND DRUG ADMINISTRATION

| PRODUCT | DATE | CHARGE |
|---|---|---|
| Electronic instrument (Theramatic model A-6 DT 40 electronic instrument) | 3/17/70 | False and misleading claims for the treatment of infections, otitis media, fractures, bone and tissue healing, smooth muscle spasm, bursitis, arthritis, low back pain, sinusitis, prostatitis, Ménière's syndrome, hypertension, certain inflammations, angina, hemorrhoids, and other diseases. |
| Respirator | 3/17/70 | False and misleading claims as to the adequacy and effectiveness of the article as a means of resuscitation for emphysema, bronchial asthma, and other therapy. Lacked adequate directions for its use and was dangerous to health when used as directed by the labeling. |
| "Provitamin B₁₅ (Pangamic Acid) capsules" | 9/29/70 | Label contained false and misleading claims that the capsules were a specific treatment for arthritis and other body toxicities; effective for treatment of bowel or kidney function, allergies, and atherosclerosis, for alleviating hypoxia, for use in coronary insufficiency, and for relieving symptoms of angina and asthma; it might well play a role in prevention of cancer. |
| Cough syrup for dogs (Dogette Cough Syrup) | 5/26/71 | False and misleading claims for relief of dry, persistent, tickling coughs of dogs, for quieting and relaxing dogs, and for suppressing coughs. |
| Vitamin E capsules | 7/23/71 | False and misleading claims: "Combats the Deadly Effect of Air Pollution . . . Lung disorders . . . holds back the ravages of emphysema"—for lung disorders, particularly emphysema. |
| "Formula LDX-33" | 12/14/71 | False and misleading claims of ability to nourish the sex organs and restore lost sexual interest, potency, or fertility. |
| Grow chest hair | 5/12/72 | False representation of a formula enabling users to grow chest hair. |
| Diagnosis of arthritis, rheumatism, and heart conditions | 5/24/72 | A Foreign Mail Stop Order placed against the Pan-American Medical Services, Monterrey, Mexico, for advertising and sale through the mails of a diagnostic service for treatment of arthritis, rheumatism and heart conditions. |

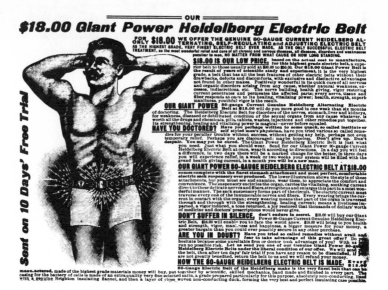

certain. Even with his guarantee, the quack is seldom known to refund any money.

*Claims of Secret Treatments.* Claims of secret machines and formulas are meaningless because the ethical physician has knowledge of all the latest treatments and has access to their use. The secret remedies of quacks, upon investigation, always turn out to be worthless.

*Testimonial Letters.* Quacks often make use of letters of testimonial; ethical practitioners seldom or never use this technique. No importance can be placed on these letters; many of them have been purchased or are written by ignorant people who really never had any disease. These people have no way of knowing why they may have felt better. Remember that 50 to 75 percent of all physicians' office visits are the result of psychosomatic complaints which will often go away through psychological suggestion, even in the absence of any effective treatment. Some testimonials are written by people who later died of the disease from which they claimed to have been cured.

*Attacks Against the Medical Profession.* The quack often loudly attacks the medical profession for its extensive use of surgery and drugs. These are, of course, the most valuable treatments for many disorders. But the quack cannot legally use drugs or surgery, so he claims the superiority of his own methods of treatment.

The quack is often very defensive and claims that he is being persecuted by the medical associations and the government. Any practitioner who makes this claim should be regarded as a possible quack since it indicates that he has used unproven methods and has probably been in legal trouble as a result.

## Public Protection

At every level of government, efforts are being made to control fraudulent health practices. The Federal Trade Commission is active in cases involving fraudulent or deceptive advertising. The Post Office Department may move rapidly in cases of mail-order fraud. The Food and Drug Administration regulates the purity, safety, and proper labeling of drugs and food products moved across state lines. Certain state, county, and city governments are also active in suppressing quackery by enacting laws that make fraudulent practices a felony.

Several privately financed groups actively participate in the restraint of health frauds. Among these are the Bureau of Investigation of the American Medical Association, the Better Business Bureau, and the Chamber of Commerce. Although these organizations have no legal regulatory powers, they can bring cases of fraud to the attention of the public and the proper legal regulatory authorities.

When a person is in doubt about the merits of a particular product or treatment, it is often worthwhile to check with a local Chamber of Commerce, Better Business Bureau, local medical society, or licensed and registered physician.

## Persistence of Quackery

How does quackery persist in spite of intensive efforts by government and individuals to suppress it? The answer is that, although the quack might not be very skilled in treating disease, he is very adept in other areas. He often operates at the very borderline of legality, perhaps obeying the letter but not the spirit of the law. When he is convicted, he usually serves a short jail sentence and pays a stiff fine (which he can well afford). Then, immediately he changes his location and perhaps his name and is back in business again.

Often, getting a conviction for a quack proves to be very difficult. Juries may be swayed by the emotional testimonies of former patients of the quack. Large corporations engaged in the sales of proprietary compounds retain excellent lawyers to fight their battles with the authorities, and the corporations often win. For example, it took the federal government 16 years to get the word "liver" removed from the name of Carter's Little (Liver) Pills on the basis that they had nothing to do with the liver.

The private citizen can aid the campaign against quackery through reporting incidents of suspected quackery to his local district attorney's office or the local medical society. It is often only through such complaints that authorities are alerted to a fraudulent operation. It is apparent, then, that today, as always, it is the responsibility of the individual to be alert to health fraud and quackery and to avoid them.

## FOR FURTHER READING

AMA Committees on Exercise and Physical Fitness and the Medical Aspects of Sports, ed., *Sports & Physical Fitness.* Chicago, Ill.: American Medical Association, 1970. *The feelings of some of the best authorities in the United States on sports and physical fitness.*

Better Homes and Gardens, *The Better Homes & Gardens Calorie Counter's Cookbook.* New York: Bantam Books, 1972. *An excellent book for the individual who wishes to change his eating habits and reduce or maintain his weight at an acceptable level.*

Cooper, Kenneth L., *The New Aerobics.* New York: Bantam Books, 1970. *Describes a complete plan of activities designed to increase total fitness.*

Crichton, Michael, "The High Cost of Cure," *Atlantic,* Vol. 224, No. 3 (March, 1970). *An exposé of how and why medical costs have become exorbitant, using the actual case histories of specific patients.*

Delmonteque, Robert, *Man's Common Sense Guide to Physical Fitness.* New York: Hippocrene Books, 1972. *A guide to safe and sane types of physical activity.*

DeLuca, H. F., J. W. Suttie (eds.), *The Fat-Soluble Vitamins.* Madison, Wisconsin: University of Wisconsin Press, 1970. *An overview of past findings and recent research concerning the actions of Vitamins A, D, E, and K.*

Geier, Arnold, *Life Insurance: How to Get Your Money's Worth.* New York: Macmillan, 1965. *Includes a useful section on health insurance which relates different types of programs to individual needs.*

Harris, W. E., William J. Bowerman, and James Shea, *Jogging: A Complete Physical Fitness Program for All Ages.* New York: Grosset and Dunlap, 1967. *The best reference available on jogging and its overall advantages for physical fitness.*

Iowa State Department of Health, *Simplified Diet Manual.* Ames, Iowa: Iowa State University Press, 1969. *The best diet manual in the field of nutrition; for a reader with a sound understanding of basic nutrition, it can be very helpful in a weight control program.*

Jones, Kenneth, Louis Shainberg, and Curtis Byer, *Total Fitness.* San Francisco: Canfield Press, 1972. *A reference explaining the interdependence of many activities which contribute to total body fitness.*

Kotschevar, Lendal, and Margaret McWilliams, *Understanding Foods.* New York: Wiley, 1969. *An excellent book on the common foods in a balanced diet; provides useful reference material.*

Magnuson, Warren G., *The Dark Side of the Market Place.* Englewood Cliffs, New Jersey: Prentice-Hall, 1968. *An exposé of modern-day quackery.*

Mayer, Jean, *Overweight: Causes, Cost, and Control.* Englewood Cliffs, New Jersey: Prentice-Hall, 1968. *A thorough discussion of all aspects of obesity; includes common questions and reliable medical answers.*

Myers, Robert J., *Medicare.* Homewood, Ill.: Irwin Publishers, 1970. *Completely explains medicare and the implications for the older American.*

Royal Canadian Air Force, *Exercise Plan for Physical Fitness.* New York: Pocket Books, 1972. *A well-recognized calisthenic program for both men and women.*

Schwartz, Herman and Michael Lipman, *Guidebook for the Hospital Patient*. North Hollywood, California: Branden House, 1968. *An excellent explanation of the costs of hospital care and how they relate to you as the patient.*

Shumaker, James M., ed., *National Health Test*. New York: Pocket Books, 1970. *See how fit you are. This book gives a person an idea of his level of fitness.*

Stare, Frederick, *Eating for Good Health,* rev. ed. New York: Cornerstone, 1969. *A practical application of nutrition principles, written in nontechnical language for the general public.*

United States Department of Agriculture, *Agricultural Handbook No. 8, Composition of Foods*. Washington, D.C.: U.S. Government Printing Office, 1963. *Gives nutrient values of a multitude of foods.*

U.S. News and World Report, *Social Security & Medicare—Simplified*. Riverside, N.J.: Macmillian, 1970. *The best guide to medical and health care and the relationship of the U.S. Government.*

Wilkenson, Bud, *Modern Physical Fitness*. New York: Barnes and Noble, 1969. *Relates enjoyable sports activities with their potential benefits in a physical fitness program.*

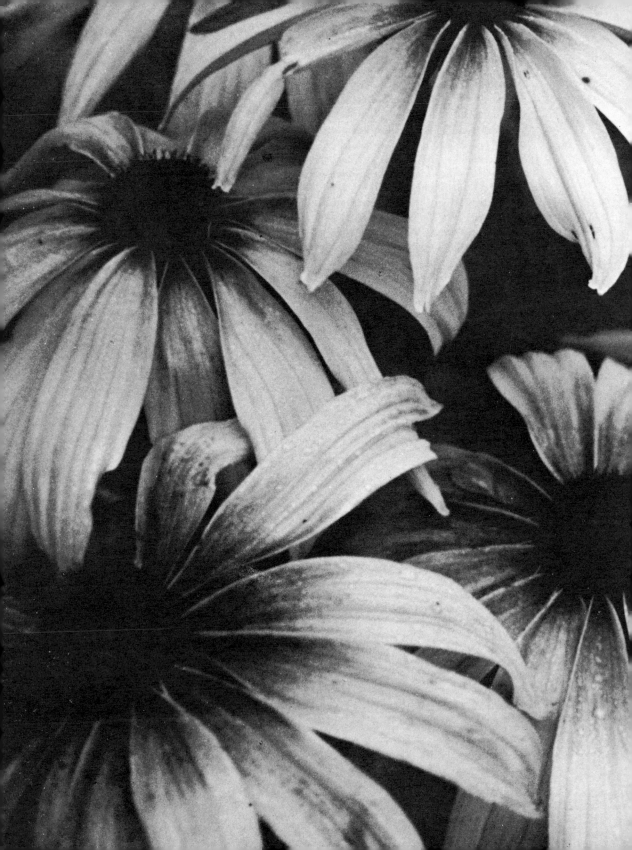

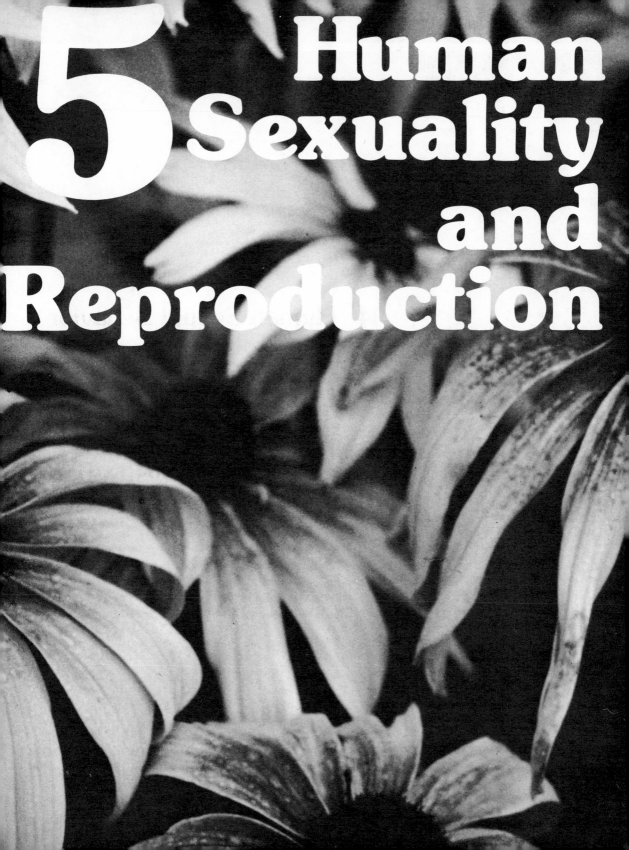

# 5 Human Sexuality and Reproduction

## 14　Human Sexual Behavior

Sex Research—A New and Needed Science • The Sexual Adjustment of the Unmarried Person • Sexual Intercourse Outside of Marriage • Extramarital Intercourse • Homosexuality • Deviate Sexual Behavior • Sexual Anatomy and Physiology • Sexual Response • Common Sexual Problems

## 15　A Personal and Social Institution

Deciding to Marry • Society's Interest in Your Marriage • Adjusting to Marriage • The Decision to Have a Child • Alternate Life Styles

## 16　Human Reproduction

Heredity • Fertility Control • Infertility • Pregnancy and Childbirth • The Sex Education of Children

# 14
# Human Sexual Behavior

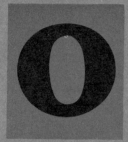

Only in recent years has human sexuality begun to emerge as a "respectable" field for physiological and behavioral research. Prior to this time, little objective research was accomplished, due to a variety of obstacles. For example, some people felt that sex was "dirty" or "sacred" or that its "mystery" was best preserved as such. Any of these attitudes would tend to discourage sex research. Another problem has been that those scientists who should have been studying sex were often inhibited in their studies by their own sexual insecurity or prudishness. Finally, since sexual inadequacy is not a major cause of death, massive research grants for its study have not been readily available.

## SEX RESEARCH—A NEW AND NEEDED SCIENCE

Sex research on a large scale was first popularized by the Kinsey group in the late 1940s and 1950s. Their work at that time consisted mainly of interviewing large numbers of persons regarding their sex history and habits. It became immediately obvious that unlike other subjects of scientific and medical research, the judgments made in sex physiology and psychology are not accepted at "face value" by society. Rather, each portion of society, each religion, and each social class imposes its own values on this research and the conclusions it presents. The same mixed reception awaited Masters and Johnson (now Dr. and Mrs. Masters) when their excellent works on human sexual response and human sexual inadequacy were published in 1966 and 1970.

Objective sex research is of value to society in several respects. It places sexuality in its proper perspective as a normal healthy part of human physiology and behavior. It removes the cloak of secrecy from sexuality, helping to reassure people that their own sexual feelings, responses, practices, and problems are typical of millions of other people, or if not, how they differ. It helps to dispel anxiety-producing misconceptions and inhibitions. And it provides a sound basis for overcoming sexual problems.

Much of the information in this and the following two chapters has been established relatively recently as a result of modern sex research programs. We have tried to avoid imposing our own behavioral standards over this information. Rather, we have attempted to provide the reader with the factual basis upon which he may make sound personal decisions about nonmarital, premarital, marital, and extramarital sexual relations, contraception, abortion, and so forth. Distinctions are made between various types of sexual relations. "Nonmarital" indicates those outside of marriage in which the persons have no direct plans for marriage. "Premarital" implies that the relations include the anticipation of marriage. "Marital" are those relations between spouses during marriage. "Extramarital" are those relations carried on by either spouse with someone outside of the marriage during the time it is in effect.

## THE SEXUAL ADJUSTMENT OF THE UNMARRIED PERSON

The sexual behavior of the unmarried person has been a source of interest throughout history. A traditional approach to sexual development and adjustment was to pretend that sexual tensions, if ignored, would somehow just go away. This attitude, of course, was unrealistic because the biological sexual drive of the unmarried person is no different from that of the married person of the same age. But the traditional attitude has been to condemn any form of sexual satisfaction outside of marriage.

Another serious flaw in this traditional attitude is that it ignores the gradations and many facets of human sexuality which cover a wide range across years of development, cultural patterns, normality, and abnormality.

### Petting

We shall define "petting" as all relations more intimate than kissing, but short of actual sexual intercourse. Petting typically includes fondling the breasts and sexual organs and may or may not lead to orgasm in either the male or female.

Any value judgment regarding petting should be based on such considerations as the age and emotional maturity of each individual, their attitudes and backgrounds, and the sincerity of their relationship. Petting can serve as a transitional step between immature and mature sexual attitudes. In this respect, it can be an important preparation for marriage.

Petting serves more as a stimulus for sexual desire than as a relief from sexual tensions. The natural tendency in petting is to gradually become more and more intimate until it culminates in sexual intercourse. Consequently, the sexually aroused couple finds it very difficult to stop short; it is such unplanned intercourse that most often results in pregnancy outside of marriage, since adequate contraception may not be readily available. Many couples develop techniques of petting to mutual orgasm as an alternative to intercourse. If this is to be done, it is important that no semen be allowed near the vaginal opening, since pregnancy can occur even without vaginal penetration by the penis.

### Masturbation

Masturbation is the production of orgasm by self-manipulation of the sex organs. In the past, masturbation was thought to lead to insanity, impotence, acne, and any number of major and minor problems. Today, masturbation is recognized as perfectly harmless and a part of normal sexuality in both the male and the female. Over 90 percent of all males masturbate at some time in their lives, as do over 60 percent of all females.

Most individuals resort to masturbation only as a substitute for sexual intercourse when the latter is unavailable. As a result, masturbation is most common among unmarried individuals, though married men and women occasionally masturbate when their partners are pregnant, menstruating, or unavailable for intercourse.

The old wives' tale that masturbation leads to insanity probably originated from the fact that emotionally disturbed individuals sometimes masturbate excessively. The fear of impotence was based on the erroneous notion that the lifetime supply of semen was limited and could be exhausted through masturbation.

Masturbation may begin at 10 to 18 years of age; the average age of first orgasm is about 14 years. The frequency of masturbation among normal unmarried males varies considerably, from about once a month to several times daily. Females typically masturbate less frequently than males.

If parents keep in mind that masturbation is a normal occurrence, they can prevent their children from developing guilt feelings about it. Girls should be warned, however, against inserting objects into the vagina for self-stimulation; such objects may cause infection.

### Nocturnal Emissions

Noctural emissions, commonly called "wet dreams," are involuntary discharges of semen, often accompanied by sexual dreams. Almost all males experience these emissions at some time. They are perfectly harmless and serve to relieve the pressure of fluid in the seminal vesicles if no other sexual outlet is available.

### Prostitution

Prostitution, though it exists in all areas, plays a minor role in the sexual adjustment of the typical college student. A few college males regularly patronize prostitutes and a few others occasionally buy their services. But the typical customer of the prostitute is older (36 to 40) and poorly educated. The obvious reasons to avoid prostitutes include their high incidence of venereal disease, the chance of getting robbed, and the chance of arrest. The state of Nevada, which has legalized prostitution in certain licensed, controlled instances, has been able to control some of these harmful effects.

## SEXUAL INTERCOURSE OUTSIDE OF MARRIAGE

Sexual intercourse before or outside of marriage is a subject of considerable interest today. It is apparent that in the last few years there has been some increase in its prevalence and a great increase in its discussion. Sexual relationships between persons are now entered into more openly than in any time in the recent past. Despite improved contraceptive methods, the illegitimacy rate is at an all-time high, a possible indication of increased sexual activity.

As with petting, there is no universal answer to the question of whether or not to engage in intercourse outside of marriage. Many individual factors must be considered. For some, religious beliefs dictate a definite NO, if the tenets of the religion are to be followed. For others below the age of consent, state laws proscribe such behavior. But, for the young adult of legal age and holding no strong religious beliefs, it becomes a highly individual question, to be decided on the basis of personal values and philosophy, giving due consideration to all possible (positive and negative) results of such action. The following are some of the considerations which should be kept in mind for those making this decision.

### *Physical Considerations*

*Pregnancy.* The basic motivation behind most of the laws and religious and social regulations pertaining to sexual behavior is to provide a stable family environment for the child and to determine who is responsible for his support. Historically, our society has held contempt for the illegitimate child and his mother. The fear of pregnancy has, therefore, traditionally been the greatest deterrent to intercourse outside of marriage. Even today, though attitudes towards sex have changed considerably, pregnancy out of marriage is usually regarded as a serious problem by even the more liberal thinkers.

Modern contraceptive methods can reduce the chance of pregnancy to a very low level if they are used properly and consistently. Anyone engaging in unmarried sexual relations should choose a highly effective contraceptive method and be certain that it is used properly. Even when a normally foolproof method (such as the "pill") is chosen, there should be a definite plan and agreement on the action to be taken in case accidental pregnancy should occur. If a couple is not mature enough to discuss this problem realistically, then it is questionable whether they are mature enough to engage in sexual relations at all.

Some of the paths available to the unmarried parents are:

*Abortion.* According to the U.S. Supreme Court, every woman in the United States has the same right to an abortion during the first six months of pregnancy as she has to any other minor surgery. In other words, during this period of time *any* pregnant woman is entitled to abortion on demand. As with all forms of surgery, whether minor or major, all abortions should be performed by qualified physicians in well-equipped facilities.

When a woman wants an abortion, this is the best way to end her unwanted pregnancy. For many, given time to analyze their own feelings, an abortion presents fewer problems than the prospect of an unwanted pregnancy or child. However, a woman should be certain that an abortion is philosophically and ethically acceptable to her. Due to religious or personal philosophical viewpoints some find abortion untenable. Abortion should be avoided if it is going to cause feelings of guilt or emotional recrimination. Regardless of her decision, a woman may still have questions. This is natural. She must make what is the best decision and then let the matter rest.

*Illegitimacy.* The prospect of keeping and raising a child out of wedlock is not pleasant to most women, although in recent years increasing numbers of unmarried women are taking this option. It is probably preferable for both mother and child over the option of marrying just "to give the child a name," then divorcing after a few years of bitter marriage.

*Marriage.* Though pregnancy is one of the most common reasons for getting married, it may be one of the poorest. A high percentage of forced marriages turn into disasters, leading to divorce or, perhaps even worse, to meaningless, bitter relationships. Unless both parties truly want to marry, it is far better to take one of the other options.

*Adoption.* In many cases adoption is the best course of action, because it should assure the child of a loving home where he is welcomed rather than resented.

*Venereal Disease.* The risk of venereal disease depends on the pattern of previous sexual relationships. If the only relationship involves a mutually faithful couple then, of course, there is no risk of infection (assuming neither is infected to start with). If a person has casual sexual contacts or has intercourse with anyone who does have such contacts, then the risk of venereal disease is greatly increased, as syphilis and gonorrhea are presently at epidemic proportions in our country.

### Psychological Considerations

*Motivation.* The individual considering sexual intercourse outside of marriage should consider his own motivations and those of his partner. Is it to be a mutual expression of love, with each truly concerned with the welfare of the other? Or, is it a case of exploitation, with one member interested only in his own sexual or ego satisfaction? The woman who allows herself to be sexually exploited repeatedly may develop negative attitudes toward sex which can adversely affect her future sexual adjustment and which may have a detrimental effect on her self-image.

*Effect on Future Marriage.* It is difficult to isolate any one factor, such as sexual activity before marriage, and then determine its exact effect on total marriage success. There are so many factors related to unhappy marriages that it is almost impossible to determine direct cause-and-effect relationships. A traditional point of view has been that premarital sex is detrimental to total marriage adjustment. But recent studies have indicated that women who enjoy full sex lives before marriage usually continue to have satisfactory sexual relationships in marriage, as determined by orgasm attainment. But, individuals with premarital sexual experience are also more likely to engage in extramarital sex. Thus, there are two significant qualifications to information of this type. One is that it does not establish any cause-and-effect relationship; it is quite possible that those

women with satisfactory premarital sexual lives were also psychologically or biologically predisposed toward sexual success. The person who is more sexually adventurous before marriage is likely to continue to be so after marriage. The other qualification is that the frequency with which the wife attains orgasm is not the only indicator of the degree of happiness of marriage. In any case, it seems that premarital sex is neither essential to nor precludes happiness in marriage. It should be noted, however, that while inexperience in sex may not contribute to marital problems, ignorance of sex certainly might.

## EXTRAMARITAL INTERCOURSE

Of no less interest today is extramarital intercourse. Although most people look upon marriage as a monogamous relationship, the simple fact is that with many couples, one or both partners are unfaithful to some extent at some time during the marriage. Views toward marital infidelity differ. Some look upon marital infidelity as a useful modifier of the marriage contract rather than necessarily a repudiation of it. The unfaithful, rather than having long-lasting extramarital love affairs or a continuous string of minor affairs, usually tend to engage in more scattered episodes lasting a relatively brief time. Such episodes may actually represent a small portion of their total married life.

Recent sex researchers examining the unfaithful tend to agree on several points. The unfaithful are not necessarily dissatisfied with their marriages or with their mates and may be relatively happily married. A minority of them, perhaps as few as one-third, seem to seek out extramarital sex for neurotic motives. Few of the unfaithful appear to feel that either they or their mates have been harmed. Some, in fact, say that their infidelity has helped to make their marriages more tolerable. However, the need for a "shot in the arm" for the marriage may imply some basic weakness in the relationship.

Infidelity, though, may not be without some risks. The faithful husband or wife, upon learning of their mate's infidelity, may respond with resentment and anger. They may feel the need for revenge. Infidelity is still singled out as one of the commonly stated causes for seeking a divorce. To avoid such consequences the unfaithful mate may seek to disguise his behavior to his spouse. On the other side, the deceived partner, not knowing of the affair, may not be perceptively affected by it.

While infidelity may remain disguised to the spouse, some husbands and wives may knowingly consider it the right of the other to develop outside relationships. The risks to the marriage of such arrangements may be somewhat greater. In spite of promises to the contrary, what assurance can the husband or wife have that the other man or woman may not present greater appeal or promise? The fear of such a possibility may tend to create jealousies if the marriage has any degree of meaning to the married partners.

As with premarital or nonmarital affairs, extramarital intercourse demands sexual responsibility. Sexual intercourse without affection or human concern for the other person is just as wrong outside of marriage as it is in marriage. Such concern should be manifest not only for the extramarital partner but also for the married mate. Or to quote Erich Fromm: "Whenever a decision or a choice is to be made concerning behavior, the (right) decision will be the one which works toward the creation of trust, confidence, and integrity in relationships. It should increase the capacity of individuals to cooperate, and enhance the sense of self-respect in the individual. Acts which create distrust, suspicion, and misunderstanding, which build barriers and destroy integrity are (wrong). They decrease the individual's sense of self-respect, and rather than producing a capacity to work together they separate people and break down the capacity for communication."*

All sexual intercourse outside of marriage must be protected by effective contraception. Knowing that the extramarital relationship will probably be temporary, the sexual partners should be determined not to exploit their partner by threat, bribe, or coercion. To do so is a betrayal of their expressed concern for each other. Extramarital intercourse may not always be satisfactory and may, for some, result in feelings of guilt and even of recrimination. For these reasons, a thorough understanding of oneself and of the extramarital partner is the only fair approach in order to avoid undesirable consequences.

## HOMOSEXUALITY

Homosexuality is the sexual attraction to members of one's own sex. Significant numbers of both males and females experience it to at least some degree during their lifetime.

While different authorities give somewhat varying figures on the incidence of homosexuality, a fair estimate based on a consensus of opinions seems to be that about 2 percent of American men and a similar percentage of American women are exclusively homosexual during adult life. A considerably larger group of both males and females (variously estimated at 25 to over 50 percent) passes through a transient period of homosexual

*L. A. Kirkendahl, *Premarital Intercourse and Interpersonal Relationships,* New York: Julian Press, 1961.

feeling and/or activity during the preadolescent or adolescent years before settling into exclusive heterosexuality.

Many homosexuals give no obvious indication of their true sexual nature. Since the opinion of the general public is still strongly against homosexuality and the chance of arrest is still great, there are valid reasons to be guarded in its display. The outward signs of homosexuality are often so subtle as to be noticed only by other homosexuals, if at all. The few male homosexuals who do make an obvious display of homosexuality may either adopt an effeminate mode of dress and action or, to attract other male homosexuals, develop a very masculine image, with strong muscular development, leather clothing, motorcycles, and similar symbols of masculinity. Female homosexuals may similarly range in appearance from very feminine to masculine.

### Homosexual Behavior Patterns

The typical pattern of homosexual relationships differs considerably between male and female homosexuals. The female tendency is to establish long-term homosexual relationships lasting for months, years, or even a lifetime. In these female relationships, one member often assumes a more dominant, masculine role, in both dress and actions, while the other member assumes the feminine role. Since there is very little open solicitation for sexual activity by lesbians, they very seldom encounter any difficulty with the law.

The typical pattern of male homosexuality is quite different. The emphasis among males is generally toward variety in sexual partners. Exclusive relationships are unusual and seldom last for any length of time. Instead, the male homosexual is often engaged in a constant, seemingly desperate, search for new sexual encounters. He spends much of his time visiting "gay" bars and similar homosexual gathering places. Because of the laws against homosexual behavior, open solicitation of partners makes the male homosexual liable to arrest. It has been estimated (Gebhard, et al. 1965) that the average number of different sexual partners of the active homosexual male is close to 200 per year. This constant search for new sexual partners exposes the male homosexual not only to the possibility of arrest, but to the venereal diseases as well. The VD rate among male homosexuals is extremely high.

Among the practices used by male homosexuals to achieve orgasm are mutual hand manipulation of the penis, oral-genital contacts, and anal-genital contacts. Techniques used in female homosexual contacts include kissing, manual and oral stimulation of the breasts, and manual or oral stimulation of the genitalia.

Some homosexuals enter into heterosexual marriages. There are several possible motivations behind these marriages. Sometimes the individual is truly bisexual and enjoys relationships with both sexes. Sometimes, the marriage is an attempt by the homosexual to live a "straight" life, thinking the marriage may solve the problem of homosexuality (it seldom does). Or marriage can be a "front" for homosexual activity, an attempt to appear socially acceptable while secretly engaging in homosexual activities. The mates in these marriages are often relatively "sexless" individuals who will make few heterosexual demands on the homosexual.

### Causes of Homosexuality

Homosexuality is thought to be the result of emotional rather than biological causes. Homosexuals are physically no different from heterosexuals; their hormone levels are no different; they do not respond to hormone treatments. Homosexuality is an emotional phenomenon, an indication of fixation or regression in emotional development. Most homosexual people do not know why they are homosexual; in fact, it may be difficult for the trained psychiatrist to know the definite cause. What may cause one person to become homosexual may not hold true for another. It is generally agreed that the influences leading to homosexuality take place during childhood. In fact, whether an individual is going to be homosexual or heterosexual is so strongly determined by the time he or she is 20 years old that without therapy the chance of a change in sexual attraction after that time is remote.

The relationship between the child and his parents is often implicated as a contributing factor in the development of homosexuality. Failure to identify with a parent of the same sex is a common finding in homosexuals. The homosexual male is often found to have had an unusually strong attachment to his mother or sister. There may be an association between the father's personality and the development of homosexuality in the son. If he is distant, unaffectionate, and generally non-nurturing the frequency of homosexuality increases. His extensive absence from the family may also have this influence. An important determining influence in the development of homosexuality can be the realization by a child that his sex was a disappointment to one or both of his parents, especially if their disappointment leads them to treat the child as if he were of the opposite sex. Occasionally a mother is found to have used a boy as a husband-substitute, showering love on him and preventing him from developing a normal attraction to girls by sheltering him from contact with them and by making derogatory remarks about girls and normal heterosexual relationships. The causes of female homosexuality are apparently more diverse and often more difficult to perceive than those of male homosexuality. It is not generally the case that girls become lesbians as a result of being too closely attached to their fathers. Actually, most girls who have close relationships with their fathers remain completely heterosexual. Lesbians typically report disruptive and unstable family backgrounds and poor relationships with either or both parents. Various emotionally traumatic experiences have generally led to a deep sense of insecurity and inadequacy, a belief that they cannot get along well with males, and strong prejudices against (or fears of) male-female relationships. It appears in some cases that the girl's parents have given her reason to fear womanhood.

Some authorities stress masochism (sexual pleasure in being abused) as an underlying cause of homosexuality. They see the entire personality structure of the homosexual as filled with an unconscious wish to suffer. Homosexuality can often fulfill this desire through arrest, imprisonment, venereal diseases, beating, and other problems which homosexuals encounter.

Isolated incidents of homosexual behavior usually result from temporary needs and drives rather than from any deeply rooted homosexual attitudes. Sexual play between children of the same sex is common and does not usually lead to any adult homosexuality. Occasional episodes of homosexual experimentation in adolescence similarly do not necessarily mean that the individuals will become homosexual adults. Even adults, when isolated from the opposite sex, such as in prison and in the military, may engage in homosexual activities without being regarded as true homosexuals. The same may be true of isolated cases of homosexual behavior while under the influence of alcohol or drugs.

### *Treatment of Homosexuality*

There is considerable controversy among psychologists, sociologists, and law enforcement officials about the most appropriate classification of homosexuality. Is it an illness, a life style alternative, a crime, or a pattern of emotional development? We see evidence of each of these explanations in our society's varied, and at times contradictory, response to the homosexual. There is interest among some psychologists for a reassessment of the present definition of homosexuality as an illness requiring treatment.

During 1972, the National Institute of Mental Health's Task Force on Homosexuality published its final report. The complexity of the question is revealed in the composition of the committee; it included social historians, sociologists, psychologists, judges, and lawyers. Clearly, the resolution of the question will not come from one area of expertise. A valid viewpoint will be reached only through further debate and research in each of these fields.

Perhaps the classification of homosexuality as either a disorder or life style should depend on the degree of satisfaction and fulfillment the individual homosexual finds in his own life. If the homosexual life is productive and personally fulfilling, there is no obvious rationale for attempting the difficult transition to heterosexualism. If, on the other hand, the individual homosexual is unhappy, anxious, depressed, or dissatisfied with his homosexuality, then it should rightfully be classified as a problem for which he should seek treatment.

As previously mentioned, homosexuality is thought to have emotional rather than physical causes. Its treatment therefore revolves around psychotherapy. Unfortunately, the rate of success in treating homosexuality has not been as great as that for many other types of emotional problems. There are two essential requirements for success. The first is that the homosexual must really want to change to a heterosexual life. The second is a therapist who understands homosexuality and has experience in its treatment. In such cases the success rate is about one-third.

Much has been said and written regarding the attitude that society and the law should assume toward homosexuality. Opinions range from those favoring strict enforcement of laws against all forms of homosexuality to total permissiveness toward homosexual behavior. It is generally agreed that punishment of the homosexual by jailing him does not change his sexual orientation or result in any subsequent change in his behavior. In fact, those who support the masochistic theory of homosexuality would say the threat of jail reinforces homosexual behavior. Unfortunately, we know very little that is helpful toward anticipating the effect of total permissiveness of homosexual behavior on the family structure. Because the family provides the major foundation for stability in a society, the implications warrant serious consideration. We feel that there must be continued legal restrictions to discourage adult homosexuals from soliciting homosexual acts from children or adolescents just as heterosexual child molestation is forbidden. Many youths spend several years wavering between homosexual and heterosexual feelings. Anything that would push them toward the homosexual life should be discouraged. We make this statement not from a moral or religious viewpoint, but rather because the homosexual life is seldom as happy or rewarding as the heterosexual life. Many of the arguments given by homosexuals in favor of their mode of living are merely a series of rationalizations to justify their unhappy lives. There is a small, but growing and vocal, movement within the United States to recognize the homosexual as a member of a minority group and to accord him or her the same civil rights as the heterosexual majority. Homosexuals currently face discrimination in housing and employment; in addition, they are frequently the targets of unfortunate stereotypes in the media and legal intrusions into their life styles. Surely, many of the homosexual's emotional problems stem from the persecution and harassment he or she suffers, and from the homosexual's resulting alienation from the mainstream of heterosexual society.

## DEVIATE SEXUAL BEHAVIOR

There are many patterns of sexual behavior which are contrary to the standards of at least some members of our society. Some forms of sexual behavior are condemned by almost everyone. Other sexual practices are condemned by some and accepted by others. For example, if a truck driver eating lunch in a truckstop café pinches the waitress, she may typically wink at him and promptly forget the incident. If a diner in a hotel dining room pinches the waitress, she will tell him to "watch it" or maybe even call the manager to talk to him. If a man pinches an attractive but unknown woman on the street, she is apt to call a policeman and have him arrested. As another example, if a man peeks through a bedroom window at a partially dressed woman, he may be arrested and convicted of a sex offense. But looking at even more scantily clothed women in a nightclub act is perfectly acceptable behavior to many members of our society. In these two examples, the major factor seems to be the context, rather than the details of the act itself.

### Forcible Rape

A detailed study of men convicted of forcible rape (Gebhard et al., 1965) indicates that they fall into several distinct groups. The most common type of rapist was found to be a man whose entire way of life includes the use of unnecessary violence. This type of rapist does not commit rape because of a lack of willing sex partners. Instead, he prefers rape to conventional sex. For this type of individual, sexual intercourse is maximally gratifying only if it is accompanied by physical violence or the serious threat of violence. This indicates a strong sadistic element in the personality of this most common type of rapist. This rapist dislikes women and gains satisfaction from punishing them. Often more violence is used than would be necessary to complete the rape. In some cases, the violence seems to substitute for sexual release or at least render the need for it less. In fact, these rapists sometimes become impotent and are unable to complete the sex attack.

A second type of rapist is the amoral delinquent. These men pay little attention to normal social controls and operate purely for their own gratification. They are not sadistic—they simply want to have intercourse, and the wishes of the female are of no importance. They are not hostile toward females, but look upon them solely as sexual objects whose role in life is to provide sexual pleasure to men.

A third type of rapist is the drunken variety. The drunk's aggression ranges from uncoordinated efforts at seduction to hostile and truly vicious behavior released by his intoxication.

A fourth type of rapist is the explosive variety. These are previously normal individuals who have suddenly snapped into a psychotic state as a result of emotional stresses. An example might be a mild-natured college student who suddenly rapes and kills.

A final category of rapist is the "innocent" male who in attempting to gain a voluntary relationship has misinterpreted the true feelings of the woman. He may be accustomed to the socially approved pattern of behavior in which a girl says "no, no" but means "yes, yes" and not realize that this particular woman really means no. Some women want to be forced into a sexual relationship. In this way an inhibited woman can enjoy sexual activity without feeling guilty about it. They tell themselves, "He made me do it." Unfortunately this excuse can have disastrous consequences if it is offered by the girl, not only to herself but to her parents, husband, or other responsible parties. Thus, the man who has attempted a "nonviolent" seduction can wind up charged with forcible rape.

### Pedophilia

Pedophilia is sexual involvement of an adult with a child. It may be either homosexual or heterosexual. Pedophilia is probably the least acceptable form of sexual behavior in our society. Since the deviation lies in the sexual immaturity of the child, the natural break-off point for classifying an act as pedophilia would be the onset of puberty, as determined by the presence or absence of secondary sexual characteristics. Since children gain sexual maturity gradually, there are, of course, many borderline cases of pedophilia.

Pedophiles are usually characterized psychologically as suffering from an arrested development (fixation) in which the offender has never grown psychosexually beyond the immature pre-pubertal stage or from a regression back to this stage of development. As a result, the great majority of sexual acts in pedophilia consist of the sex-play type found in children, such as looking, showing, fondling, and being fondled. The nature of the sexual act usually corresponds to the maturity expected at the age of the victim rather than at the age of the offender.

In the vast majority of heterosexual pedophilia cases (Mohr et al., 1964) the offender belongs to the close environment of the child. The offender is usually known to the child and the family of the child. The offenders are most commonly neighbors, family friends, or relatives. Less than one-fifth of the offenders are strangers or only casual acquaintances. In homosexual pedophilic offenses, the offender is more often a stranger.

Parents, police, and the courts can minimize the harmful effects on victims of pedophilic offenses by skillful handling of these cases. It has been found (Mohr et al., 1964) that the child is often damaged more by the events following the offense than by the offense itself. The effect on the child depends greatly on the reaction of parents and other adults upon discovery of the offense. If the parents react with obvious fear, anger, disgust, or hysteria, the child is more likely to suffer lasting effects. An additional problem is the appearance of the child as a witness in court. Interrogation and cross-examination can be far more damaging than the offense itself.

### Exhibitionism

Exhibitionism is the purposeful exposure of the penis to an unsuspecting female as a final sexual gratification without any intention of further sexual contact. This is a rather restrictive definition intended to fit a specific type of behavior pattern. The exposure must be intentional and not incidental as in the case of a drunk urinating. The object of the act must be female, either child or adult. Exposure to other males is commonly an overture to homosexual activity and is not related to this offense. The penis may be flaccid or erect and the exposure may or may not include masturbation.

The intention of the act is to arouse an

emotional expression in the victim. According to Mohr et al. (1964) it is not always clear just what the desired reaction is, since most exhibitionists cannot give a valid account of their feelings at the time of exposure. The most common intention of the exhibitionist seems to be to evoke fear and shock rather than pleasure from his victim. An amused reaction often sends the exhibitionist into a state of depression. It is important to note that the exhibitionist is not soliciting further contact with his victim. On the contrary, he is afraid of any closer contact. If a woman approaches him for sexual contact, he is likely to run away. The exhibitionist is one of the most harmless of sex offenders.

The most significant psychological finding in exhibitionists is a deep feeling of inferiority and sexual inadequacy. Thus, through exposing themselves, they seek a feeling of power, dominance, and sexual adequacy—the reaction they are striving for is shock at the large size of their sex organs. This probably explains why they often expose to children, who are more likely to be shocked than adults. In addition, this is probably the reason why an amused reaction can be so crushing.

The female victim of the exhibitionist should consider him to be a nuisance rather than a danger. She should realize that no further contact is desired and that there is no danger of rape.

### Voyeurism

A voyeur is a person who attains sexual gratification by looking at sexual objects or situations. One of the complications in studying voyeurism is the fact that almost all males have some degree of voyeuristic tendency. Society accepts such forms of voyeurism as viewing "topless" shows at bars, reading *Playboy* magazine, and watching pretty girls in brief bathing suits. The true sexual deviate is the peeper or "peeping Tom" who looks into a private room or area with the hope of seeing nude or partially nude females without their knowledge or consent. The peeper wants to see the female behaving in presumed privacy. A few peepers call attention to themselves by such actions as tapping on a window, but the vast majority of peepers try to avoid detection.

The goal of the peeper is to see an attractive female nude or engaged in some kind of sexual activity. Gebhard, et al. (1965) report that peepers prefer to watch females who are strangers to them. They do not find their sought-after satisfaction in women they know. Gebhard also reports that a substantial number of peepers masturbate while watching.

Gebhard's studies of peepers showed that the most common type are the sociosexually underdeveloped. These are men who are unusually shy with women and who have strong feelings of inferiority. Their interests are heterosexual but their overwhelming fear of being rejected keeps them from seeking normal heterosexual activity. These men develop a pattern of peeping while masturbating, which becomes a truly compulsive activity carried out over long periods of time.

Other convicted peepers include a variety of types. Some are men who quite by accident came upon the opportunity to observe a nude woman and happened to get "caught." Some were drunk at the time of their arrest. A few are mentally deficient. It is unusual for a peeper to become a rapist.

### Incest

Incest is sexual intercourse between individuals too closely related to marry legally. The relationship can be father-daughter, father-stepdaughter, mother-son, mother-stepson, or brother-sister. Incest is one of the most ancient and widespread of the sexual taboos.

Most incidents of incest develop either

within a subculture, which takes a less strict attitude toward such behavior, or as a result of the mental incompetence of one of the partners. Even in the contemporary United States, there remain certain subcultures in which incest is thought of as unfortunate, but not a grave or unexpected situation. Gebhard et al. (1965) found that incest is most common among impoverished, unintelligent, uneducated individuals living in rural surroundings. They come from a cultural background wherein sexual morality is publicly emphasized, but privately breached with impunity.

When an incestuous relationship exists within a subculture that more strictly enforces its taboo against incest, there is generally an element of alcoholism or drunkenness, low mentality, or emotional illness.

### Fetishism

Fetishism is sexual arousal from perception of inanimate objects. Fetishism is a displacement reaction, a sexual response not to a living object, but to a symbol of that object. A certain amount of fetishism is entirely normal—certain items of clothing, such as black lace panties, have so universally been equated with sex appeal that some sexual arousal from the sight of them is neither surprising nor abnormal. At what point, then, does a fetish become abnormal? Some possible criteria for fetishism are (1) the fetish item is used in masturbation; (2) the fetish item is necessary for erection for intercourse; (3) sexual partners are chosen on the basis of possession of the fetish item; (4) the fetish item is collected (through purchase or theft).

As one might expect, the most common fetish items are lingerie, such as panties, brassieres, and stockings. More surprising is the rather common fetish with shoes. There is a thriving mail-order industry offering items of fetish through advertisement in certain sex-oriented magazines. A fetishist en-counters legal problems only if he is caught stealing his fetish item.

Fetishism, like voyeurism, is thought to indicate sociosexual immaturity. The heterosexual adjustment of the fetishist is generally poor. There is often a history of other sexual deviations as well, including homosexuality, peeping, and transvestism.

### Transvestism

Transvestism is wearing the clothing of the opposite sex. The practice exists among both men and women. Transvestism usually indicates a distorted and confused sociosexual life which often, but not always, includes homosexuality. There are several possible motivations behind transvestism.

First, there is the true homosexual. He or she dresses in garments of the opposite sex as an outward sign of homosexuality (to attract persons of the same sex) and as a symbol of the wearer's preferred role in homosexual acts. In this case, the clothing has no emotional or sexual value to the wearer. It is a means to an end, not an end in itself.

Second is the true transvestite who wears the clothing of the opposite sex for the emotional or sexual gratifiction it provides. This type of transvestism is an end in itself and often involves fetishism.

Finally, there is the transsexualist. This is a man or woman who would prefer emotionally to be a member of the opposite sex. The entire life pattern of the transsexualist is generally that of a person of the opposite sex. The transvestite clothing has no sexual value in itself, but only symbolizes the social and/or sexual role to which he or she aspires. These are the persons who occasionally undergo sex-transformation surgery. It should be emphasized that their original problem is emotional, rather than physical; but in some cases the sex-role transversion is so deeply ingrained that psychiatry has been unable to change their outlook. Their trans-sexual attitudes can usually be traced back to childhood. Apparently, they had parents whose sexual roles were unclear or who were disappointed that the child was not of the opposite sex.

### Sadism and Masochism

Sadism is the attainment of sexual gratification from the infliction of cruelty upon another person. The sexual sadist is often unable to achieve orgasm without the use of some form of violence. There are both male and female sadists and heterosexual and homosexual sadism. As was mentioned in the discussion of forcible rape, sadism is often a motivating factor in rape. The rapist frequently uses more force than is necessary to complete the rape, and elements of torture are sometimes involved. Many men use sadistic cruelty in their relationships with prostitutes or even with their wives, being unable to gain satisfaction without this cruelty. Sadism can take forms which have no apparent relationship to its sexual basis. According to some authorities, such forms of violence as child-beating, wife-beating, and professional boxing have a sadistic basis.

Masochism is the attainment of sexual gratification from suffering physical pain. There are men and women who must be physically punished in order to gain sexual arousal or orgasm. The punishment often involves beating, whipping, biting, pinching, scratching, burning, and similar painful treatments.

Various psychological explanations have been offered for masochism. It has been interpreted in terms of the destructive impulses carried in the unconscious mind. It has also been related to subconscious guilt feelings from which the masochistic punishment gives temporary release.

### Bestiality

Bestiality is engaging in sexual contact with animals. Studies have shown this practice to be rather common among rural boys. Kinsey et al. (1948) reported that about 17 percent of farm boys at some time have sexual contact with animals to the point of orgasm. Yet this is one of the most taboo forms of sexual outlet. Even in rural areas, bestiality is the object of both condemnation and ridicule.

There are apparently no important psychological motivations behind typical bestiality. It is usually engaged in only as a substitute for more normal sexual relationships. The animal is generally used as an aid to masturbation, rather than as a sexual stimulus in itself.

## SEXUAL ANATOMY AND PHYSIOLOGY

Reproduction of the whole individual in humans is achieved by the sexual process —the fusion of the female sex cell, the egg (ovum), and the male sex cell, the sperm. This fertilized cell (zygote) then develops into an adult individual.

The singular significance of sexual reproduction to humans can be seen when we compare ourselves with our parents. Each fertilization of an egg by a sperm brings together new genetic combinations. No one of us is exactly identical to either of our parents. Throughout the history of man, this type of reproduction has made possible the mutations which, over thousands of years, have permitted adaptation to changing environment.

This form of reproduction contrasts with the asexual process found among more primitive plant and animal forms, where reproduction is by a mere division of a single cell or organism into two smaller, but similar, cells. Such a process involves no genetic re-combining.

### The Female Organs of Reproduction

The female genital organs are both internal and external. The internal parts of the system include the ovaries, fallopian tubes, uterus, and vagina. The external organs consist of the hymen, labia majora and minora, and clitoris.

### The Internal Organs

*Ovaries.* The production of sex cells, eggs (ova), is accomplished by the ovaries (the female gonads). They are situated deep in the pelvic cavity, one on either side of the uterus. The ovaries serve a dual function, producing both eggs and hormones. Within the ovary are many vesicles called ovarian follicles. At the time of birth, it is estimated that the ovaries contain about 400,000 immature follicles. Beginning with puberty these immature follicles mature at the rate of 1 about every 28 days and develop into a graafian follicle. Each month, usually midway between menstrual discharges, a graafian follicle ruptures and releases a mature egg. Since the reproductive life of the female extends about 35 years (ages 12 to 47) and about 1 egg per 28 days is produced (or 13 a year), only about 450 eggs out of a possible 400,000 ever mature.

The graafian follicle begins development near the center of the ovary. As it enlarges it moves toward the surface until it finally appears like a little blister on the surface. Near the midpoint between menstrual discharges it ruptures and releases the egg enclosed within it, a process called *ovulation.* Actually ovulation may occur as early as the eighth day and as late as the twentieth day. After ovulation, the blood clot is soon replaced by yellow-colored cells and is called the corpus luteum. This body remains about 14 to 15 days after which it degenerates into a fibrous body or corpus fibrosum.

*Fallopian tubes.* The fallopian tubes, or oviducts, are about 4 inches long and extend from the uterus out to the ovaries. The outer end of each tube is fringed (fimbriated), and these finger-like fringes are adjacent to each ovary. When the egg ruptures through the wall of the graafian follicle the fimbria catch the egg and pass it into the tube. The inner lining of the fallopian tube is covered with minute, hairlike structures called cilia. Once inside the fallopian tube the egg is propelled toward the uterus by the movement of the cilia and contractions in the walls of the tube. The egg has no powers of movement of its own.

Once the egg is released from the ovary, it can be fertilized by any sperm which may be present. Three to four days is normally required for the transport of the egg from the ovary through the fallopian tube to the uterus. An egg is believed to remain viable for about 24 hours, after which it begins to degenerate. Since both the egg and the sperm have a limited life, fertilization must take place within about 24 hours after ovulation if conception is to occur that month.

Usually fertilization occurs within the fallopian tube. Although the ovum is normally picked up by the fallopian tube on the same side as that on which the ovulation occurred, it has been clearly shown that eggs have, on occasion, migrated across the pelvis to be picked up by the opposite tube. Sperm present around the ovary at the time of ovulation (from a recent insemination) have been known to fertilize an egg outside of a fallopian tube in the pelvis. In the event such a fertilized egg is not picked up by a fallopian tube, it might develop in the pelvis completely outside the uterus.

*Uterus.* The uterus (womb) is a hollow, pear-shaped organ located in the pelvis. It is slightly above and behind the bladder, but in front of the rectum. It is loosely suspended in position by several ligaments. Its normal position is a forward tilt. Loosening of these ligaments due to childbearing may cause it to tilt backward. Other causes of misplacement can be pelvic diseases (such as cancer) and congenital deformity. In the adult it may be about 3 inches long and 2 inches wide. Its walls are thick and very muscular. In pregnancy it stretches to over 12 inches in length as it expands to accommodate the growing baby. The upper half of the uterus is the corpus (body), the lower half is the cervix, and the lower opening is the os.

The inner layer of the uterus, the endometrium, is richly supplied with blood vessels and glands. Following ovulation, the egg descends through the tube into the uterus. If the egg has been fertilized, it becomes embedded in the endometrium within 3 to 4 days.

*Vagina.* The vagina is a tube extending from the external genitalia to the uterus. This muscular tube is 4 to 6 inches long, and lies between the bladder and the rectum. It serves as the excretory duct for the uterus, the female organ for intercourse, and the birth canal. The mucous tissue lining it contains glands which give off a viscous secretion during sexual arousal. The rhythmic contractions of its muscular walls during the climax of intercourse produce an intensely pleasurable sensation called orgasm.

### The External Organs

*Hymen.* In young girls the external opening of the vagina may be partially closed by a membrane called the hymen. This membrane varies in size and thickness, and may remain intact until the first sexual intercourse. It may, however, be greatly reduced in size before mating as the result of the use of tampons (vaginal insertions used during menstrual discharge), by a physician as a part of a medical examination, or through participation in active sports. In a few cases it may need to be surgically cut or stretched by a physician before intercourse can be accomplished. Contrary to common belief, its rupture may not involve bleeding. Its absence should not be taken as a sign of lack of virginity.

*The Labia.* Two pairs of liplike structures surround the external opening of the vagina. The outer and larger pair are the labia majora; the inner and smaller pair are the labia minora. The space between the labia minora into which the vaginal passageway and the urethra open is the vestibule.

*Clitoris.* Directly ventral to the vestibule is a small erectile organ called the clitoris. Somewhat similar to the penis in the male, it is rarely longer than 1 inch. As with the penis, the clitoris has many nerve receptors. During sexual play it becomes erect and is the chief site of sexual excitement in the female. Unlike the penis, the clitoris does not contain the urethra.

The fatty cushion on the surface of the body directly anterior to the labia majora is the mons veneris. During the time of puberty it becomes covered with curly hair.

### Menstruation

Menstruation is the periodic discharge of blood, mucus, and cellular fragments from the uterine endometrium, occurring at more or less regular intervals (except during pregnancy and lactation) from the time of puberty to the menopause.

The onset is commonly between the twelfth and thirteenth year, but may occur as early as the tenth year or as late as the sixteenth.

The onset of the first menstruation is referred to as the menarche. Since puberty is the broad range of physical changes that occur between childhood and maturity, menarche represents just one sign of puberty.

The cessation of menstruation, menopause, commonly occurs between 45 and 50 years of age. As the menarche represents just one sign of puberty, so menopause is just one sign of the climacteric, sometimes referred to as the "change of life."

Although menstrual discharge most commonly occurs every 28 days, women vary considerably in the length of their menstrual cycles—the interval of days between discharges. Some women are known to have cycles as short as 21 days, and others as long as 38 days. In fact, with many women the length of the menstrual cycles varies from cycle to cycle.

The duration of the menstrual flow is usually 4 to 6 days, but periods ranging from 2 to 8 days in length may be considered normal for some women. For a given woman, the duration of the flow is commonly similar month after month.

Usually the blood is liquid, although clots may appear if the flow is excessive. The average amount of blood lost ranges from 25 to 60 milliliters (about 2 to 4 table-spoonsful) each menstruation. Some women report a weight gain of 1 to 3 pounds just before the beginning of menstrual discharge. This is retained water rather than fat. The average weight gain, however, is only about ¼ pound.

### The Menstrual Cycle

The cycle of events in the uterus from the beginning of one menstrual discharge until the next is called the menstrual cycle. Four distinct phases occur during the typical 28-day cycle:

1. *Proliferative or follicular phase*—after menstruation has stopped (days 3–5 of the cycle), the endometrial lining is thin. The glands contained within the endometrium are straight, short, and narrow. In the ovary the graafian follicle is maturing. During this phase, which lasts about 10 days, the follicle produces a hormone, estrogen, which causes active growth in the endometrium. The endometrium becomes quite thick and dense.

2. *Ovulatory phase*—ovulation usually occurs between days 12 and 16, but most commonly on day 14. During the day of ovulation, there is little change in the endometrium. As soon as the ovum ruptures through the graafian follicle, the remains of the follicle become a corpus luteum.

3. *Secretory or luteal phase*—under the influence of hormones given off by the corpus luteum, the endometrium continues to increase in size. The glands in the endometrium become quite enlarged and tortuous (twisted) and become very active. This phase of the cycle lasts 13 to 14 days. In the event the egg is not fertilized, the corpus luteum disintegrates. With the disintegration of the corpus luteum the hormones it has been producing decrease, and the cells and glands of the endometrium begin to die, causing the destructive phase, or menstrual flow. In the event the egg is fertilized, it becomes embedded in the thick endometrium, where it continues its development.

4. *Destructive or menstrual phase*—this phase occurs because of the death of endometrial cells. This layer has a very rich blood supply. With the tissue disintegration, both blood and cell fragments are discarded together. This phase usually lasts 4 to 6 days.

### Hormones and the Ovarian Cycle

The ovarian cycle is under the control of two sets of hormones, those from the anterior

## GONADOTROPIC HORMONES

| HORMONE | EFFECT |
| --- | --- |
| Follicle-stimulating hormone (FSH) | FSH directs the development and activity of the graafian follicles. It causes the follicle to secrete causing it to secrete estrogen. |
| Luteinizing hormone (LH) | LH helps to prolong estrogen production. It triggers ovulation, thereby initiating formation of the corpus luteum and causing it to secrete both estrogen and progesterone |
| Luteotropic hormone (LTH) | LTH, also called prolactin, helps to prolong estrogen and progesterone production by the corpus luteum. It causes milk secretion by the mammary glands after the birth of a baby |

pituitary gland, called gonadotropic hormones, and those from the ovary. The table on gonadotropic hormones names and describes the effect of the three hormones.

*Ovarian Hormones.* Under the stimulation of the gonadotropic hormones, the ovaries secrete two hormones, estrogen and progesterone.

*Estrogen* is produced by the graafian follicle before ovulation and by the corpus luteum after ovulation. It brings about the maturation of the secondary sex characteristics. These are changes that occur during puberty and include the development of the breasts, the deposition of fat around the hips, a change in hair distribution, the maturing of the reproductive tract, and the female sexual drive. Complete removal of the ovaries (oophorectomy) before puberty prevents the development of secondary sex characteristics and the sexual organs remain immature. Removal after puberty causes the cessation of menstruation and causes the body to become masculine.

Estrogen also stimulates the growth of the endometrium during the proliferative phase of the cycle. Increased amounts of estrogen through the combined action of the follicle-stimulating hormone (FSH) and the luteinizing hormone (LH) feed back to the pituitary gland causing it to slow down FSH production and speed up LH production. As seen in the figure of events in a typical menstrual cycle, this occurs during the proliferative phase.

*Progesterone* is produced by the corpus luteum. These are its effects: it prepares the endometrium for the implantation of a fertilized egg. In pregnancy, it maintains the endometrium in good condition. During pregnancy, it is produced by the corpus luteum during the first 2 to 3 months and by the placenta thereafter for the course of the pregnancy. If there is no pregnancy, increased amounts of progesterone in the blood feed back to the pituitary gland causing it to slow down LH and LTH (luteotrophin) production.

It should be apparent by now that the ovarian hormone estrogen is antagonistic to the pituitary hormone FSH. FSH initiates

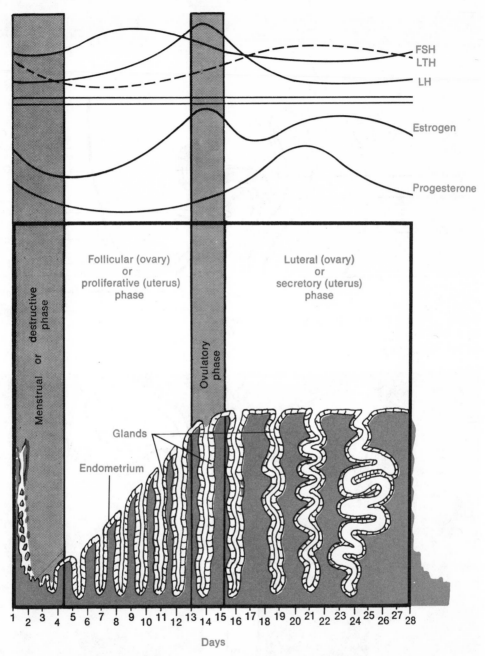

The menstrual cycle. The upper portion of the graph shows the hormone levels through the average 28-day cycle. The lower portion shows the changes in the endometrium that are occurring simultaneously in response to differing amounts and combinations of these five chemicals.

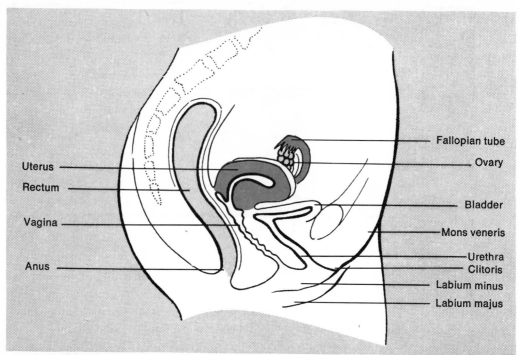

Uterus

Rectum

Vagina

Anus

Fallopian tube

Ovary

Bladder

Mons veneris

Urethra
Clitoris
Labium minus
Labium majus

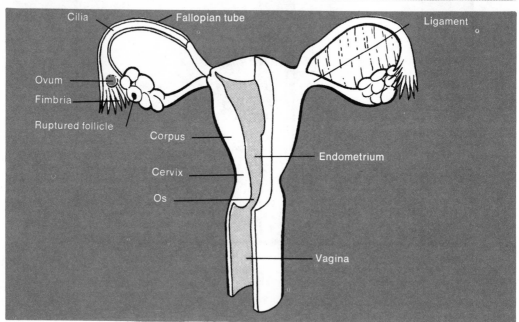

Cilia

Fallopian tube

Ligament

Ovum

Fimbria

Ruptured follicle

Corpus

Cervix

Os

Endometrium

Vagina

The female reproductive system (top).
The uterus and related organs (bottom).

292

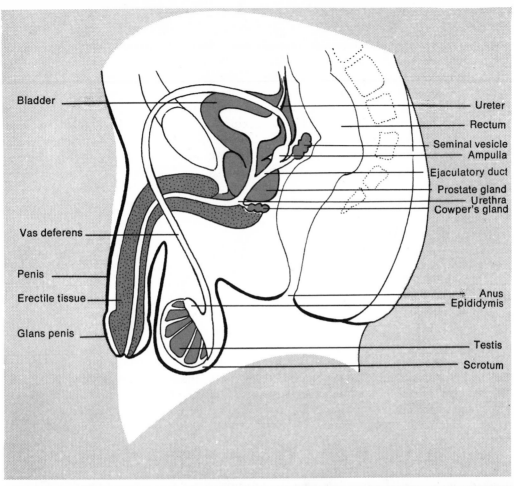

Bladder

Vas deferens

Penis

Erectile tissue

Glans penis

Ureter

Rectum

Seminal vesicle
Ampulla

Ejaculatory duct

Prostate gland
Urethra
Cowper's gland

Anus
Epididymis

Testis

Scrotum

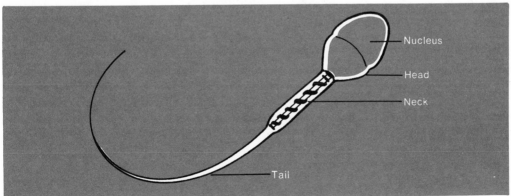

Nucleus

Head

Neck

Tail

The male reproductive system (top).
A human sperm cell (bottom).

293

and stimulates the ovary to produce estrogen, but then estrogen inhibits further FSH production. FSH cannot be abundant again until the amount of estrogen in the body drops off. Likewise, the ovarian hormone progesterone is antagonistic to the pituitary hormone LH. LH stimulates the corpus luteum in the ovary to produce progesterone, but then progesterone feeds back to the pituitary and inhibits further LH production.

This raises a question. If progesterone is essential to maintaining the endometrium, but if progesterone can be cut off (and the endometrium discharged) by the action described above, how does a pregnant woman maintain her pregnancy? The answer is that in the event an egg is fertilized, the outer cells of the developing embryo (which by this time is implanted in the endometrium) give off a new hormone which serves the same function as did LH and LTH. This new hormone, chorionic gonadotropin, serves to keep stimulating progesterone production by the corpus luteum, thus maintaining the endometrium and retaining the pregnancy. The corpus luteum continues to produce progesterone until about the thirteenth week of pregnancy. At this point the corpus luteum "gives out." The massive amounts of progesterone needed to maintain the endometrial lining for the remaining weeks of pregnancy must be supplied by the placenta.

### The Male Organs of Reproduction

The male genital organs are less complex than those of the female. The male does not need to provide for the fate of the fertilized egg. The sole task of the male genital organs is to see that sperm cells are produced and introduced into the female tract. Thus the male genital organs are more external and more obvious.

### Sperm Production

Sperm cells are produced in the testes (testicles, male gonads). Each testis is an oval gland about 1½ inches long. The testes are suspended from the under side of the body in a bag, the scrotum. Sperm production cannot occur at normal body temperatures. The scrotum allows the testes to be suspended from the body; thus their temperature is 3 to 4 degrees lower than normal body temperature, which appears to be ideal for sperm production. In cold temperatures, the thin scrotal muscles contract and pull the testes closer to the body wall; in hot temperatures the muscles relax allowing the testes to be suspended farther away from the body.

Not only do high temperatures prevent sperm production, they also may destroy sperm cells, causing infertility (temporary inability to reproduce) or even sterility (permanent inability to reproduce). Low temperatures inhibit sperm production, but do not destroy sperm cells.

During pregnancy, the testes of a male fetus are formed in the abdominal cavity. About the eighth month of pregnancy, the testes of the fetus migrate from the abdominal cavity into the scrotum. Failure of this descent to occur leads to sterility. Such a condition is called cryptorchidism (crypt meaning "hidden" and orchid meaning "testis"). This condition can be corrected surgically.

The testes serve as endocrine glands as well. The male sex hormones they produce begin to flow in large amounts at about 13 years of age. This occurs with the onset of puberty and marks the beginning of the physical changes leading to sexual maturity. Such changes (secondary sex characteristics) include the development of broad shoulders, lowered voice, the growth of hair on the face, chest and pubis, and the development of the male sex drive.

Within each testis are a great number of very small tubes called seminiferous tubules. Sperm cells are formed inside these tubules. Beginning during puberty, these sperm cells are produced without let-up for the lifetime of the male. Initial production starts slowly, then increases, until, in the sexually mature male, the incredible number of 10 to 30 billion sperm cells are produced each month. The number of sperm produced during a man's lifetime defies imagination.

Each sperm cell is microscopic in size. The length of each cell is about 50 microns (it would take 480 of them end to end to cover an inch). Each cell consists of a head, neck, body, and tail. One set of chromosomes (23) is carried in the head.

### Sperm Release

*Epididymis.* As the sperm mature they move out of the seminiferous tubules and collect in a coiled tube called the epididymis. It lies on the upper side of each testis and would be about 20 feet long if uncoiled. Here sperm are stored until released from the body by ejaculation or until they disintegrate and are reabsorbed by the tubules.

*Vas deferens.* The vas deferens is a duct about 18 inches long which carries sperm from the epididymis to the ejaculatory duct. Near the ejaculatory duct is an enlarged section called the ampulla which, like the epididymis and vas deferens, serves for the storage of sperm. During ejaculation, the walls of the deferens contract, propelling sperm cells through the duct.

*Seminal vesicles.* The seminal vesicles are a pair of glandular structures located at the base of the bladder in front of the rectum. They empty into the vas deferens to form the ejaculatory duct. During ejaculation, the vesicles contract and add their glandular secretions to the semen.

*Prostate gland.* This large organ is located directly below the bladder. It surrounds the urethra (the duct carrying urine from the bladder to the end of the penis). The ejaculatory ducts pass through each side of the prostate gland to join the urethra. During ejaculation the gland contracts to add its secretions to the semen.

In older men the prostate gland commonly enlarges so that it obstructs the urethra, thus hindering urination. This condition occurs to some degree in over half of all elderly men and can usually be corrected surgically.

*Cowper's glands.* Two small glands about the size of peas lie on either side of the urethra slightly below the prostate gland. These glands produce an alkaline secretion which precedes ejaculation and is evident at the tip of the penis as a drop of clear, sticky material. This secretion serves to remove any urine that may still be in the urethra and to lubricate the vaginal canal in intercourse.

*Penis.* The male organ for copulation is the penis. Containing the urethra, the organ is used both for urine excretion and, in the erect state, for semen ejaculation. As with other physical dimensions, its size varies. In an erect state it will average about 6 inches in length and 1 inch in diameter. Passing through the length of the penis are three columns of erectile tissue, two corpora cavernosa, side by side, and a smaller corpus spongiosum, beneath and housing the urethra. At the tip of the penis the corpus spongiosum enlarges to form the glans penis. The glans penis is richly supplied with nerve receptors, making it especially sensitive to external stimulation. A free fold of skin, called the foreskin or prepuce, overhangs the glans penis when it is relaxed. Surgical removal of the foreskin to prevent infection is known as circumcision.

The corpora of the penis are richly supplied with blood vessels, which are empty of blood when the penis is limp but engorged with blood during an erection. An erection may be brought about by physical manipulation of the penis, by sexual thoughts, by pressure from a full bladder or rectum, by wearing clothing which fits too tightly, or by any event which causes congestion of blood in the region of the penis. The inability to attain an erection is called impotence. It is not to be confused with sterility, which is either an insufficient number or total lack of sperm cells. A man may be sterile, yet fully potent.

*Semen.* Semen, or seminal fluid, is the fluid ejaculated during the male sex act. It consists of fluids from the testes, seminal vesicles, prostate gland, and Cowper's glands. The semen is a grayish-white sticky fluid, which contains 60 million to 120 million sperm per milliliter.

*Ejaculation.* Physical stimulation of the penis not only causes it to become erect, but finally results in forcible expulsion of semen, called ejaculation. Ejaculation usually results in the discharge of about 2.5 milliliters of semen. In sexual intercourse ejaculation occurs at the climax and sperm cells are placed in the vaginal canal. It is usually accompanied by a feeling of intense sexual excitement and emotional release called orgasm. Shortly after ejaculation the orgasm subsides, the penis becomes limp, and the male feels sexually satisfied.

### Male Reproductive Hormones

The male hormones are collectively called androgens. A principal androgen, called testosterone, is produced by the testes. It is formed by cells between the seminiferous tubules, called interstitial cells. It is responsible for the development of the male secondary sexual characteristics as well as the development of the reproductive organs.

Testosterone production is, in turn, under the direct control of two gonadotropic hormones from the pituitary gland, namely follicle-stimulating hormone (FSH) and interstitial-cell-stimulating hormone (ICSH). ICSH is considered analogous to luteinizing hormone (LH) produced in the female. FSH causes the seminiferous tubules to produce sperm cells. ICSH causes the testes to produce testosterone. When the amount of testosterone becomes too great, it reacts against the ICSH, which is then reduced. Testosterone can also serve to control FSH.

The absence or removal of the testes may cause hormonal deficiencies in the male. Since the production of testosterone becomes increasingly important to male sexual characteristics after the time of puberty, the effects of insufficient testosterone would depend on when the deficiency occurs. If it occurs before puberty, the male fails to develop male secondary sex characteristics. A boy who loses his testes prior to puberty is known as a eunuch. If a male loses the testes after the onset of puberty, he will retain some male secondary sex characteristics and lose others. The removal of the testes is called castration.

## SEXUAL RESPONSE

During recent years there has been a change in the climate of public opinion toward insight into human sexual response. The research and publications of Dr. Alfred Kinsey opened people's eyes to the gulf between accepted myths of sexual behavior and the actual behavior of men and women. This has been furthered greatly by the work of Masters and Johnson. Sexuality is a significant element of a person's totality and of the social setting within which that person develops. There is plainly an emerging consensus that a person's understanding of his own and his partner's sexuality is a fundamental dimension of that person's fulfillment and happiness.

### Male Sexual Response

Males can be sexually aroused by a surprising variety of stimuli. The most obvious and strongest sexual stimulus is, of course, touch.

The vast majority of men respond also to at least some additional stimuli, such as erotic literature, visual stimuli such as clothed or nude women or their pictures, erotic motion pictures, sounds of sexual activity, or just thinking about sexual activity. Any stimulus (such as a perfume or a song) that is associated with past sexual experiences can produce a sexual response.

*Response to Stimulus.* The most obvious male sexual response is erection of the penis. But there are many other manifestations of sexual arousal in the male. The heartbeat of the aroused male jumps from a normal rate of about 70 to a rate of 110 to 180 beats per minute. There is also an increase in the blood pressure and rate of breathing. There is an increase in muscular tension throughout the body, including the arms, legs, abdomen, face, and neck. There is also, of course, an increasing level of psychic excitement along with the physical changes of sexual arousal.

With prolonged sexual arousal, a few drops of preejaculatory fluid are gradually emitted from the penis. Masters and Johnson (1966) found this fluid to frequently contain live sperm cells.

The increase in sexual arousal to the point of orgasm (ejaculation) requires tactile stimulation of the penis in all but a very few males, though in a highly aroused man orgasm may follow a very brief contact. Masters and Johnson divide the male orgasm into two stages. The first stage is a period of 2 or 3 seconds before ejaculation during which the male can feel the ejaculation coming and can in no way restrain or control the process. The second stage is the actual ejaculation of semen from the penis by a series of contractions of the urethra and related muscles. The first two or three contractions expel the semen under such pressure that it may fly through the air if the penis is not within the vagina. Subsequent contractions are less forceful.

Following ejaculation the penis usually returns gradually to the flaccid stage. During the few minutes immediately after ejaculation, the glans of the penis may be painfully sensitive to any continued tactile stimulation. If the male attempts continued stimulation of his female partner or if she continues active pelvic thrusting immediately after his ejaculation, it is apt to be quite painful to him.

The minimum time interval before repeated male erection and orgasm is highly variable—among different men and for the same man at different times. It may range from minutes to days. This time interval increases with the age of the man and with general physical or emotional fatigue, but is decreased by the degree of original sexual arousal, the degree of sexual restimulation after ejaculation, and the period of sexual continence prior to the first ejaculation. If the man is young, has been without sexual release for some time, or is restimulated after ejaculation, he may be ready for further sexual intercourse within just a few minutes after ejaculation. The penis, in such cases, may not entirely lose its erection, but will still generally be too sensitive for continued thrusting for a few minutes. It should be stressed, however, that the majority of men are incapable of resumed erection for an hour or more after ejaculation.

### Female Sexual Response

Recent research indicates that women are apparently more variable in their sexual response than men. Like men, they are generally highly responsive to touch and to the sight of particular potential or actual sex partners.

Yet, unlike men, women seldom respond to pictures of attractive members of the opposite sex and in general women do respond to a narrowed range of stimuli. Their response to such stimuli as erotic movies and sounds of sexual activity are variable, but typically less intense than the responses of men to these same stimuli.

*Response to Stimuli.* The female's body responses to sexual stimulation are even more widespread than those of the male. Many organs in addition to the sexual organs are involved. The increases in heartbeat, blood pressure, and breathing rate are similar to those of the male. Bodywide muscle tension is as pronounced in females as in males. There may be widespread flushing of the skin over most of the body, which Masters and Johnson report in about 75 percent of females, but only about 25 percent of males.

The female breast response to sexual arousal may be quite definite. The nipples usually become larger, firmer, and highly sensitive to tactile stimulation. The overall size of the entire breast may increase due to engorgement of the blood vessels with extra blood.

Many changes can be observed in the female genitalia during sexual arousal. One of the first responses is the production of lubricant material by the walls of the vagina. The major labia become elevated and the minor labia become engorged with blood. The vagina becomes enlarged in both length and width. The clitoris undergoes an erection similar to that of the male penis, becoming enlarged and firm as a result of engorgement with blood. With further stimulation, there is an increased production of vaginal lubricant and the minor labia become bright red.

The period of sexual stimulation needed to bring a female to the point of orgasm varies from woman to woman, and from time to time for the same woman. The experience of most couples is that the woman needs a longer period of stimulation to achieve orgasm than does the man. But Kinsey et al. (1953) reported that the average woman can masturbate to orgasm almost as fast as the average man. They attributed the difference

in times to the fact that the masturbating woman can manipulate her sensitive areas more specifically than is possible in intercourse. This conclusion would seem to be confirmed by the finding of Masters and Johnson that the measurable physiologic intensity of female orgasm is greatest in masturbation, moderate in partner manipulation, and lowest in intercourse.

The female orgasm is more variable in intensity and duration than the male orgasm. The physical manifestations of female orgasm include a series of contractions of the vagina and uterus, roughly corresponding in number and interval to the contractions of male ejaculation. There is, of course, no emission of fluid in female orgasm. The body and facial muscles, which have become very tense by the time of orgasm, may undergo involuntary contractions and spasms.

The subjective feelings of a woman during orgasm, as reported by Masters and Johnson (1966), begin, as in the male, with a feeling that orgasm is imminent, followed by an intense sensual awareness of the pelvic region. Sensory perception of the environment is totally or almost totally suppressed. The next feeling, reported by almost every woman, was that of warmth, starting in the pelvic region and spreading throughout the body. A final feeling reported consistently was a pelvic throbbing.

The female capacity for repeated orgasm is much greater than that of the male. Many women can, with additional stimulation, repeat orgasm within a very few minutes, often until three to five or more orgasms have been achieved.

### Techniques of Intercourse

It is not the intention of this book to give detailed instructions for achieving sexual satisfaction, because attempts to follow such instructions can hinder, rather than help a couple in attaining their goal. We will, instead, give a few general comments which may or may not be useful to a particular couple. We feel that a good sexual relationship can be achieved if each partner has an adequate knowledge of sexual psychology and physiology, a positive attitude toward sex, and a concern for the sexual satisfaction of the partner. Open and uninhibited discussion of sexual desires and responses is more important than any effort to follow "rules" in a book. Each partner should feel free to tell the other which practices increase sexual enjoyment and which decrease it. An interest in sexual experimentation is good, especially after several years of marriage; but if a couple is satisfied with conventional sexual techniques, there is certainly no need to engage in the exotic and awkward positions and practices recommended by some authors.

*Preparing for Intercourse.* There is no set routine which is universally necessary or useful in preparing for intercourse. The sexual responses of individual men and women are highly variable and individual, so a technique that is ideal for one couple might have no value for another.

It is common, however, for the woman to need a longer period of stimulation before intercourse than the man in order to prevent pain upon first penetration and increase her chance of achieving orgasm. While a man can attain erection in a few seconds, a woman may need several minutes to become fully aroused and produce adequate vaginal lubrication.

Most women enjoy a few minutes of sex play before actual penetration of the vagina as it prepares them physically and psychologically for successful intercourse. Premature penetration is a complaint expressed by many women. Every woman will discover particular types of caresses and stimuli which provide her with the most intensive sensations, and

she should freely communicate this information to her partner. Among the types of sexplay which stimulate many women are kissing various parts of the body, gently fondling or tightly squeezing the breasts, lightly rubbing, pinching, pulling, sucking, or lip-biting the nipples, squeezing or lightly rubbing the buttocks, lightly stroking the insides of the thighs, and manipulation of the genital organs. Genital manipulation is mentioned last because many women prefer to become somewhat aroused before this begins. Many books recommend direct manipulation of the clitoris, but Masters and Johnson (1966) suggest that indirect clitoral manipulation by stimulating the mons area is preferred by most women as direct clitoral stimulation can be painful. There is no medical or moral reason to refrain from oral-genital contact if this is acceptable to each partner. In sexplay, any practice which is accepted and enjoyed by both partners has its place. Women who are fatigued or under emotional stress may need more than usual stimulation prior to intercourse.

One important test of whether a woman is ready for penetration of the vagina is the extent of lubrication of the vaginal walls. The fingers of the man can readily determine this. If a woman is sometimes ready for penetration before the vagina is adequately lubricated, the penis can be lubricated with one of the water-soluble vaginal jellies which are readily available in drug or grocery stores.

There are occasions when the opposite situation exists—the woman is ready for intercourse, but the man needs sexual stimulus in order to achieve erection. This situation can easily come about when a highly aroused man ejaculates before or just after penetration, leaving the woman aroused and unsatisfied. Such an event may be temporarily disappointing, but is certainly not serious. Erection can usually be restored after a few

299

minutes if the woman gently handles the penis and scrotum of the man. Few things excite a man more than having a woman touch or show interest in his sex organs. Men who are older, fatigued, or under emotional stress may need similar stimulation prior to intercourse.

*Sexual Intercourse.* There are almost innumerable different positions which have been successfully used in sexual intercourse. There has been a tendency in many of the "marriage manuals" to stress positions which place the penis in direct contact with the clitoris, based on the assumption that if the clitoris is the most sexually responsive part of the female body then it should receive direct stimulation. But the research of Masters and Johnson and the personal experience of many couples have indicated that such contact actually decreases the sexual pleasure of both the man and the woman. Sexual positions in which the clitoris receives indirect stimulation are more satisfactory for the majority of women and probably all men. Any position which allows a full penetration of the vagina by the erect penis will provide an adequate amount of indirect clitoral stimulation.

A couple who try many different positions for intercourse will probably find several which seem particularly good for them and will probably use all of these positions from time to time. Some of the more common basic positions are discussed briefly below. Each of these positions has many variations.

*The man-above position.* This is probably the most common position in use in the United States. It seems to be the most natural and comfortable position for many couples. The woman lies on her back with her legs spread apart, either drawn up or straight out. The man lies facing her, between her thighs. If guidance of the penis into the vagina is necessary, either the man or woman can give this assistance. This position allows most couples to kiss freely, but is more restrictive of breast manipulation than some of the other positions.

*The woman-above position.* In this common position, the man lies on his back while the woman lies above and facing him. Some couples roll from the man-above position to the woman-above position, or vice versa. Some women can achieve orgasm more easily in the woman-above position by controlling the pelvic thrusts while the man lies more or less passively.

*Face-to-face side positions.* There are many of these positions. They offer several advantages. Neither partner must support the weight of the other, so they are good for prolonged sexual connections. Kissing is easy, as is breast manipulation or any other type of caress desired.

*Rear-entry positions.* There are several different rear entry positions. The woman may lie on her side or face down or may kneel on her hands and knees. In any case, the man approaches from behind, passing his erect penis between her legs and into her vagina. These positions are often enjoyed by thin people, but seldom by heavier persons as it may be difficult or impossible for them to penetrate the penis deeply enough into the vagina. These positions facilitate breast manipulation, but, of course, kissing is more difficult.

*Other positions.* The variety of sexual positions is limited only by the imagination and agility of the couple. Many couples occasionally enjoy a more unusual position, for variety in their lovemaking. The sitting positions are enjoyed by some couples. In one of these, the man lies on his back while the woman sits astride him, feet forward. This position allows very deep vaginal penetration. In other sitting positions, the man may sit on a chair or the edge of a bed while the woman sits astride him. Some couples even enjoy intercourse while standing up, using front or rear entry. There is no reason why any position which affords mutual pleasure should not be used.

After the penis has been fully inserted into the vagina, a man is often at the very peak of his sexual arousal and near orgasm. In order to prevent premature ejaculation, many couples find it desirable to lie together quietly for a short time before beginning the pelvic thrusts of intercourse. By lying quietly at this time and any subsequent time that orgasm seems near, many men can delay ejaculation for some time without loss of erection.

Certain marriage manuals place a great emphasis on the importance of simultaneous orgasm. We feel that simultaneous orgasm is not an important goal in sexual intercourse and that concentration of efforts toward this goal may decrease the pleasure received by each partner, rather than increase it. Since the orgasm of the male is practically assured (except in impotence, as discussed later), all efforts should be concentrated toward helping the woman achieve orgasm.

Women vary in the ease with which they can achieve orgasm. The difference may be either physical or psychological, but it is very real. Every study made has shown that significant numbers of women can achieve orgasm only with difficulty, if at all. Kinsey's classic study (Kinsey et al., 1953) indicated that after 5 years of marriage, only 40 percent of wives reached orgasm over 90 percent of the time, and that 17 percent of wives never reached orgasm. After 20 years of marriage, 11 percent of wives still had failed to reach orgasm in intercourse. More recent studies indicate that the young women of today are more successful in achieving orgasm than

those of 1953, but that many women still reach orgasm only with difficulty.

The majority of women do not expect to achieve orgasm with every intercourse. But the woman who reaches orgasm too infrequently is likely to lose her enthusiasm for sex. The man who wants to keep his sexual relationship happy and vigorous should try to satisfy his partner as often as possible.

There is no single pattern of orgasm which is best for every couple, though many couples find, through experimentation, a pattern which seems best for them. Many couples develop a pattern whereby the woman reaches one or more orgasms first, followed by the ejaculation of the man. In other couples, the woman finds that the stimulus of the penis throbbing in ejaculation is just what she needs to push her to orgasm.

### Oral and Anal Sex

Many couples greatly enjoy oral and anal sex practices, whereas other couples never even experiment with them, perhaps feeling they might be unhealthy, abnormal, or immoral. Actually, there is no medical or moral reason to avoid oral or anal sex, and many couples or individuals who try these practices enjoy them and at least occasionally include them in their lovemaking.

Oral and anal sex are useful in adding variety and new heights of excitement to lovemaking and in stimulating a less responsive sex partner. Oral practices include fellatio (oral stimulation of the penis), cunnilingus (oral stimulation of the female organs), and "69" (combination of fellatio and cunnilingus). Oral sex may be a preliminary to genital coitus or may proceed to orgasm by either or both partners.

Anal practices include insertion of a finger into the anus of either partner, prior to or during coitus, and anal intercourse in which the penis is inserted into the female's anus (pederasty). In the latter practice certain precautions are necessary. It is usually advisable to lubricate the penis with a vaginal jelly to prevent tearing the delicate anal tissues. Many physicians also recommend washing the penis if vaginal intercourse is to follow anal penetration to avoid possible vaginal infection with rectal bacteria. As in oral sex, anal sex may progress to orgasm or lead to vaginal coitus.

Oral and anal stimulation are especially useful to middle-aged and older couples. A man reaches his peak of sexual desire and capacity at about age 18 and gradually declines thereafter, while a woman may not reach her peak of sexual desire until about the ages of 35 to 45. Thus, in middle age the desire of the woman may exceed the capacity of the man to fulfill, especially if he is several years older than her. In such cases, the woman's skillful oral and hand stimulation of the man's penis, scrotum, and anus will often assist him in attaining and maintaining an erection at times when he might not otherwise.

### Frequency of Intercourse

The frequency of sexual intercourse is a source of conflict in many relationships. In almost any marriage, there will be times when one partner would like sexual intercourse and the other partner is either not interested or incapable of responding. Such situations may place a great burden on the marital relationship unless both partners are understanding and tolerant. Some of the marriage manuals have portrayed the ideal marriage as being a continuous sexual spree with each orgasm coming bigger and better than the previous one. In reality, sex is only a part of the total marriage relationship, and the success of a couple's sexual relationship is often a reflection of their total marital relationship.

It is very difficult to make direct comparisons of the basic sex drive of men and women, due to the different nature of these drives. In a man, the accumulation of fluids within the seminal vesicles and prostate gland acts as an internal sexual stimulus. The longer these fluids build up, the greater becomes the need for their release. The man who has not ejaculated for an extended period of time may experience a level of sexual tension seldom, if ever, known by a woman. Yet, the sexually awakened woman does experience compelling sexual drives which demand release, particularly if she becomes sexually aroused, with blood engorging her sex organs. In past years, when "nice" women were not really expected to enjoy sexual intercourse, it was assumed that the sexual desire of women was much less than that of men. Since cultural and psychological factors so greatly influence the sex drive of women, it seems likely that the average woman of the nineteenth century was sexually more passive than the average woman of today.

Various research projects have indicated that the average husband would like to engage in intercourse a little more often than would his wife. Of course, in a particular couple there may be a great similarity in sexual desire or a very great difference, with either the man or his wife having the greater desire.

There is no particular frequency of intercourse which is most desirable. Among happily married and physically healthy couples, the frequency of intercourse ranges from once a month or less to several times a day. The average frequency, though it should not be interpreted as a goal for an individual couple, is between two and three times a week. A young, recently married couple is likely to exceed this frequency, whereas an older couple would probably not engage in intercourse that often. According to Kinsey et al. (1948), the average frequency for 60-year-old men is about once every three weeks.

If disagreement over frequency of intercourse is creating conflict within a marriage, each partner should try to evaluate the situation, rather than just fighting about it. Let us first consider the more likely situation—a couple wherein the man desires intercourse more often than does the woman. First, there are several things the man should ask himself: Am I keeping myself physically attractive? Am I pleasant and loving with my wife at all times, or just in bed? (Women generally need much more psychological preparation for sex than do men.) Do I spend enough time in precoital sex-play? Do I seriously try to help her reach orgasm as often as possible? (The woman who is too often disappointed soon learns to avoid frustration by avoiding sex.) Are the conditions right for privacy and freedom from interruption during intercourse? Is she inhibited by fear of pregnancy? (Many women fail to respond because either consciously or subconsciously they fear pregnancy. A change in contraceptive method may be helpful.) Am I expecting too much of her? Few men can appreciate the amount of energy the modern woman must spend on childcare, housework, community activities, and perhaps a career. There is often just too little energy left for sexual activity. In the past, the tired woman often took a passive role in sexual intercourse, but today many men expect their wives to take an active part. The woman, herself, may expect to reach orgasm if she engages in intercourse and may be reluctant to begin intercourse if she feels she lacks the energy to achieve orgasm.

The woman in this situation might ask a few questions of herself: Why do I refuse him? Am I trying to punish him for something which is beyond his control? Are my attitudes toward sex positive and healthy? Would I be more confident with another contraceptive method? Have I honestly explained to him why I sometimes refuse him? When I am tired, do I offer to take a passive role in intercourse to relieve his sexual tension?

The situation in which the woman wants intercourse more often than the man is more difficult, since the man must attain an erection and generally take a fairly active role in order to satisfy her. Again, the woman might consider possible reasons for his reluctance. Does she try to be sexually appealing? Are her demands excessive? As a man grows older, his biological capacity for sex diminishes. The man in this situation is in a particularly bad emotional position. He is faced with the demands and perhaps derision of his wife, in addition to his own feelings of inadequacy. One of the most important needs of the male ego is a sense of sexual adequacy. This man may easily develop anxieties which will increase his sexual problems. The man who feels sexually inadequate is often reluctant to make any attempt at intercourse, for fear of impotence. He avoids the risk of ego-damaging impotence by avoiding sex. This situation becomes worse with the passage of time, so prompt efforts should be made to remedy it. A physician should be first consulted to rule out the possibility of any physical cause. If no physical cause is found (most impotence is psychological), then a qualified marriage counselor should be consulted.

### Penis Anxieties

Many young men suffer needless anxiety regarding the size of their penis. Some worry that it may be too small to satisfy a woman; some fear that it may be too large to be accommodated by the vagina. All of these fears are made needless by the nature of the vagina and of female sexual sensitivity. The size of the penis and whether or not it is circumcised has nothing to do with the sexual satisfaction of the man himself or of the woman. Sexual technique and experience are the important things.

The diameter of the vagina stretches to fit the size of the penis. Even after several babies have been born, the vagina usually remains small enough in diameter to tightly contain even the smallest penis. On the other hand, the vagina is capable of stretching enough to allow the passage of a baby, so a large penis will certainly create no problem.

As far as the length of the penis is concerned, there are very few sensory receptors in the deeper part of the vagina. These receptors are concentrated in the clitoris and labia and outer vagina. As a result, it is difficult or impossible for a woman to feel the difference between a long penis and a short one.

Some young men even worry about the fact that their penis seems to curve (most of them do curve) or have some other irregularity. Every man should realize that the size or shape of the penis is of negligible importance in sexual intercourse.

### Sex in Menstruation, Pregnancy, and Old Age

There is no important medical reason for refraining from sexual intercourse during menstruation. Most couples do, however, avoid intercourse during the 2 days of heaviest flow for aesthetic or practical reasons. But during the 2 or 3 days of limited flow which follow, intercourse may be enjoyed by both the man and the woman. Some women seem to especially enjoy intercourse at this time due perhaps to their hormone levels or the freedom from fear of pregnancy.

Sexual intercourse can usually be continued in pregnancy until about 4 weeks before delivery, unless some condition arises

which causes the physician to recommend against it. Some women find their sexual drive increased during pregnancy, while others find a decrease. Intercourse should definitely be discontinued as soon as it causes the woman any pain or discomfort. Intercourse is usually prohibited for 6 to 8 weeks after delivery to allow for adequate healing of the sexual organs. During the period before and after delivery when intercourse is prohibited, an understanding wife may wish to provide her husband with periodic sexual release by petting him to orgasm.

Old age need be no barrier to an active sexual life and, according to Kinsey et al. (1948, 1953) and Masters and Johnson (1966), many older persons continue to be sexually active, though the frequency of activity drops considerably. Those individuals who were most sexually active in their youth are generally more active in their old age. In both sexes, a continuity of sexual activity is important. It is easier to remain sexually active than it is to resume sexual activity after a long period without it.

## COMMON SEXUAL PROBLEMS

The sexual relationships and even the marriages of many couples are damaged or destroyed by problems of sexual function. Most of these problems are actually of psychological origin and can be overcome through mutual understanding, open communication, factual knowledge, and, if necessary, professional help. In this section, we will consider a few of the more common sexual dysfunctions.

### Female Orgasmic Dysfunction

The variety of problems related and unrelated to female sexual function has long been known, and incorrectly, as "frigidity." The term has been used as a catch-all. At one extreme it describes the woman who, though responsive, never displays or feels any sexual interest or arousal. At the other extreme it could describe the woman who does not attain orgasm on every occasion of intercourse, or the woman who does not respond instantly to a man's sexual advances. Frigidity has been used both for the woman who is rarely sexually aroused as well as for the woman who is easily aroused, but seldom or never to the point of orgasm.

Masters and Johnson have thus discarded the rather meaningless word frigidity for the more descriptive phrase *female orgasmic dysfunction.* According to them, the phrase should be used for the woman who is not able to achieve orgasm in her sexual response.

The nonorgasmic woman can be placed in one of two categories. One, the woman who has never achieved an orgasm in her life through any method of sexual stimulation, suffers from *primary orgasmic dysfunction.* Two, the woman who has experienced at least one orgasm in her life (by coitus, masturbation, or some other form of sexual stimulation), but who no longer experiences orgasm, suffers from *situational orgasmic dysfunction.*

When orgasmic dysfunction seems to be a problem, the first step taken should be a physical examination to rule out any physical cause of interference with sexual pleasure. While such cases are not common, a physical problem such as a tough, intact hymen can make intercourse painful or impossible. Such physical problems can usually be easily corrected. Another problem with which a physician can help is fear of pregnancy. Many women are inhibited in their sexual responses by conscious or unconscious fear of pregnancy. The change to a birth control method in which a woman has greater confidence can often improve her sexual responsiveness.

Many women (and men as well) suffer from long-term residual sexual inhibitions as carryovers from childhood indoctrination by parents, religious groups, and even other children that sexual pleasure is in some way wrong or immoral. If such inhibitions are deeply ingrained into the personality, professional counseling may be necessary.

But many women who do not suffer from obvious conflicts still do not respond adequately. For example, a woman may find that she is "turned off" by her husband, yet is highly "turned on" by other men. In such a case, the cause must lie either in some trait or traits of the man to which she does not respond, or in the quality of the total relationship between them. Certainly, when the relationship between a man and a woman starts to deteriorate, the sexual responsiveness of the woman toward that man is often quickly extinguished.

Many men are highly proficient at turning off their partner. The most common complaint of women regarding men is "lack of consideration." This blanket term can include anything from premature ejaculation to body odor. The male's role in turning on or off women may be roughly divided into two categories. The first is that the very fact of being male arouses a host of positive and negative emotional reactions in a woman. Whether the positive or negative reactions prevail depends on the characteristics of the man in relation to the past experiences of the woman. The second category is the behavior of the man, including both what he does and does not do.

In considering the first category (maleness), we must be aware of the important aspects of the father-daughter relationship. When a small girl starts to turn away from her mother as her most important love object and, so to speak, falls in love with her father, the father's attitude and behavior toward his daughter can be crucial. To give a little girl a good start toward healthy womanhood, a father must be able to show affection for his child, high regard for her femininity, and the appropriate behavior expected of a mature parent.

A woman's indifference toward a man may sometimes be attributed to his failure to live up to her expectations (whether realistic or not) of what a man should be. These expectations are largely shaped through positive and negative experiences with various males, especially those in her family as she grows up.

Another common complaint of women is that "the romance is gone." The various media of communications have led many women to believe that marriage should be all youth, beauty, glamour, and excitement. This picture does not match well with the man who comes home from work wanting his dinner, the newspaper, and his favorite television program. He wants to go to bed, have intercourse, roll over, and go to sleep. As a result, many women complain of a lack of intimacy, feeling used and useless, and resent being merely a sexual object. The outcome is that they are no longer sexually responsive (at least to that man). Their anger and resentment is expressed in withdrawal.

### Impotence and Premature Ejaculation

Impotence is the inability to attain or maintain erection of the penis. Premature ejaculation is male orgasm and loss of erection before the reasonable sexual desires of the female are satisifed. Impotence and premature ejaculation are the most common forms of male sexual dysfunction. These problems are often related to one another and, according to some definitions, premature ejaculation is a form of impotence.

Impotence, like frigidity, is generally the result of emotional, rather than physical causes. In cases of severe or persistent impotence, however, a physical examination should be obtained to rule out possible physical causes.

Impotence exists in all degrees. In its most severe form, called primary impotence, the penis never, under any circumstances, becomes erect nor has it ever, during the life of the man. This is the form of impotence that is most likely to have an organic (physical) cause. This is especially true if the penis is never erect during the rapid eye movement (REM) or dream phase of sleep or on awakening from REM sleep.

Much more common is a transient or secondary form of impotence in which erection sometimes occurs, though not necessarily when intercourse is desired, or ceases to occur in a formerly potent male. This form of impotence is almost always the result of emotional factors. There are probably few men who escape having at least a few episodes of transient impotence at some time during their lives. Guilt, anger, conflict, anxiety, jealousy, depression, fear, and hostility are among the emotions that commonly result in impotence.

The incidence of transient impotence increases with age, though younger men are certainly not immune from this problem. The first incident of impotence usually occurs during a period of emotional stress, and is especially likely to occur following heavy drinking. Any kind of emotional problem may be involved, but job problems and love conflicts are very common causes of transient impotence. Also, fatigue must not be overlooked as a cause of temporary impotence. Other frequent causes of impotence are anxiety growing out of fear of sex as something bad and immoral which may be punished (a common problem in extramarital affairs); feelings of inadequacy as a man; and excessive fear of or hostility toward women.

The reaction of a woman to a man's impotence will greatly influence his success in that and future attempts at intercourse. Her immediate feelings may be those of hurt and rejection and her natural impulse may be to hurt in return, perhaps making fun of the man, ridiculing him, or accusing him of having an affair. Such a reaction will produce enough feeling of anxiety and inadequacy to practically insure that the next attempt at intercourse will also fail. On the other hand, a reassuring female response, perhaps including gentle hand or oral stimulation of the male organs, may result in immediate potency or in any case will not interfere with future efforts at lovemaking.

Premature ejaculation, while seeming to be just the opposite of impotence, may have similar emotional causes. Even fewer men are likely to get through life without ever experiencing an incident of premature ejaculation. In fact, under certain conditions, premature ejaculation must be considered an entirely normal and predictable event. For example, it is unrealistic to expect a young man who has been without sexual release for many days to withhold ejaculation while a woman thrusts vigorously in efforts to achieve her own orgasm. Similarly, the first attempt at intercourse with a new and highly exciting woman may be normally expected to result in premature ejaculation.

How do we define premature? Certainly, ejaculation before penetration of the vagina is premature, as is ejaculation immediately thereafter. But what about ejaculation after the woman has had one orgasm when she would really like to have three? What about the woman who takes an hour to reach orgasm? Obviously, there can be no clear-cut definition of premature ejaculation.

How do you distinguish "normal" premature ejaculation from the "problem" variety? The distinction here is that if a man has regular and frequent intercourse with the same woman, and it often ends in premature ejaculation, it is a problem. In such a case there may be underlying psychological causes, which may be quite similar to those of impotence. Examples: hostility toward the woman, in which premature ejaculation is used to deny her sexual satisfaction; guilt about sex, in which premature ejaculation is used to "get it over with"; feelings of sexual inadequacy, in which there is a rush to prove that the penis is still working; fear; and love conflicts.

A variety of solutions for the problem of premature ejaculation are available. Of prime importance, as in impotence, is for the woman to minimize the problem, rather than making a big issue of it. If the premature ejaculation is of one of the "normal" types described, then the male is likely to be young enough and highly enough aroused that a second erection will soon follow the first and, with seminal pressure reduced, prolonged intercourse should be possible. Regular sex partners can learn to delay male orgasm by both holding very still when premature ejaculation threatens. This is especially useful just after penetration when premature ejaculation is most likely to occur. Some doctors recommend that a topical anesthetic ointment be applied over the glans (head) of the penis to delay ejaculation. The stimulus to the penis can similarly be reduced by wearing a condom (rubber). Masters and Johnson, in *Human Sexual Inadequacy,* recommend an "exercise" for premature ejaculation in which the woman's hand stimulates the male penis almost to the point of orgasm, then, with the thumb and forefinger, tightly squeezes the shaft of the penis about an inch below the glans. Done repeatedly, this often solves long-term problems of premature ejaculation. A more basic approach is psychotherapy. Since the more persistent cases of premature ejaculation are of psychological origin, this is sometimes the only method of treatment that can produce lasting results.

# 15
# A Personal and Social Institution

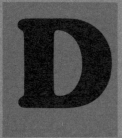

**D**espite a liberalization of attitudes toward sex outside of marriage, the majority of individuals today still find the most satisfactory sexual expression and personal happiness within a good marriage. Over 90 percent of all men and women in the United States eventually marry. Many of these find great happiness in their marriages; others find misery. What makes the difference? Individual readiness for marriage and choice of a mate greatly influence the chance of attaining happiness in marriage.

## DECIDING TO MARRY

Success in marriage demands considerable emotional strength and maturity. Many marriage failures can be traced to inadequate emotional development of one or both of the partners.

### Age at Marriage

The age at which a person marries is influenced greatly by such individual factors as educational goals, military duty, and social and cultural background. The national average age at the first marriage is just over 23 years of age for men and just under 21 years for women. Many people, girls in particular, feel pushed to marry at a fairly early age to avoid getting "left out" and becoming "old maids." Such fear is not warranted because at any age, numerous individuals eligible for marriage will be found. In fact, some of the best marriage prospects delay marriage for several years in order to reach educational or career goals.

Many studies have shown that the average happiness level in marriage increases with the age of the couple at the time of marriage. Emotional conflict, sexual maladjustment, money problems, in-law trouble, and divorce are all much more common among those couples who marry in their teens. Marriages where the husband was in his teens are particularly unhappy.

One of the sources of problems with young marriages is that many people greatly change their value systems and life-styles sometime between the ages of 16 and 22. During this period one's interests, tastes, ideals, standards, and goals usually undergo a complete change. If people marry before this change, there is a strong possibility that they will have little in common a few years later.

A related problem is that early marriage often interferes with the development of a mature philosophy. There is a tendency for the intellectual growth of an individual to stop at the time of his marriage. This can be prevented, of course, but many young married people fall into a deep philosophical and intellectual rut from which they never escape.

### Emotional Maturity

The emotional demands of marriage are much greater than those a couple experiences during dating. Thus, an important requirement for marriage is emotional maturity. This generally increases with age, but some individuals remain emotionally adolescent even though they have legally become adults.

Before marriage, a person should be as free as possible of emotional maladjustments, such as moodiness, jealousy, anxiety, depression, and insecurity. Their presence in a marriage can be disastrous. A person who is subject to such maladjustment should seek qualified professional counsel.

The truly mature person has skill in establishing and maintaining good interpersonal relationships. He recognizes the needs of others and is willing to assume some responsibility for meeting these needs. Each partner in a marriage must have such a concern for the other if happiness is to result.

### Social Maturity

Social maturity develops through social interaction. Before marriage, social maturity should be built through dating many different individuals. This gives a better basis for the selection of a marriage partner and helps satisfy social curiosity. The person whose dating is more restricted may later,

after marriage, feel he has missed something and try to compensate through extramarital affairs.

Many people feel a need for a period of single, independent life before marriage. They want a time of freedom between the bondage of childhood and the bondage of marriage. Most people appreciate this freedom to a point, after which they feel ready for marriage. A few find this freedom permanently satisfying and prefer not to marry. There is no reason why these people should feel any obligation to themselves or to society to marry.

### Financial Resources

Money is conceded by many couples to be a source of conflict, even in successful marriages. The minimum amount of money a couple needs to live on is highly variable. Most young couples enter marriage without great amounts of money. But if the husband is to be a student, there must be a careful evaluation of the marriage situation to avoid the unfortunate situation of an education terminated for financial reasons.

Often the parents of student couples offer some financial help. But the couple should evaluate this possibility in terms of their sense of independence. If such help is going to be a source of conflict, then some other financial arrangement must be developed. If the couple is to rely on the earnings of the wife, then obviously it is important that a highly reliable method of contraception be used. A pregnancy in this situation would be a serious financial and emotional burden.

Because few couples ever have what they consider to be enough money, a couple's attitude toward money and how to use it is likely to be more important than the size of the paycheck. A given amount of spendable income for one couple may be sufficient to meet common interests, while the next couple

309

may be suing for divorce because the same amount of money is not enough. The relation of income to happiness must be relative to expectations. When a couple feels committed to an occupational field where income is lower, they can be happy if they are content to live on that level. If, however, their expectations run higher than income, their marriage may be troubled.

### Selecting for Happiness

Your chances of a happy marriage are determined by your own personal traits, those of your partner, and how these traits act upon each other. Let us consider, then, some of the traits to look for in a potential mate. Right away, let us dispel the notion of "the one and only" or the "marriage made in heaven." For every person there are thousands of potentially good mates. If the person you might be considering for marriage seems to have a serious deficiency in some respect, just keep looking. On the other hand, if no one seems to fit your ideal for marriage, you might well be overcritical or just not ready for marriage.

### Personality

The personality of your marriage partner can make the difference between your own happiness and misery. Traits which help produce happiness in marriage include the ability to adjust to changes in conditions, optimism, a sense of humor, an honest concern for the needs of others, and a sense of ethics.

### Hereditary Traits

Some individuals carry obvious hereditary defects. Others seem perfectly normal, but come from families in which such defects are known to occur. These individuals may or may not be carrying undesirable hidden genes. If there is any question regarding the possibility of transmitting defective genes, it is wise to seek genetic counseling, either from a physician or a specially trained genetic counselor recommended by a physician. Any decision to marry and have children, marry and not have children, or not to marry should be based upon such advice and not on the advice of uninformed, but well-meaning, friends and relatives.

### Genuine Mutual Love

You might be surprised to find that love is not listed first among the major criteria for selecting a marriage partner. This, of course, is not because we do not consider it of prime importance, but rather because it is a difficult thing to evaluate. The distinction between genuine love and infatuation is not always clear. Infatuation is frequently associated with immaturity, a "puppy love." It is a kind of substitute for love until a person has the capacity to love someone fully and deeply. It tends to involve sexual attraction more than personality attraction. Infatuation is unrealistic, a fantasy. The object of the infatuation is seen as a "dream mate," lacking any undesirable traits. It usually wears off quickly; yet it may, with time, develop into mature love.

A person truly in love is concerned with his loved one's happiness and well-being. He is tender, protecting, and loyal. He is willing to sacrifice some of his own pleasures in order to bring pleasure to his loved one. There is a desire to share ideas, emotions, goals, and experiences. Love continues to grow with the passage of time.

There should definitely be a strong sexual attraction between any persons considering marriage. It would be an unusual couple who would want to marry in the absence of a sexual attraction. However, many people mistake sexual attraction for love, when it is actually just a part of love. A couple can have a very good sexual relationship without loving each other, but such a relationship would make a poor basis for a happy marriage.

Now let's get back to the point about love as a factor in deciding to marry. Obviously, it is difficult to tell you what love is, though we have tried to demonstrate what love is not. Above all else, true mature love is the one factor that will inspire a couple to look at all the factors conducive to a happy marriage with care, and with respect for themselves and each other.

### Agreement on Parenthood

Any couple considering marriage should reveal their feelings about having children. Ideally, they should agree on whether they want children and, if so, how many. It is always unfortunate when a person who wants children marries one who would rather remain childless. Automatically, one or the other of them is destined to be unhappy. If there is serious disagreement on this matter, it would be well for each individual to look for another mate.

If neither person wants children, there is no reason to feel guilty about a decision to remain childless. Studies have shown that children are not essential to happiness. In fact, they have been shown to place additional strain on an already unhappy marriage. A couple need feel no obligation to themselves or to society to produce children.

### Similarity in Background

It is important for any couple considering marriage to take a critical, objective look at their differences in personality and family background. These differences may be minor and insignificant or major and have a great bearing on the marriage. Many studies have shown that the more similarities between two individuals, the greater their chances of marital success. Significant differences may involve age, nationality or race, economic status, education, intelligence, religion, or previous marital status. Most marriages can be successful despite these differences, if the

couple is willing to work out the special problems involved.

*Age.* When there is a wide difference in age, the individual must examine why he wants to marry a person considerably older or younger than himself. Is it the desire for immediate economic security? Is it a feeling of flattery at commanding the attention of a more mature or more youthful person? Is the older person seen as a "father" or "mother" figure? Does the older person need to dominate or the younger to be dominated? Is it just an infatuation? On the average, marriages are happiest when the man and woman are within a few years of each other in age. However, if the marriage with a wide age gap fulfills a great need for each person, then such a marriage may also be happy.

*Race and Nationality.* Marriage between members of different races or nationalities face the most difficult problems of any type of mixed marriage. Not only can there be problems within the marriage, but the couple may experience resentment and prejudice from family members and unenlightened members of society.

The internal problems in these marriages may revolve around customs, standards, and points of view. For example, the attitudes toward women and their rights, duties, and status may be quite different. Family patterns of authority and the role expected of each member may conflict. Attitudes on raising children and care of elderly relatives may be another area of disagreement. These are not always problems in mixed marriages, but such topics should be discussed objectively before any marriage between different races or nationalities takes place.

The problems caused by prejudices of family members and society are particularly frustrating, because they should not exist in a democratic society. The source of many of these problems is the ethnocentric attitude of groups which guard their ethnic heritage to excess and often sincerely believe in the supremacy of their group over all others. The elders of some of these groups encourage their youth to maintain a distance from outsiders, to continue to respect the traditions and customs of the group, and to marry within the group. The young man or woman who marries outside the group may experience total rejection by even immediate family members.

Other problems may arise in finding housing and employment, especially in black-white marriages. There may even be problems in finding friends who will fully accept both partners. The amount of social prejudice felt by the interracial couple will vary from city to city and with the part of the country. Interracial couples may find their best acceptance today in college towns, where the general attitude is usually more enlightened and liberal than in many other places.

It is likely that the number of interracial marriages will continue to increase, if the trends of the past few years can be projected into the future. The breakdown of social prejudices is painfully slow, but it can be hoped that the need for a discussion such as this will eventually be a thing of the past.

*Economic Status.* Even though our society has always claimed that one of its goals is social equality regardless of economic status, patterns of behavior do vary greatly with the economic status. Behavior that is "correct" at one economic level may meet with disapproval at another level. Attitudes toward authority, freedom, ethics, education, and other values may differ. Marriage of individuals of different economic backgrounds may require some adjustment of these attitudes.

A problem area in a marriage involving different economic backgrounds may be in-law relationships. The wealthier set of in-laws may not entirely accept the son-in-law or daughter-in-law who comes from a less affluent background.

Other problems can arise when a girl who has been raised in affluence marries a young man of limited income. This couple has two choices. One is to accept financial aid from the girl's family (if it is offered), which may be psychologically damaging to the young man; or they can live within their income, which may require a difficult adjustment for the girl, if her values are materialistic. There may be no problem at all, but this is another area that should be discussed and agreed upon before marriage.

*Education.* Even with the increasing educational opportunities available today, it is not unusual for a couple to have a wide difference in level of education. Along with more education usually goes a change in reading tastes, personal goals, and social sophistication. A better educated partner may be interested in entirely different recreational activities. Compatibility in marriage is largely a matter of common interests. Differently educated persons are likely to have few common interests. There is a tendency for boredom to develop and for each to go increasingly his own way. Yet, there are individuals who, though short on formal education, have horizons that are wider than many college graduates who confine their interests to a specialized major field of study.

*Intelligence.* Perhaps a similarity in level of intelligence is even more important than similarity in level of education. In marriages in which there is a wide contrast in basic intelligence, there is a tendency for the partners to drift apart. Not only may the more intelligent partner long for stimulating exchange of ideas with someone else, but also the less intelligent person may develop feelings of inferiority. Each may grow lonely.

These marriages can be successful if each partner recognizes the other's strong points and allows each to excel in his own way. Common interests can be found and cultivated.

*Religion.* Religious differences can be one of the most disruptive influences in a marriage. The important factor is not simply the fact of difference in religious affiliation, but the significance of religion to each of the partners. To some, religion means nothing. To others, it is the unifying force in their lives. A religion shared in marriage can form a powerful bond between man and wife. Religious conflict can act as a powerful wedge, forcing them apart.

Most of the differences we have discussed prior to religion can be worked out satisfactorily. However, in certain combinations of religious beliefs, if each person remains faithful to his religion, there may be constant conflict throughout the marriage. Such marriages should be entered into only after mutually acceptable answers to all possible questions and problems of mixed marriage life have been reached. Nothing should be left to chance or to be settled after marriage. Following these decisions, the couple should go together and discuss them with the parents and the clergy of each faith. Their decisions should be clearly in mind and well stated (in writing, if necessary), so there can be no possibility of misunderstanding. This last point is particularly important in regard to the religious education of any children they might have. If, after such discussions with parents and clergy, there still seem to be conflicts, it would probably be better for each to look for someone else whose religious beliefs are more similar to his own. This may seem to be a pessimistic view of the problem, but it does seem that the best way to avoid the problems of a religiously incompatible marriage is to avoid such a marriage.

*Previous Marital Status.* One out of every four marriages today involves a person who has been married before. The chances of falling in love with a divorced or widowed person are not remote. Marrying a person who has been divorced or widowed is not the same as marrying one who has never been married before. A past marital experience affects the attitudes a person brings to a second marriage. These attitudes may be the product of memories of a happy marriage or the bitter aftertaste of marital disappointment.

Second marriages can turn out to be very desirable and happy. Or the problems that were causes of trouble in the first marriage may reappear. Before marrying a previously married individual, there must be definite answers to several questions, such as, "Has the divorced or widowed person recovered sufficiently from the feeling of loss to make a wise choice or is he desperate? If the former mate is still living, what are his attitudes toward that person? What are the chances of the former mate coming between the new partners? Can the new mate be content to live in a home previously occupied by the former partner? Are the real causes of the divorce, rather than simply the legal grounds, known to the new mate? (Remember that you have just heard one side of the story.) Is there any assurance that the same problems will not recur? Has the person been divorced more than once? (Third and subsequent marriages are usually poor risks.)

If the divorced or widowed person has custody of children from a prior marriage, a prospective mate should want to be assured of acceptance by them. Also, one's own attitude toward these potential stepchildren should be honestly appraised. In the event there are children born into the second marriage, in addition to children present from the first one, the parents must make every effort to avoid any showing of partiality toward one set of children.

### *Rational Selection*

In summary, a good aid for a person making a rational selection of a marriage partner would be to sit down and list all of the qualities he considers desirable in a partner. This should be done objectively and not be just a description of the current sweetheart. Out of this list he should select the ten most essential qualities for his ideal. He should then grade the person being considered as a mate. This should give some indication of the person's general acceptability for marriage.

This may seem like a harsh and unromantic way to deal with an affair of the heart, but it can prevent an unwise marriage based on emotion alone. Some people actually choose their marriage mates with less care than they choose their cars.

Finally, do not expect to find an individual who has all of the ideal traits. A happy marriage results when two imperfect people work toward the same goal, a meaningful, satisfying relationship, with all the necessary adjustments and sacrifices that it required.

## SOCIETY'S INTEREST IN YOUR MARRIAGE

In the rigid hierarchical cultures of the past, marriage was important for familial and social reasons. People married to preserve the family line, to pass on the land or the inheritance, and to have children who would maintain the status quo. The happiness of the man and woman were not of primary importance. Arrangements were made by the family.

Today such concerns are viewed as of secondary importance. The couple's goal is now personal happiness—arising from personal intimacy. This represents a shift from a social and legal control of marriage to an increasingly self-centered view of sexual and personal responsibility and accountability.

Although subject to change, the family exists in order to provide stability and protection for the group. When ignored, chaos has resulted. It is widely observed that a central reason for the eventual collapse of Rome was the family disruption resulting from the prolonged absence of its young men and fathers. Family life deteriorated, morals eroded, and Rome underwent a notorious sexual revolution.

To prevent repeating such errors, cultures have built basic codes and customs to protect marriage. Those who may or may not marry are restricted by social custom, religious tenet, and legal statute. Once married, one is expected to honor his commitments until freed legally and, for some, religiously.

### *Marriage Laws*

Every state has laws regulating marriage. Although these laws vary somewhat from state to state and are changed periodically, there are certain similarities among them.

*Minimal Age for Marriage.* Every state has a minimum age requirement for marriage. The age ranges from 14 to 17 for girls and from 15 to 18 for boys. The most common age requirements are 16 for girls and 18 for boys. Two-thirds of the states allow exceptions when the girl is pregnant or has an illegitimate child or in certain other special circumstances.

All states require parental consent for marriage if either partner is below a given age. Most commonly, such consent is required if the age of the boy is below 21 or the girl below 18.

*Physical Examination and Blood Test.* In all but a few states, a medical examination which generally includes a blood test is required. In most states, this is for the detection of venereal disease only. A few states also examine for one or more of the following: feeble-mindedness, uncontrolled epileptic seizures, infectious tuberculosis, chronic alcoholism, mental illness, and drug addiction. About two-thirds of the states require that the examination must be given not longer than 30 days before the issuance of the marriage license. In some cases, the blood test must be within 10 days of the issuance of the license.

*Waiting Period.* Most states have legislated a "cooling off" period either between the application for a marriage license and its issuance or after the license is issued but before it can be used. The purpose of these laws is to prevent marriage on a sudden impulse. Typical waiting periods are from 3 to 7 days. Thousands of unhappy marriages are believed to have been prevented by these waiting periods. Those states with no waiting periods are common marriage sites for eloping couples.

*Prohibited Marriages.* Every state prohibits marriage between close relatives such as brother-sister, father-daughter, mother-son, and marriages between step-parents and step-children. Over half of the states prohibit the marriage of first cousins and a few of even second cousins. All states prohibit the marriage of a person who is already married to one living spouse (bigamy). Marriage of a person who is legally judged to be mentally ill is prohibited in all states. Other prohibitions in some states include feeble-mindedness, epilepsy, and the "biologically unfit." No state considers a marriage valid which involves force or willful misrepresentation. To represent oneself falsely is usually grounds for annulment of the marriage.

*Common-law Marriages.* A common-law marriage is one in which both parties agree to live together as husband and wife without license or ceremony. Such marriages are now officially recognized by only a few states. Most states that do recognize common-law marriages consider them valid if they have been continued for at least 7 years.

### *Engagement*

Engagement today means the private agreement between a man and a woman to marry each other. The engagement may or may not be made "formal" by public announcement. If such a formal announcement is made, it is usually after a period of informally testing the arrangement. If there is no formal announcement, it is easier to break off the engagement if the couple later desires to do so.

### *Purposes of Engagement*

One of the main purposes of engagement, whether informal or formal, is to let each partner feel how he reacts to a prolonged relationship with the other. During this time they can test their reactions to the new relationship in a more intense and exclusive manner. Since most people still feel that marriage should involve exclusive sexual fidelity between the couple, it is important that a similar fidelity exist in engagement. It is very unlikely that the individual who is unfaithful during engagement will be faithful in marriage. Yet, during engagement, the two people need not seal themselves off from society. If, for example, one of them is away in school or military service, the other should be allowed the liberty to date. Such dating should be limited to pleasure and convenience without serious interest or sexual activity, and should not be limited to one person. Such dating can relieve some of the loneliness of separation and can be a good test of a couple's devotion. If their love can withstand

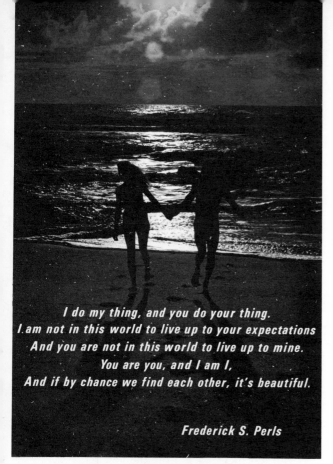

I do my thing, and you do your thing.
I am not in this world to live up to your expectations
And you are not in this world to live up to mine.
You are you, and I am I,
And if by chance we find each other, it's beautiful.

*Frederick S. Perls*

how much money should be spent on it? Do the partners adequately understand sexual intercourse and contraception? Are they going to want children, and if so, how many? What are their attitudes on the use of contraceptives? Where is the husband going to derive his income and how much will it be? How will their money be spent? Does the wife plan to work? Where do they plan to live? Will either be continuing with college? These questions and many more require definite answers before marriage.

### Sexual Relations during Engagement

Engagement should be a time of increasing intimacy, leading toward unrestricted sexual expression in marriage. The extent of intimacy during engagement is a matter for each couple to decide. Expression of affection through petting is normal and is helpful preparation for marriage. Each partner can learn the sexual responsiveness and reactions of the other, aiding in a smooth transition into marital intercourse.

Some couples feel that sexual intercourse during engagement is desirable and engage in it without any apparent problems. Other couples question the advisability of intercourse at this time, agree on definite limits to their lovemaking, and then respect these limits. The training of other couples places them in a dilemma—they want to have intercourse, but do not think they should. If intercourse is going to result in guilt feelings, then it is probably better to wait for marriage. That is, after all, one of the reasons for marriage.

Some people approaching marriage worry about the effect that past sexual experiences may have on their marriage. They may wonder if their own sexual adjustment will be difficult or if they will experience rejection by their partners. The best way to avoid any such problem is to minimize the past and

a minor test like this, the chances are better that it can withstand the tests of marriage. If the relationship cannot stand such a trial, and either jealousy or a new love interest develops, then it is good to discover before marriage, as the same thing would likely happen after marriage. It is always far easier to break an engagement than a marriage.

Other purposes of engagement are to allow time to answer the many questions essential to a successful marriage. Often the attempts to answer these questions will indicate that no marriage should take place. Some of these questions include: When and where will the wedding be held? Who will be invited to attend? Where should the honeymoon be and

316

build on the future. What is done is done. The past should not be allowed to interfere with the present and the future.

There may be a question of how much should be told about past sexual experiences. There certainly is no need to confess everything. Uncalled for confessions may only arouse basic suspicions and create doubts. Minute details regarding the past are better left untold. However, anything that could affect the marriage should be told before, not after, the wedding.

Some things that should be told because they can affect the marriage and would probably be revealed with time anyway include previous marriages and how they terminated; any serious health defects, particularly if they relate to childbearing; any record of felony convictions; any financial debts or obligations. Again, these should be revealed before marriage, not after.

### Length of Engagement

There is no definite length for an engagement. It should, of course, last long enough so that all of the functions we discussed can be carried out. It is well documented that the divorce rate is very high among couples who know each other for only a short time before marriage. As a general rule, it is good to have at least one year of close relationship before marriage. Countless poor marriages would be prevented if all couples were to know each other well for a year before marriage.

### Breaking Engagements

Although broken engagements can be unpleasant, they are much preferable to broken marriages. If a partnership is incompatible, it is far better to admit it before marriage than after. If, at any time, either partner wants to break an engagement, it should be broken. Once a person makes up his mind to break an engagement he should act promptly and kindly. He should not allow the opinions of family or friends, the fact that the wedding plans are underway, or embarrassment or pride to prevent him from acting on his decision. He should disregard any pleas, promises, or threats the other person might make. The wishes of the other party should not be "given in to" out of pity or fear. In time, both parties will get over the experience and an unhappy marriage will have been avoided. No person should ever assume a "this one or nobody" attitude. There are thousands of good marriage partners available to anyone who will seek them out. To the jilted party, this advice: do not act "on the rebound" to hastily start another serious relationship, either for spite or to salvage your own hurt feelings. Such swift actions can lead to an even worse marriage than was avoided.

### Premarital Counseling

Increasing emphasis is being placed on premarital counseling to assist couples in making an adequate marital adjustment. It has been found that the probability of happiness in marriage can be predicted by examining certain background factors, personality traits, engagement relations, engagement adjustment, and other anticipated factors.

The counselor may be a professional marriage counselor, a clergyman, or a physician. Some marriage counselors use personality tests to indicate a person's suitability for marriage or the likely compatibility of a couple. If either member of the couple has inadequate knowledge of sexual intercourse and reproduction, he or she may be counseled by books or discussions. The couple should be prepared to discuss with the counselor any fears or inhibitions they may have regarding normal sex life. He should question them regarding financial plans, housing, budgets, and any other phase of marriage that may be a subject of adjustment.

In 1971 the state of California passed legislation requiring premarital counseling for couples seeking a marriage license whenever one or both of the individuals were under 18 years of age. The amount and type of counseling given the young people was left to each county. Some counties require that the minor verify that he has received counseling from a qualified counselor (marriage counselor, pastor) and that he is considered ready to accept the responsibility of marriage.

## ADJUSTING TO MARRIAGE

### Beginning a Marriage

Starting a marriage should be one of the most pleasurable and memorable stages in life. There is the excitement of setting the date, looking at homes, making wedding plans, the actual ceremony, and the honeymoon.

*The Wedding Ceremony.* The particulars of the wedding ceremony are usually determined by the couple and their families. The role of the parents of the couple can be small or large. Although many couples want their weddings to be something they and their friends will remember, no wedding should place a heavy financial burden on either the couple or their families. The central idea in planning a wedding and honeymoon should be to minimize the stress-producing factors, and financial burden is one of the greatest stress producers.

A wedding is merely the beginning of a relationship and is not an end in itself. It does not need to be a big "production." Plans should be made carefully so that, in the effort to carry out an impressive ceremony, the couple does not become so nervous, confused, and fatigued that the setting for a good hon-eymoon adjustment is lost. The wedding should fit the desires of the couples, not the social aims of their parents.

The wedding rite may be a brief statement before a judge or justice of the peace or a modest-to-elaborate church ceremony. The wishes of the couple should be respected. Many religious groups have typical ceremonial forms that are followed, some being more symbolic than others. Regardless of the form chosen, the ceremony should fit the social and emotional needs of the couple, affirming their goals and pledging their commitment in terms that are meaningful to them.

*Elopement and Secret Marriage.* An elopement is a kind of "runaway" wedding in which the fact of the marriage is made known only after the wedding. In a secret marriage both the fact of the wedding and the marriage are kept secret for an extended period. There may be valid reasons for elopement. Parents may have an unjustified opposition to the marriage, in spite of the reasonable age and maturity of the couple. Family factors such as illness, recent death, or parental disharmony may make elopement more desirable. Many couples elope to save the high cost of the typical wedding ceremony and reception.

There are also arguments against elopement and secret marriage, especially the latter. The couple may be acting too hastily because of fear or pregnancy. They may be by-passing some of the important functions of engagement (the divorce rate is much higher after elopements and secret marriages). Parents, friends, and relatives, whose support is needed during married life, are sometimes hurt and alienated. If the marriage is to be kept secret for a period of time, the couple faces frustration in keeping it quiet, and yet fulfilling their marriage. If the wife becomes pregnant, the explanations become rather awkward and unconvincing.

*The Honeymoon.* A honeymoon is a special period during which, in privacy and isolation, a couple takes the first steps of adjustment to shared living. Although not every couple can or does have a honeymoon, it can help smooth the transition from single to married life. A honeymoon should be well planned to make the adjustment as easy as possible. Ideally, it should allow the partners to concentrate on each other, sexually and socially, rather than on business, extended travel, or crowded activity schedules. The place chosen for the honeymoon should be one that both can enjoy, but the cost should not create an undue burden. The honeymoon should last long enough to allow for adjustment, yet not so long that it leads to boredom.

### Marital Sexual Adjustment

The sexually inexperienced bride and groom will very likely have some anxieties about their wedding night. Each partner hopes for a mutually satisfactory sexual experience, but has many doubts. Much of this anxiety can be reduced with proper preparation. The bride's premarital consultation with a gynecologist can help considerably. At that time, a contraceptive method should be prescribed which minimizes the fear of pregnancy and which will not interfere with total freedom in sexual expression. Oral contraceptives are ideal for this purpose. The gynecologist should also check the virginal bride-to-be for the presence of an unusually tough hymen. Such a hymen can make her sexual initiation painful and unpleasant. It is a simple matter for the gynecologist to dilate or cut the hymen, thus eliminating the possibility of an unpleasant introduction to marital sex.

Even with these precautions, the virginal couple should not expect their first efforts at sexual intercourse to be entirely successful. Actually, the wedding night may not be the best possible time to start a satisfactory sexual relationship, after the usual multitude of problems in organizing a wedding and too much to drink at the reception. The inexperienced groom may seldom have adequate sexual control and, on the first attempt at intercourse, may ejaculate and lose erection almost immediately after vaginal penetration, or even before. But after a few minutes, he should be able to attain erection once again and, with seminal pressure reduced, delay ejaculation for some time.

An inexperienced bride may be disappointed in her failure to achieve orgasm on her wedding night. But many studies have shown that the virgin bride often does not reach orgasm through intercourse for a matter of several days, weeks, or even months. In fact, a significant number of woman achieve orgasm only after a year or more. Marital adjustments take time. Time is required to break down fears and inhibitions and to learn sexual techniques. The sexual happiness of the wife depends greatly on her husband. His attitudes toward sex and toward her will considerably influence her sexual responses. The sexual adjustment of the wife is made easier when her husband is free in his expressions of love and tenderness toward her. His attitude of patience with her is also critical.

Sexual satisfaction is not the only aim of marriage. Placing too high an expectation on sex can be disappointing. The success of a marriage cannot be measured by the number of orgasms per month as some of the "marriage manuals" seem to indicate. Sex must be viewed only as a part of marriage, but a couple should not neglect working toward a satisfying sexual adjustment.

### Extramarital Sexual Relations

Most people enter into a marriage with the

idea of sexual exclusiveness. They plan to remain sexually faithful and expect their new mate to do the same. Within the American culture, sexual exclusiveness in marriage is still considered an important value. Of course, extramarital affairs do occur in many marriages. But it is interesting to note that even the parties who engage in such affairs often show their disapproval of their own conduct by offering elaborate justifications for their actions or by feeling guilt.

There are, certainly, some marriages in which one spouse overlooks, forgives, or even encourages the extramarital affairs of the other. There are even marriages in which each partner openly carries on affairs with the knowledge and approval of the other. But in no way can these qualify as happy marriages. The individuals involved are usually quite unhappy and desperate in their search for sexual and/or ego satisfaction. Despite the surface appearance of mutual understanding in these marriages, there are generally deep undercurrents of guilt, jealousy, and resentment.

Sexual unfaithfulness by one partner can be just a single brief affair, a series of occasional short affairs, or a chronic situation. When the husband is unfaithful, he usually gives such reasons as his wife is unloving, or that intercourse with his wife is uninteresting due to her lack of enthusiasm, or that she is unwilling to have intercourse as often as he wishes to. Reasons given by unfaithful wives are similar: lack of affection or skill or interest in lovemaking on the part of her husband, or his failure to help her achieve orgasm. It is likely that in most cases these are merely surface indications of deeper marital problems. Persons entering into serious affairs outside of their marriage are generally reacting to unfulfilled nonsexual needs instead of, or in addition to, unfulfilled sexual needs. For example, there is very

commonly a need for ego gratification, a longing for the pleasure of sharing mutual interests with a loved and loving person, or a need for intellectual stimulation not supplied by the marriage partner. Adultery is not a basic cause of unhappy marriages, but rather a symptom of trouble in a marriage. Therefore, it is unwise to label one party as "innocent" and one as "guilty," as divorce courts have so often done. In many cases, no one is guilty; there are just basic incompatibilities between the marital partners. In other cases, the innocent party is rather directly responsible for the adultery of the guilty party.

Qualified professional marital counseling can often find the underlying cause of marital difficulties. If both partners are willing to "forgive and forget" and work to correct their deficiencies, then even a very rocky marriage may be returned to happiness.

### Divorce

In some marriages it becomes apparent that because of unresolved conflicts there is no longer a basis for trying to continue the relationship. The relationship of marriage can be broken either formally or informally. It may be broken informally by desertion, in which one partner simply disappears, or by separation, in which the couple agrees to live separately. Neither desertion nor separation constitutes a legal divorce nor terminates the marriage. A marriage can be legally terminated by annulment if it can be established that some legal requirement for marriage was never met (due to fraud, deception, illegal age, bigamy, or some other violation). Or divorce can be obtained if it can be established that one partner violated the marriage rights of the other. Technically, divorce usually must be based on such grounds rather than just on mutual agreement.

Grounds for divorce among the various

states include adultery, cruelty (physical or mental), irreconcilable differences, desertion, nonsupport, alcoholism, drug addiction, impotence, insanity, pregnancy at time of marriage, bigamy, fraud, force or duress, felony conviction, and imprisonment. A particular state might recognize many or few of these grounds. Persons seeking divorce often go to extremes to establish complaints within these categories, even though the actual cause of marital failure was something entirely different. This practice is so common that the number of decrees awarded in certain categories tells very little of the true nature of the marital conflicts among the couples involved.

The majority of divorce decrees are awarded to women for several reasons. Generally, women have access to more grounds for divorce than men. The courts tend to be more sympathetic to the divorce suits of women and tend to award alimony more readily to them. It is also more common for the woman to be awarded custody of the children, if any, than the man. The man typically makes child support payments to his ex-wife until the children reach a given age.

The first major divorce reform in the nation, California's Family Law Act, became effective in 1970. It is expected that other states may follow California's lead. This act eliminated the term "divorce" and substituted "dissolution of marriage." Its most important reform changed the legal termination of marriage from an adversary action in which one party must be found "guilty" and one "innocent" to a neutral petitioning requiring no finding of misconduct. Cruelty, adultery, and other previous grounds for divorce were eliminated. A marriage may be dissolved now only on a finding of irreconcilable differences or incurable insanity, the latter being the only grounds remaining from

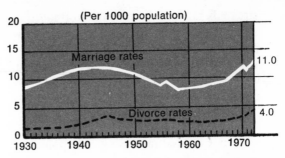

Marriage and divorce rates in the United States, 1930–1972. (*Source: Public Health Service, U.S. Department of Health, Education, and Welfare.*)

the old law. The act also details more enlightened child custody rules, emphasizing the quality of the parent-child relationship instead of the personal vices of the parent, as in the past. Finally, the interlocutory period was shortened from one year to six months.

*Incidence of Divorce.* The divorce rate, as shown in the next figure, has been both higher and lower than it is today. The high point occurred during the readjustment period following World War II. The trend in recent years has been a gradual rise in the divorce rate. In 1972 the divorce rate was 4.0 divorces per 1000 population, compared with 2.2 in 1957. There were 790,000 divorces in the United States during 1972. This represented one divorce for every three marriages.

The incidence of divorce can be correlated with several characteristics of the marriage. Divorce occurs more frequently in cities than in rural areas and more often among those of lower income than those of higher income. It is more common during the first five years of marriage than later. Marriages in which one or both parties were less than age 20 at the time of marriage are more likely to end in divorce.

It must be remembered that divorce rates

are only a partial indication of marriage failure. There are many couples whose marriage has failed but who have not obtained a divorce for economic or religious reasons, fear of loss of social or professional standing, the presence of children in the home, or fear of admitting failure. The increase in divorce rates is due to many factors, which may or may not include increasing unhappiness in marriage. The evolving criteria for success in marriage place a greater importance on love and companionship, without which a marriage today is more often considered to be a failure. Public opinion toward divorce is increasingly liberal. More and more people are deciding that the temporary pain of divorce is better than living in the continuing turmoil of an unhappy marriage. The increasing independence and freedom of women to be self-supporting has probably been influential also. On the other hand, a woman who is not prepared to enter the labor market, who has not developed marketable skills, may find the loss of financial security a greater threat than is the undesirable relationship. This is perhaps more relevant for the female reared with marriage as the only adult goal. The older female or male may also have health problems that further threaten the prospect of being alone or able to remarry.

*Effects of Divorce upon Partners.* The emotional effects of divorce are greater than the average person who has never been through it realizes. Both parties involved usually find it a painful experience, emotionally, socially, and financially. It usually does not solve the basic human problems that were its true cause. New problems are created for both the divorced couple and any children they might have had. There is often a mixture of feelings of guilt and resentment. For some, the readjustment demanded is severe enough to call for the outside help of friends, clergymen, or a psychiatrist.

*Effects of Divorce upon Children.* Particularly bewildering is the effect of divorce upon children. They are in a no-man's land, being pulled in two directions. The best affection the divided parents can bestow is not compatible to the security a child should feel in a warm home relationship. He is helpless in resolving his position with each of his parents, since he feels loyalty to both of them. Any court battle over custody only aggravates the damage. Some children become so emotionally disturbed that their attitudes toward their school work and friends are noticeably affected. Their world has collapsed. The child often develops a feeling that somehow he was responsible for the divorce. As the child matures, it becomes necessary for him to achieve an outlook on the matter which does not warp his own chances for a successful marriage. He must be convinced that his parents' problems do not reflect upon him. Most of all, he must learn from his parents' experience so that he does not make similar mistakes.

*Divorce Prevention.* The most effective divorce prevention takes place before marriage. This includes the development of desirable attitudes toward marriage and the selection of the right marriage mate. There is a need for a re-emphasis of the place of stable marriage as the basis of the social order in this country. One's success in marriage influences the success with which he can creatively accomplish goals of all kinds. For many of us, a successful marriage is essential to personal fulfillment.

*Remarriage.* Divorce need not be the end of marital pleasure. The remarriage rate among divorcees is high, indicating that few of them are completely soured on the idea of marriage. According to the U.S. Bureau of the Census, a divorced man or woman of any age is more likely to remarry than the never-married person of the same age is to get married. The bureau reports, for example, that at age 30 a single woman has a 50 percent chance of marrying, while a divorcee of that age has a 94 percent chance of remarriage.

The divorce rate among second marriages is somewhat higher than in first marriages, but the divorce rate soars in third and subsequent marriages. On the other hand, a remarriage may result in much greater happiness than the original marriage. Remarriages can turn out well if the new partners earnestly try to avoid the problems that destroyed the first.

## THE DECISION TO HAVE A CHILD

Whether or not a couple wants children is a crucial decision. To have children represents a long-term commitment that will be most demanding on the couple in all ways.

There are some excellent reasons for deciding not to have a family. Children are not needed to perpetuate the species. The world is already suffering from the effects of enormous overpopulation. Many well-adjusted couples feel sufficiently rewarded with their understanding of themselves, each other, and their professions to more than compensate for the emotional rewards of children. Children, particularly when infants, place heavy demands on a couple. A person may not be prepared emotionally or physically to provide these. Some couples see that it may be impossible to raise children the way they feel they should be raised because costs are too high, congestion too great, and resources too few.

Yet, many couples desire children despite these conditions. As they assess themselves and their resources they are willing to provide, or sacrifice, for a child. They look forward to the emotional rewards that come from creating a new person and from helping this child reach his emotional and intellectual potential.

The decision to have or not have children is as important as is the decision to marry. Questions the couple should answer in reaching this decision should include: Is our marriage stable enough to bear the stresses of a family? Do we love children enough to sacrifice for their welfare? Do we both agree on wanting a child or will it create hostility in one of us? (An unwanted child may not only lead to a disturbed parent, but to an emotionally disturbed child.) Rather than making a decision to *not have* a child, couples should assume they are not going to have a child until they decide *to have* one.

## ALTERNATE LIFE STYLES

Increasing numbers of people are choosing to live in other than the traditional marriage arrangement. They are generally motivated by a search for individual freedom and fulfillment. Actually, most of the life styles being adopted are not really new at all, but have long existed in various forms and at various periods of history. In many cases, though, the motivations behind these alternate life styles are new, and in almost every case the openness of these arrangements and their acceptance by society is growing.

Certainly the simplest alternate life style is just to remain single and live alone. If a person is satisfied with this arrangement, then there is no psychological or sociological reason why he should not pursue it.

Long-term homosexual "marriage" is another possibility and for many individuals proves to be a satisfactory life style. As is true for several other life styles, persons choosing homosexual marriage should be strong enough to withstand the stigma, however unwarranted it may be, that some elements of our society still direct toward certain life styles.

The alternate life style that has attracted the greatest following in recent years is the common practice of "living together," which in many respects resembles the old-fashioned common-law marriage. In this arrangement, a heterosexual couple sets up housekeeping in a fashion that greatly resembles marriage, the principal difference being the absence of license or ceremony. The motivations for living together are what distinguishes this as a separate life style. While old-fashioned common-law marriage is often associated with lower income levels and is usually motivated by economic expediencies, living together is a middle- and upper-class phenomenon with various motivations. It may be based on a philosophic rejection of marriage as being too confining and restrictive for individual growth and "personhood." It may be motivated by the romanticist view that the love relationship remains stronger when it is maintained voluntarily, rather than enforced by the legal contract that marriage represents. In still other cases, living together is viewed as a trial period which, if successfull for a period of time, will lead to legal marriage.

Most couples living together expect of each other the same degree of fidelity as is typically expected by marriage partners, with neither person free to engage in sexual relations with anyone else or even to date anyone else. Thus, the degree of freedom in the relationship of living together is really little greater than in marriage, with the exception of the legal ease with which the relationship can be terminated. Of course, the emotional trauma in breaking up can be as great as in terminating a marriage.

Even among the strongest advocates of living together, there are many who feel that legal marriage should accompany the birth of children. The commitment involved in legal marriage, while not guaranteeing a lasting relationship, at least indicates an intention on the part of each person to make a stable partnership. In addition, the great majority of people in our society still stigmatize the child born of unmarried parents. While this stigma is terribly unfair to the child, it is a reality and will probably continue to be so for some time.

The most revolutionary of the alternate life styles is group marriage—a catch-all term applied to a wide variety of polygamous living arrangements in which small groups of adult males and females, and their children, live together under one roof or in a close-knit settlement, calling themselves a family, tribe, commune, or community. All property is generally collectively owned and all the members work for the common good. Many group marriages represent utopian mini-societies largely opposed to the mores and values of contemporary American society.

The collectivism of group marriages usually extends to their sexual relationships. While some communes consist of conventionally faithful married couples, more commonly there is some degree of sexual sharing.

Most group marriages, as well as most other utopian schemes, are destined to fail. Many of the problems of traditional marriage are merely multiplied in group marriage. Considering the difficulty in finding just two people who can live together compatibly, it becomes a near impossibility to find larger groups of people who can live harmoniously and lovingly together. A marriage of one man and one woman involves one interrelationship, which we all know is difficult to keep in working order. But the smallest possible group marriage, three people, involves 3 interrelationships; four people makes 6 relationships; and fifteen people results in 105 relationships. Jealousies and love conflicts are similarly multiplied in group marriages, and considerable individual freedom must be sacrificed in the process of coordinating and scheduling many lives. Thus, most group marriages are unstable and typically last for only a few months.

# 16
# Human Reproduction

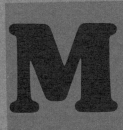

ost people have at least a practical interest in heredity as shown by their frequent attempts to associate traits of a child with similar traits of his parents, grandparents, aunts, uncles, and so forth. But recent advances in the scientific study of heredity have made it important for the enlightened person to have some basis for understanding the actual mechånisms whereby hereditary information is stored in cells, is passed on to offspring, and works to create desirable or undesirable hereditary traits. Many authorities believe that the science of genetics is reaching the point where it may be eventually possible to modify human heredity—perhaps eliminating undesirable traits and increasing the frequency of desirable ones. Parents may someday (perhaps soon) have considerable control over the genetic makeup of their children. It is possible that even the genetic material of the adult may be alterable. The entire course of human evolution may be changed. Thus, genetics will become not a matter of curiosity, but a topic of vital concern and, most likely, of controversy. Let us therefore consider some of the basic mechanisms of heredity.

## HEREDITY

### The Cell

The key to the whole matter is in the cell and its contents. All plants and animals are made up of the microscopic units of living material which are called cells. A human being, for example, contains about 2 trillion $(2 \times 10^{12})$ cells.

Cells from the diverse tissues of the body may appear to be quite different from one another. Although all cells are similar in the first day of embryonic life, as they develop into different kinds of tissues, they become differentiated in order to carry out their specialized tasks, such as carrying oxygen in the blood, transmitting nerve impulses, contracting on signal, or supporting the mass of the body.

However, most cells of the body maintain a similar structure (see figure of "typical"

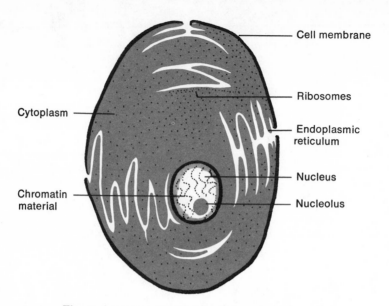

The major parts of a "typical" human body cell.

cell). The cell consists of a nucleus surrounded by cytoplasm, all of which is enclosed within a cell membrane. Within the cell are yet other, less obvious structures.

*The Nucleus.* Located within the cell, often near the center, is the spherical nucleus. Suspended within it are twisted filaments called chromatin material. These filaments carry the genes, which bear the information necessary to direct the construction of a new individual. Here and there within the nucleus may be seen one or several spherical bodies called nucleoli.

*Cytoplasm.* The material outside the nucleus but within the cell membrane is often referred to as cytoplasm. This material is fluidlike and mobile. Suspended in it are less obvious structures, some living (organelles) and some nonliving (inclusions). As seen in the figure, within the cytoplasm is a system of canals, called the endoplasmic reticulum, through which materials move. Lined up against the outside walls of the endoplasmic reticulum are small bodies called ribosomes. The ribosomes control the making of types of cell proteins (enzymes) which in turn direct the development and activity of the cell.

*Chromosomes.* At the time of cell division, the twisted chromatin strands compress together and condense, appearing as rodlike structures, which are referred to as chromosomes. The number of chromosomes within the nucleus varies with different species of organisms.

The 46 chromosomes normally found within the nucleus of each human cell actually represent two similar sets of 23 chromosomes each. Each set of 23 chromosomes is referred to as the haploid number (or $1n$); two similar sets are referred to as the diploid number (or $2n$). The diploid number is found in almost all cells of our body. Only the sex cells (sperm and eggs) possess the haploid number. The logic of this is that when a sperm unites with an egg, the new united cell (the zygote) will contain the same number of chromosomes as all other cells. (If the sex cells possessed the diploid number, the zygote would possess 92 chromosomes and would thus double with each generation.)

Each of the chromosomes in a haploid set (23) is different from the others in shape and size, but all haploid sets of human chromosomes are similar. In other words, each chromosome in one haploid set matches a similar chromosome in any other haploid set (there is one exception in the male which we will explain later).

On fertilization each sex cell (sperm or egg) contributes a haploid set. If we wanted to, we could think of one set as being the paternal set (from the sperm) and one set as being the maternal set (from the egg). The two comparable chromosomes from each haploid set can be thought of as a pair. We could think of each diploid set of chromosomes as consisting of 23 comparable pairs.

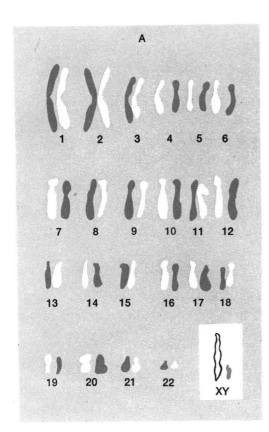
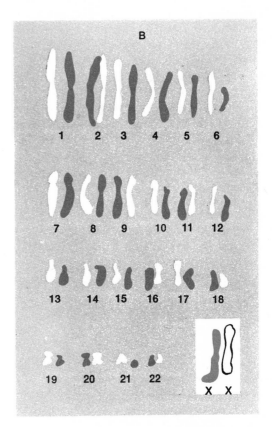

A schematic view of human chromosomes: (a) normal male; (b) normal female. Note the XY pair in the male; these are each diploid sets. In each pair of chromosomes the dark chromosome represents that contributed by the father (paternal set), and the light represents that contributed by the mother (maternal set).

Fertilized eggs receiving an abnormal number of chromosomes (more or less than 46), tend to develop abnormally and die early. In the event that the embryo fully develops and the child is born, it may be abnormal, such as in the case of mongoloids (who may possess 47 chromosomes).

### The Genetic Code

Chromosomes are made up of theoretical parts called genes, which determine hereditary traits. It is known that genes consist of a substance called deoxyribonucleic acid (DNA). Each molecule of DNA, if magnified sufficiently, would look like a twisted ladder, called a double helix. (See figure showing structure of DNA.) The most important parts of the ladder are the rungs. Each rung consists of a pair of nitrogen bases (simple compounds containing the element nitrogen). Four different nitrogen bases are used to construct the rungs: adenine (A), thymine (T), guanine (G), and cytosine (C). Each rung is made up of one or two combinations, A with T, or C with G. The rungs may read A–T, T–A, C–G, or G–C. The trait produced by a gene is determined by the sequence of these pairs as they appear in specific groups of three, called triplets. Each DNA molecule is made up of thousands of rungs. This allows for considerable variation in nitrogen-base sequences and thus variation in human traits.

Most important is how the DNA molecule acts. What must it do? It possesses the genetic code; now there must be some way to translate the molecule's information into action within the cell.

*Replication.* First of all, in order for the DNA molecule to do its work, it must be present in each cell. Therefore, each time a cell divides the DNA ladder must duplicate itself so that there is a precise copy of it within

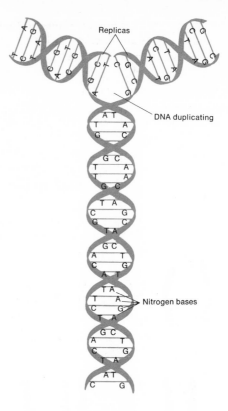

A replicating DNA molecule.

each new cell. The DNA molecule does this by "un-zipping." As shown in the diagram, the DNA ladder splits down the middle, dividing each rung in half. The half of each divided rung stays attached to its side of the ladder. Then, from materials available within the cell, each half of the DNA molecule reconstructs a complete ladder: A attracts T, C attracts G, and two completed ladders are formed. All of this occurs before the cell itself divides, so that when division takes place, each of the two new cells formed receives complete DNA molecules.

*Translating the Code.* The function of DNA molecules is to serve as a pattern for the construction of proteins. Proteins are essential to the cell because they direct most of the chemical reactions occurring within the cell. Accordingly, the characteristics of living organisms are determined by the kinds of proteins present within the cell.

The sort of protein constructed depends on the kinds of amino acids present in the cell and the order in which they can be put together. But at this point, a problem arises. The DNA molecules are confined inside the nucleus. The amino acids are out in the cytoplasm. In some way the DNA information must be carried out of the nucleus to the protein construction sites (ribosomes) alongside the endoplasmic reticulum.

The chemical messengers are molecules of ribonucleic acid (RNA). These molecules resemble DNA except that they are single stranded, and one of their typical nitrogen bases is different from those found in DNA. There are several types of RNA; the one we want here is messenger RNA (mRNA). These molecules are formed inside the nucleus against one strand of the DNA molecule. Once formed, the mRNA moves outside the nucleus, locates ribosomes in the cytoplasm, and hooks on to them.

At this point, another kind of RNA, transfer RNA (tRNA), moves through the cytoplasm, locates single amino acids, attaches them, and leads them to the mRNA. Once the tRNA finds the right spot on the mRNA for its amino acid, it unloads it and moves away to look for another amino acid. (See figure on formation of protein molecules.) These amino acids at the mRNA are

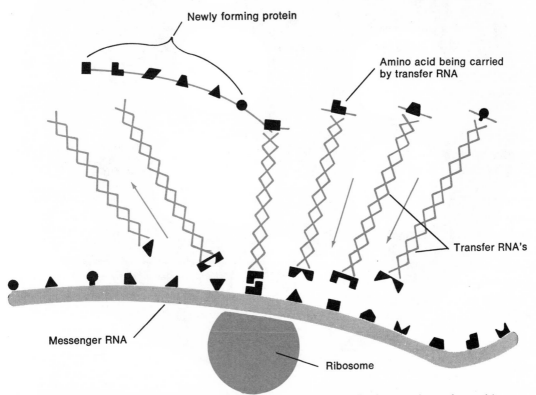

Newly forming protein

Amino acid being carried by transfer RNA

Transfer RNA's

Messenger RNA

Ribosome

The formation of protein molecules. Note that the transfer RNA deposits amino acids according to the "blueprint" carried by the messenger RNA.

arranged according to the pattern of the *m*RNA (which was determined by the arrangement of the DNA). The amino acids now attach sideways to each other, forming a new protein. Once formed, the protein unhitches from the *m*RNA and moves off into the cytoplasm where it serves to direct the cell's chemical activities.

### Cell Division

Once the sperm and the egg have united to form a new cell, this cell must divide a fantastic number of times to form a human being. There are two forms of cell division.

*Mitosis.* The most common process of cell division is mitosis. The chromosomes dupli-

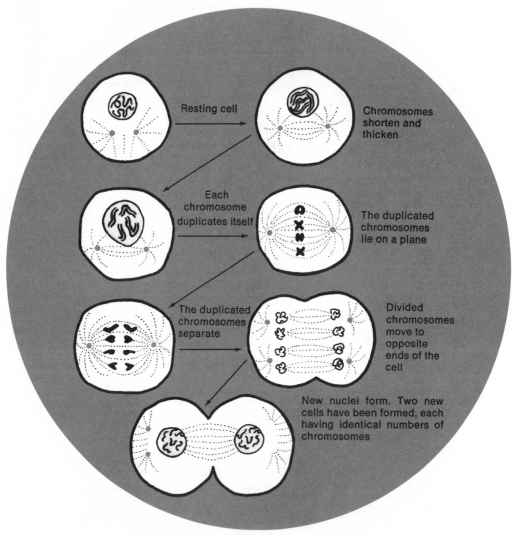

Resting cell

Chromosomes shorten and thicken

Each chromosome duplicates itself

The duplicated chromosomes lie on a plane

The duplicated chromosomes separate

Divided chromosomes move to opposite ends of the cell

New nuclei form. Two new cells have been formed, each having identical numbers of chromosomes

Mitosis, the production of two genetically identical cells.

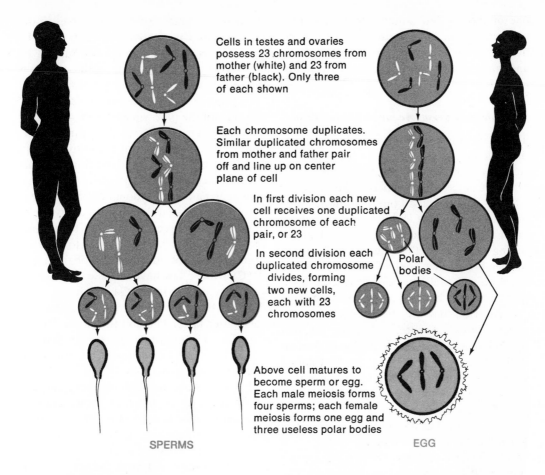

Cells in testes and ovaries possess 23 chromosomes from mother (white) and 23 from father (black). Only three of each shown

Each chromosome duplicates. Similar duplicated chromosomes from mother and father pair off and line up on center plane of cell

In first division each new cell receives one duplicated chromosome of each pair, or 23

In second division each duplicated chromosome divides, forming two new cells, each with 23 chromosomes

Polar bodies

Above cell matures to become sperm or egg. Each male meiosis forms four sperms; each female meiosis forms one egg and three useless polar bodies

SPERMS

EGG

Meiosis, the production of sperm and egg cells. Note: the number of pairs of chromosomes shown here has been reduced to 3 (6 chromosomes) for simplicity. Remember that each body cell in a human has 23 pairs (46 chromosomes) and that a germ cell has only one member of each pair (23 chromosomes).

cate themselves exactly (see figure on mitosis), giving each of the new cells precise copies of the DNA information found in the original cell (see DNA replication). This way each new cell is identical to the parent cell.

*Meiosis.* Another type of cell division is meiosis. This process takes place exclusively in the testes and ovaries; thus, you might correctly assume that this process reduces the number of chromosomes from the diploid number to the haploid number.

There is no way of determining which chromosome will go to which new cell during reduction. It is strictly a matter of chance, or what is called random assortment. The original maternal-paternal sets will be split up. One maternal chromosome may go to one of the sex cells and the next maternal one may go to the opposite sex cell. Each new sex cell will contain some of the father's and some of the mother's traits. (See figure on meiosis.)

## Inherited Versus Acquired Characteristics

There are some women who, during pregnancy, make certain that they listen to classical music or meditate on famous works of art or read best-selling books. Some make efforts to not look upon one-eyed individuals or other sorts of physical deformities, believing that what they experience or think about during pregnancy affects the fetus. Nothing of the sort is true. Sons of lumberjacks are not born with well-developed muscles. Even though Jewish boys have been circumcised for centuries, they are still born with a prepuce. The old practice of binding the feet of Chinese girls had to be repeated anew with each generation. Traits that are developed through diligent effort and in response to a person's environment are described as acquired characteristics.

Such physical traits as sex, intelligence, height, color of skin, and blood type are inherited characteristics. These traits are not influenced by "maternal impressions." The full expression of certain physical traits will depend on one's education, medical care, and diet; thus, both inheritance and environment are important in development. But, the physical traits as such are determined by chromosomes.

## Actions of Genes

Chromosomes are made up of genes which in turn are composed of DNA. Genes express themselves as traits. Since each body cell contains two sets of chromosomes, each cell possesses two genes for each characteristic. These genes occupy the same position on each chromosome. The two genes for a given

characteristic may express themselves in the same way or differently. If the action of the gene pair is alike, the genes are said to be *homozygous* for that trait; if the action is different, they are said to be *heterozygous*.

In the event the genes are heterozygous, one gene of the pair will commonly be dominant over the other, and the trait it determines will be apparent in the individual. In such a case, the gene not creating a visible effect is recessive, or concealed. A homozygous gene pair may be dominant or recessive.

An example of a dominant-recessive relationship can be seen in the trait for tasting. Most individuals have the ability to taste the organic compound phenylthiocarbamide (PTC), while a few have no taste for it. Those who have a taste for PTC know it, for when they get some in their mouths they sense a very bitter taste. The ability to taste PTC is the effect of a dominant gene. A person can taste PTC either by possessing two dominant genes for the trait (homozygous dominant) or by possessing one dominant gene and one recessive gene for the trait (heterozygous). Any person who is not a taster of PTC would possess two recessive genes for the trait (homozygous recessive).

In the example selected, the usual trait is expressed by a dominant gene and the exception by a recessive gene. It is considered normal for a person to be able to taste PTC. However, dominant genes do not determine only normal traits. The table on inherited traits shows that some dominant traits can also be abnormal.

## Undesirable Genes

Traits determined by genes may be desirable or undesirable. Undesirable genes cause physical development which obviously deviates from the norm. If the deviation is slight the person may be able to survive in spite of the abnormality. If the deviation is severe,

## SOME HUMAN TRAITS KNOWN TO BE INHERITED ACCORDING TO DOMINANCE AND RECESSIVENESS

| DOMINANCE | RECESSIVE |
|---|---|
| **Hair and Skin** | |
| early baldness (dominant in male) | normal |
| pigmented skin, hair, eyes | albinism |
| ichthyosis (scaly skin) | normal |
| dark hair | blond hair |
| non-red hair | red hair |
| **Eyes** | |
| brown | blue or gray |
| congenital cataract | normal |
| nearsightedness | normal vision |
| farsightedness | normal vision |
| astigmatism | normal vision |
| glaucoma | normal |
| **Features** | |
| broad lips | thin lips |
| large eyes | small eyes |
| long eyelashes | short eyelashes |
| broad nostrils | narrow nostrils |
| **Skeleton and muscles** | |
| polydactyly (more than 5 digits on hands and feet) | normal |
| syndactyly (webbing of 2 or more fingers or toes) | normal |
| brachydactyly (short digits) | normal |
| progressive muscular atrophy | normal |
| **Circulatory system** | |
| blood groups A, B, and AB | blood group O |
| hypertension (high blood pressure) | normal |
| normal | hemophilia (X-linked) |
| normal | sickle cell anemia |
| **Excretory system** | |
| normal | diabetes mellitus |
| **Nervous system** | |
| tasters (PTC) | nontasters |
| normal | congenital deafness |
| normal | phenylketonuria (PKU) |
| Huntington's chorea | normal |

the person may be unable to survive. In other words, the effects of the gene are lethal, but they are lethal only if their effects are manifest. Dominant genes that are lethal are easily spotted and can perhaps be counteracted. There is greater concern with lethal genes that are recessive. Such recessives will not be noticed unless they are present in the homozygous state. It is possible for undesirable recessives to be concealed for a number of generations. They need be of little concern as long as they are masked by a dominant gene.

Concealed recessive genes may become visible when close relatives produce children. If one possesses a given recessive gene that is concealed, since they have similar hereditary backgrounds, it is likely that the other also carries the same concealed recessive. Therefore, there is a great chance that their offspring will be homozygous for these recessive genes. The only biological problem in the marriage of close relatives is that their children might inherit and manifest undesirable homozygous recessive genes that were concealed. An example of a condition in which a person possesses two particular homozygous recessive genes is phenylketonuria (PKU), which usually causes permanent neurological damage.

### Other Gene Actions

Not all genes operate according to the rules of dominance and recessiveness. In some cases a gene pair that is not alike will cause a blending effect; each gene having equal effect. Some traits are the effect of two or more pairs of genes. In other cases, a given gene pair may affect several different traits. The actions of genes is varied and complex, and there are many traits whose gene mechanism is not fully understood.

### The Determination of Sex and X-Linked Traits

As previously mentioned, one haploid set of chromosomes is similar to any other set. This is true for chromosomes pairs 1 through 22. In the male, pair 23 is not well matched; in the female pair 23 appears to be matched. In the female these two chromosomes are both called the X-chromosomes. In the male there is only one X-chromosome; the odd mate is called the Y-chromosome. Although different in shape and size, in meiosis this pair acts as though it were similar.

As already seen, in meiosis only one chromosome of each pair goes to one egg or sperm. When the female produces an egg, it gets only one X-chromosome. When the male produces sperm, the X-chromosome goes to one sperm, the Y to another. Thus, while all eggs possess an X-chromosome, this is not true for all sperm. There will be both X- and Y-sperm cells. When an X-egg unites with an X-sperm, an XX-zygote is formed; this develops into a female. When an X-egg unites with a Y-sperm, an XY-zygote is formed; this develops into a male. Sex is thus determined by chromosomes.

By this system, we could expect males and females to appear in about equal numbers. Actually, records show that more male than female babies are born. In the United States, the proportion is about 106 to 100 among whites; about 103 to 100 among blacks. Among Koreans, it is 112 to 100; among Cubans, 101 to 100.

Being determined by chromosomes, the sex of a child is fixed at the moment of conception. As seen, this determination is the work of the father, not the mother. Although the chance of producing males to females is about one to one when thousands of cases are considered, the sex of the children in a given family may not be so well divided. There are some families in which there are four or five girls and no boys, or vice versa. The father of an all-girl family should not consider himself effeminate or lacking in virility. It is simply a matter of chance.

### Other Effects of X-Chromosomes

As with other chromosomes, the X-chromosomes are made up of hundreds of genes. The Y-chromosome, on the other hand, appears to be almost without genes. Those genes appearing on the X-chromosomes are said to be X-linked. Since the X- and Y-chromosomes relate to the sex of a person, we can expect the presence or absence of certain genes on these chromosomes to create certain visible effects.

Since the male lacks the effects of a second X-chromosome, any gene appearing on the single X-chromosome, whether recessive or dominant, becomes apparent. In order for the female to manifest the effects of a recessive X-gene, the recessive must be homozygous. An example would be red-green color blindness. It is caused by a recessive X-linked gene. For purposes of illustration let us look at some real-life situations.

*Example 1.* The father is red-green colorblind and the mother carries two dominant genes for normal color vision. As evident in the figure on X-linked traits the father can transmit colorblindness only to his daughters. The daughters will not be colorblind but will carry the gene as a "hidden" recessive.

*Example 2.* The father has normal vision, but the mother is a carrier. Any daughters from these parents receiving the mother's gene will be carriers with normal vision. Any daughters receiving the mother's dominant gene will carry only genes for normal color vision. Any sons receiving her dominant gene

will have normal color vision. Any sons receiving her recessive gene will exhibit colorblindness.

The frequency of red-green colorblindness in males is about 1 in 12; in females about 1 in 144 (12 x 12). The number of female carriers (normal vision but carrying the recessive) is about 1 in 12. There are other examples of X-linked characteristics such as:

1. Ichthyosis (a rough, scaly skin condition)
2. Brown teeth
3. Rickets due to vitamin-D resistance

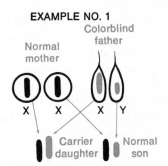

EXAMPLE NO. 1

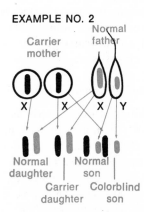

EXAMPLE NO. 2

The pattern of inheritance involving X-linked traits. The black chromosomes represent dominant genes for normal color vision; the striped ones represent recessive genes for color blindness.

335

4. One type of muscular dystrophy
5. Hemophilia
6. Two types of diabetes insipidus
7. Ocular albinism (Absence of eyeball pigmentation)
8. Atrophy of the optic nerve
9. Male toothlessness and hairlessness

It is even suspected that some X-linked recessives may be lethal, but to date, such evidence is incomplete.

### Congenital Defects

Gross structural deformities present at the time of birth are called congenital defects. The incidence of these is relatively high. About 1 in every 16 babies born in this country is born with a serious physical defect. Some defects cause physical or mental handicap, disfigurement, shortened life, or death. Of the 200,000 babies born each year with serious congenital defects, about 15,000 die before they reach their first birthday. Some malformed embryos do not reach full development but are aborted before birth. Some authorities estimate that about one-third of all "miscarriages" are due to malformed embryos.

### Kinds of Congenital Defects

Many kinds of defects have been observed. Some of the more common include birthmarks, cleft lip (harelip), cleft palate, clubfoot, congenital heart disease, congenital urinary tract defects, diabetes, mongolism, hydrocephaly, missing limbs, extra fingers and toes, cystic fibrosis, open spine, sickle cell anemia, galactosemia, PKU, and erythroblastosis.

*Erythroblastosis Fetalis.* There is a blood factor called the Rh (Rhesus) factor which is found in the blood of about 5 out of 6 Americans. Those having it are called Rh-positive; those lacking it, Rh-negative. If an Rh– person receives Rh⁺ blood (through transfusion or because an Rh⁻ mother is pregnant with an Rh⁺ child and some blood seeps across the placenta) the foreign Rh⁺ blood stimulates the production of an antibody, anti-Rh. This antibody can travel across the placenta. Produced in the body of the Rh- person, it can enter the bloodstream of the Rh⁺ and cause the destruction of the red blood cells.

This reaction usually does not take place the first time Rh⁺ blood gets into the bloodstream of the Rh⁻ person, such as on the first transfusion or with the first pregnancy. The destructive action of the antibody may occur upon a second mixing and thereafter.

The Rh-factor may be a problem in pregnancy only where the father is Rh⁺ and the mother who is Rh– is carrying an Rh⁺ child. The anti-Rh antibodies produced by the mother's body destroy the fetus' red blood cells causing a severe type of anemia (inability of the blood to carry oxygen) and jaundice. To compensate, the bone marrow releases erythroblasts (immature red blood cells). In severe cases the infant may be born dead or may die shortly after birth. He may survive but be mentally retarded.

Today a physician can make tests indicating a dangerous anti-Rh level during pregnancy. Damage can often be prevented by an exchange blood transfusion immediately after birth or even before birth. An injection (RhoGAM Immune Globulin) has been available since 1968 for administration to the Rh- mother within 72 hours after giving birth to an Rh⁺ child. This product. a concentration of anti-Rh antibodies, neutralizes any Rh-antigen that might contaminate the blood of the mother during the birth process. This, of course, is of no benefit to the child that has just been born, but it does very effectively reduce the chances of an Rh-incompatibility in the next pregnancy.

### Congenital Heart Disease

Congenital heart disease causes more deaths during the first year of life than any other congenital defect. Infants with severe malformations often die shortly after birth.

A number of malformations involving the heart and large blood vessels may occur. The heart develops through a number of important steps during the pregnancy. The blood of the unborn child travels through the umbilical cord to the placenta, where it exchanges gases and wastes in its blood with gases and foods in the mother's blood. The blood entering the child's body from the placenta is rich in oxygen. It passes to the liver and into the right side of the heart. Since the fetus is not yet breathing, its lungs do not require the great amount of blood required after birth. The heart of the fetus therefore has two bypasses, the foramen ovale and the ductus arteriosus, which allow much of the fetal blood to pass through the heart quickly and out into the body. (See figure on fetal circulation.)

After birth, when the child starts breathing, these by-passes normally close. But it is estimated that these closures may be incomplete in as many as 20 percent of all children, resulting in types of congenital heart defects.

Many other types of heart defects may occur. The common symptom of such defects is a blue skin color (cyanosis). This is due to inadequate oxygen in the blood. A baby with such a condition is often called a "blue baby." Many heart conditions can be repaired during infancy with surgery.

### Causes of Congenital Defects

Faulty genes cause about 20 percent of all birth defects; a faulty environment in the uterus another 20 percent; and combinations of the two 60 percent. Hereditary defects may cause chemical disturbances in the fetus which may result in conditions such as phenylketonuria, galactosemia, and cystic fibrosis.

The uterine environment includes those things that happen to the mother during pregnancy and the things that take place in the uterus around the fetus. Virus infections in the mother, particularly during the first three months of pregnancy, may cause defects. One such infection is rubella (German measles). Most dangerous during the first 4 weeks of pregnancy, it may cause deafness, heart and eye defects, and even mental retardation.

Drugs the mother takes during pregnancy may cause abnormalities. Such was true with thalidomide, a tranquilizer-sedative, which was available in Europe during the early 1960s. It may cause severe deformity of the long bones, so that children are born with both arms and legs missing. The deformity occurred when mothers took the medication during the second month of pregnancy.

Most defects start during the first 90 days of pregnancy. Drugs (sedatives, tranquilizers, and other drugs) that might be safe to take under most circumstances may be dangerous in light of the rigorous demands of early pregnancy. This is especially true with the unplanned pregnancy in which damage may be done before the woman even knows she is pregnant. Knowing that there may be other causes for a missed menstruation, a woman may take insufficient precaution in her exposure to x-rays, virus infections, or drugs. She may not see a physician for several months, by which time she has already passed the time of greatest fetal damage.

### Prevention of Congenital Defects

Here are some simple suggestions on how prospective parents may reduce the chances of birth defects in their children.

1. Do not marry a close relative; this increases the risk of producing a defective child.

Such increased risk is the basis for state laws prohibiting close relatives from marrying each other.

2. All married couples should have a family physician. He should be made aware of any known history of family defects or sources of complication such as an Rh-incompatibility so he can correctly counsel the couple. They should both seek his counsel before planning a pregnancy, and then the woman should see him at regular intervals during the pregnancy. Since premature babies are more likely to be defective than full-term babies, medical care during pregnancy is essential to avert premature delivery.

3. The physician treating other conditions should be told of any suspected pregnancy, even though the woman may only think she is pregnant. A woman who either is pregnant or apt to become pregnant should take only those medications prescribed by her physician.

4. The pregnant woman should avoid contact with diseases. If there has been known contact, she should inform her physician.

5. Except in emergency, x-rays should be avoided during the first 90 days of pregnancy.

6. Smoking should be avoided during pregnancy. The more a mother smokes during pregnancy, the less her baby will weigh. The weight of a baby at birth can relate to its chances of survival, especially if it is exceptionally small.

7. The age of the mother must be considered. A high correlation exists between birth defects and the age of the mother, and in some cases, the father. Mothers under 18 and over 40 produce a greater percentage of defective children than those between the ages of 18 and 40.

8. Since diet affects growth, women should learn to eat properly. Diet must be thought of both in terms of the woman's own health and the future growth and development of her children. The fetus depends entirely on the diet of its mother.

## FERTILITY CONTROL

There are two significant problems that face many couples. One is insuring the conception of children that are wanted. The other is preventing the birth of children that are not wanted.

A couple has the right to the greatest degree of personal richness and satisfaction possible for them from their relationship. The number of children they will have and when they will have them are all-important in this attainment. The thoughtful couple desiring children wants the assurance they will be ready for them in terms of family stability, personal and emotional adjustment, physical health, finances, and living conditions. Just as important for the couple not wanting children is the prevention of birth. Family planning is parenthood by choice, rather than by chance.

Methods of controlling birth can be divided into four categories: sexual abstinence, contraception, sterilization, and abortion. Within each of these categories there are one or more methods commonly in use today. Each method has its advantages and disadvantages.

In selecting the method which is right for a given woman, the most important factor is safety. The ideal method must be relatively harmless to use. It must neither be harmful to a woman's normal health nor reduce her ability to have a child in the future, if she wants one. A second consideration is its effectiveness. A woman should have the assurance that the selected method will guarantee against an unwanted pregnancy. Other considerations are whether a certain method is medically suitable in terms of a woman's medical history and whether it can be used with physical comfort. Another factor is the matter of convenience. The preferable method would be one requiring the least change in a woman's habits and attitudes. It should conform to a couple's aesthetic attitudes toward sexual relations and their religious convictions. The price of the method should be a factor. Most methods are relatively inexpensive in this country, at least in comparison with the medical bills incurred in any single pregnancy. Even so, the somewhat lower costs of some methods may make them more attractive than others. A last consideration may be the matter of personal taste. It simply remains for a couple who want to limit the size of their family to study the facts and choose the method that best suits them.

### Sexual Abstinence

Abstinence requires that a couple restrain themselves either from the sex act entirely or from certain aspects of it, especially at those times of the woman's menstrual cycle when fertilization is most likely. This will prevent the sperm from meeting the egg.

*Withdrawal (Coitus Interruptus).* This method of preventing the sperm from getting inside the woman involves the withdrawal of the penis from the vagina just before the male ejaculation occurs. This is an ancient technique and is mentioned in the Old Testament. It was a common method prior to the development of mechanical and chemical contraceptives.

To be effective this method requires that the man be alert to the first signs of orgasm and be prepared to terminate intercourse at any moment. For some couples this does not seem to produce any ill effects. For others this interruption of intercourse just before the moment of greatest pleasure may disturb the entire sexual relationship.

In terms of its effectiveness, withdrawal presents a serious problem. As seen from the table on the effectiveness of various fertility control techniques, for every 100 couples practicing withdrawal for a full year, 18 women are likely to become pregnant. One reason for this is that some of the first fluids emitted from the penis, even before orgasm, may contain sperm. Another reason is that any mistake in timing withdrawal may permit some semen to be deposited in the woman. One drop of semen may be sufficient to cause pregnancy. The first drops of semen discharged by the male contain a higher concentration of sperm than later semen. For couples desiring to be successful in limiting their family size, this method would be used only in an emergency or as a last resort.

*The Rhythm Method.* This method is based on the fact that a woman usually produces a mature egg once a month with some predictability. If the egg fails to meet a sperm within 24 hours, it begins to degenerate. Sperm inseminated into the woman's body and kept at normal body temperatures can remain alive for 24 to 72 hours after intercourse and still fertilize an egg. Conception can occur only if intercourse takes place slightly before or during the time in which the egg is alive. Thus, there should be a single 3-day period each menstrual cycle during which pregnancy might result. This is all simple enough. The big question each month is when does this period occur?

Ordinarily a woman produces a ripe egg about 14 days before the start of the next menstruation. Ovulation seems to be tied more closely to the next onset of menstruation than to the last one. But assuming that a woman has menstrual periods that are invariably 28 days apart, the mature egg may

| EFFECTIVENESS OF FERTILITY CONTROL TECHNIQUES | |
| --- | --- |
| METHOD | PREGNANCY RATE |
| Douche | 31 |
| Rhythm | 24 |
| Jelly alone | 20 |
| Withdrawal | 18 |
| Condom | 14 |
| Diaphragm | 12 |
| Intrauterine devices | 5 |
| Sequential steroids | 5 |
| Combined steroids | 0.1 |
| Sterilization | 0.003 |

SOURCE: Based in part on a report by Gregory Pincus in *Science*, 153, No. 3735 (July 29, 1966).

be released anywhere from the 17th to the 13th day before the next menstruation begins (see figure on rhythm method). Even for a woman with such menstrual regularity there is no way of predicting in any given cycle when it will occur. To be safe, such a woman must refrain from intercourse on these 5 days. Intercourse 2 days prior to earliest ovulation could still leave live sperm to fertilize the egg, and intercourse a day after the latest possible ovulation could mean an egg was still present to be fertilized. Thus, for a regular 28-day woman using the rhythm method, it is recommended she refrain from intercourse from the 19th to the 12th day before her next menstrual discharge, or from the 10th to the 17th day after the beginning of

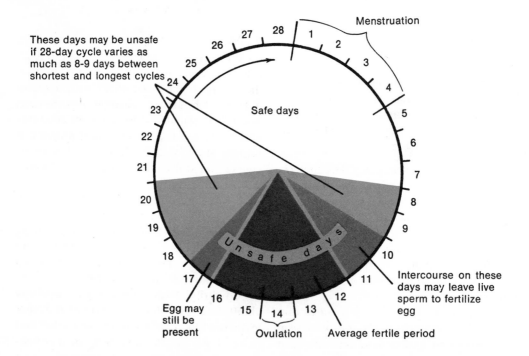

The theory of the rhythm method. The shaded sections indicate days of greatest chance of pregnancy (the darker the shading, the greater the chance). This chart is based on an average 28-day menstrual cycle.

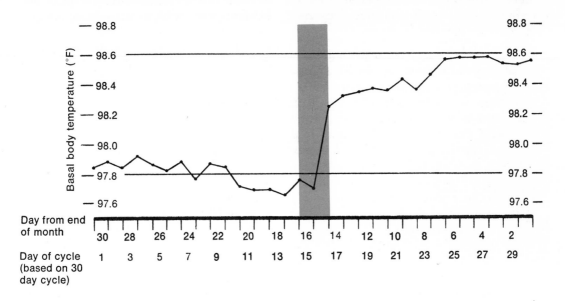

Basal body temperature (BBT) during typical menstrual cycle. Ovulation will commonly occur 14 days before the end of the cycle. Since the length of menstrual cycles varies, the days on the chart are listed in reverse order.

her last discharge. For a period of 8 days each month she must not have intercourse.

Unfortunately, most women do not menstruate with such clocklike regularity. Some women have menstrual cycles as short as 21 days and others as long as 38 days. The average woman may vary as much as 8 to 9 days between her shortest and longest cycles. Many women do not realize how irregular their menstrual cycles are.

The major drawback to the rhythm method is detecting the day of ovulation. On or about the day of ovulation about 25 percent of women sometimes experience a low abdominal pain called *mittelschmerz,* occurring as a result of irritation from the ruptured follicle. Few women experience this with every cycle.

Another clue to the approximate day of ovulation is the shift in basal body temperature (BBT). This is measured with a special thermometer which shows tenth-of-a-degree graduations relatively far apart. The readings are based on the fact that ovulation causes changes in the normal body temperature of a woman each month. The BBT figure shows the typical pattern as a function of the day of cycle.

This method of calculating sex life each month is a major disadvantage to many couples. Regulating sex according to the calendar rather than to the way a person feels does not appeal to most young couples. Even faithful adherence is not totally effective in preventing pregnancy. Twenty-four out of one hundred women practicing this method for a year could be expected to become pregnant.

### Contraception

Contraception today amounts to one of two things. It may either prevent fertilization or prevent ovulation. The types of contraceptive methods available fall into three categories: mechanical, chemical, or hormonal.

*Mechanical. The condom.* The condom is usually a synthetic rubber sheath worn rather tightly over the erect penis. There is a rubber ring at the open end to help hold it in place. The function of the condom is to prevent the sperm from reaching the vagina. It is about as effective as the diaphragm in preventing pregnancy, and its effectiveness can be increased if it is used in conjunction with a contraceptive jelly applied to the outside of the condom or foam inserted into the vagina before intercourse.

The condom is used widely around the world both for the prevention of venereal disease and the control of pregnancy. It is one of the handiest methods to use and can be purchased almost anywhere. Until the availability of the contraceptive pill and the intrauterine device, it was one of the most effective methods of birth control.

The main disadvantages are that the condom interferes with the full enjoyment of the sexual act by dulling the sensations and that it requires interruption of the sexual relationship in order to be put into place. Neither of these objections need be of great significance to the couple seeking protection.

The failure rate of the condom can be reduced by taking several precautions in its use. Only high-quality condoms should be used and careful handling is required to prevent tearing. It should be placed on the penis well before orgasm since preejaculatory fluid may contain sperm cells. If the erection subsides before the penis is removed from the vagina the condom no longer fits tightly and sperm may seep over the top or the condom may slip off, in either case allowing sperm to enter the vagina, and pregnancy may result. Like other contraceptives, the condom should be used throughout the woman's menstrual cycle, rather than just when the woman's fertility seems most likely. Otherwise, a couple is, in effect, taking the same risk of pregnancy as if the rhythm system were used.

*The diaphragm.* The vaginal diaphragm, used widely in the United States, is a shallow rubber or synthetic cap designed to cover the neck of the uterus and thus prevent sperm from entering. It has a flexible metal spring or coil to hold it in place. It ranges in size from 2 to 4 inches in diameter to allow for variations in the size of the vagina. A woman must be fitted for a diaphragm by a physician; it can then be purchased by prescription at a drugstore. Since a woman's vaginal dimensions change as a result of the beginning of intercourse and childbirth, the diaphragm size should be checked when necessary.

The diaphragm is usually used with a spermicidal cream or jelly which provides additional protection. The spermicide is applied to all surfaces of the diaphragm.

When a diaphragm is properly fitted and inserted, the woman should not feel its presence. It does not impair sexual sensation for either partner and apparently has no physical side effects.

Although the diaphragm was once popular, its effectiveness is not great. Out of one hundred women using it for one full year, about twelve are likely to become pregnant.

*Intrauterine devices.* The intrauterine device (IUD) has been used for a long time. It has been known for centuries that a foreign object in the uterus prevents pregnancy, though the mechanism of this prevention is not completely understood. Physicians tried placing devices in the uterus, but were not highly successful because of the body's rejection of foreign matter. This problem has been largely solved with newer materials.

The devices vary in shape, size, and kind of material. Common shapes include rings,

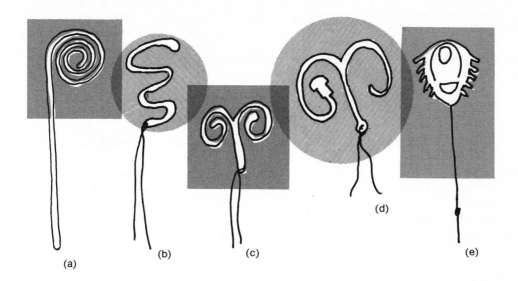

(a)  (b)  (c)  (d)  (e)

Intrauterine devices commonly available. (a) Margulies spiral (with stem); (b) Lippes loop; (c) Saf-T-Coil; (d) Saf-T-Coil nullip; (e) Dalkon shield.

spirals, loops, bows, shields, and springs. They range in size from 7/8 to 1 3/8 inches. They may be made of stainless steel, preformed plastic, or copper. The plastic devices, shown in the figure on intrauterine devices, are inserted by being pushed through a small tube into the uterus. All must be inserted by a physician or specially trained nurse. Once in place, the device can remain for many years without any harmful effects to the patient. No other contraceptive protection is necessary and the woman wearing it should be totally unaware of its presence.

There may be some unpleasant side effects from the use of the IUD. Pelvic cramps, irregular and unusually heavy menstrual bleeding, and spontaneous expulsion are reduced by decreasing the size of the device. The overall safety of an IUD depends upon two factors: the style selected and the training and experience of the person inserting it. If the side effects are severe, and the woman cannot tolerate the IUD, it should be removed. Some women, especially those who have not had children, are unable to retain the devices and expel them. It is estimated that about one-third of the users suffer complications (particularly excessive bleeding and backache, which are relieved when the IUD is removed).

Although the effectiveness of the devices varies with their shape and size, out of one hundred women using the device for one year, about five could expect to become pregnant. In the event a pregnancy occurs while the device is still in the uterus, it does not interfere with the normal development or delivery of the child. There is great hope for the worldwide use of the IUD today in terms of its low cost, ease of insertion, and long-term effectiveness once in place.

*Chemical. The douche.* Some women believe that pregnancy can be prevented by washing away the semen after intercourse by douching, or washing out, the vagina. Various douches have been used—hot water, cold water, vinegar, lemon juice, soap chips dissolved in water, or washes available in drugstores. A large rubber bulb, or syringe, is filled with the fluid and emptied into the vagina.

The douche is an ineffective method of birth control (thirty-one out of one hundred women using this method for a year would be expected to become pregnant). The reason for this low effectiveness is that the act of intercourse can result in sperm being deposited directly into the uterus. A douche can wash out the vagina, but not reach the uterus. The major usefulness of the douche is as a method of feminine hygiene, especially after the menstrual period. Frequent douching interferes with the natural cleansing actions and, therefore, is not recommended by most physicians.

*Vaginal spermicides.* Various chemical preparations kill or impede the movement of sperm. These vaginal spermicides are available in the form of creams, gels (jellies), aerosol foams, and suppositories.

The woman selecting this method uses a special applicator to insert a measured amount of the spermicide into the vagina one hour or less prior to each intercourse. One application is good for only one intercourse. The action of the preparations is twofold: the spermicide acts to kill the sperm on contact; the chemical base of the preparation forms a coating that keeps surviving sperm from reaching the egg. The plastic applicator deposits the preparation high in the vaginal tract at the opening into the uterus. The effectiveness of jellies alone in preventing pregnancy is not excellent. Out of one hundred women using this method for one year, twenty are apt to become pregnant.

Vaginal foams are a variation on the creams. They are packaged in a can under pressure and the contents are released into a plastic applicator, by which the foam is applied high in the vagina.

Suppositories are small pencil-shaped glycerin-gelatin preparations containing a spermicide which melts at body temperature. They are inserted deep into the vagina a few minutes to an hour before intercourse.

Foaming tablets dissolve on contact with the moisture in the vagina when inserted. They release a carbon-dioxide gas to produce a foam that spreads the spermicide over the upper vaginal area. A tablet should be inserted several minutes to an hour before intercourse.

*Hormonal.* The female oral contraceptive pills are designed to prevent ovulation. These pills, which are highly effective in preventing pregnancy, are composed of female hormones that usually make a woman able to conceive. The pills' basic hormone is progestin, a synthetic drug similar to the female hormone progesterone. Some forms of the pill also contain estrogen. You will recall from an earlier discussion that the pituitary gland produces the hormones FSH and LH which are necessary for the production and release of a mature egg in the ovary. The follicles in the ovary produce both estrogen and progesterone. Among other functions, the estrogen inhibits the production of FSH, and progesterone inhibits the production of LH. When the pill is taken daily starting with day 5 (the fifth day after the beginning of menstruation), the presence of progestin and estrogen inhibit the body's production of FSH and LH before they are able to produce a mature egg. Ovulation does not occur and no egg is present to unite with the sperm which are released during intercourse. The woman then fails to become pregnant. This suppression of egg production is very much like the suppression of egg production that takes place while a woman is pregnant. Under the influence of natural estrogen and progesterone, no other mature eggs are produced until after the pregnancy has terminated.

There are several types of pills produced today, as discussed below.

*The combined pill.* The first pills produced combined estrogen and progestin. Most combined pills are designed to be taken for 20 or 21 days of the menstrual cycle, starting on day 5 and ending on day 24 or 25. Then for 7 or 8 days, the pill is omitted, allowing menstruation to occur. Only one type of pill is taken. Some women experience side effects such as nausea, headache, swelling of the breasts, and bleeding. Commonly these symptoms diminish or disappear after the first several months. In addition to preventing ovulation, the combined pill also makes the uterine lining less receptive to a fertilized egg, thus making the pill even more effective than it might otherwise be. Out of one thousand women using the combined pill for one year, only seven are apt to become pregnant.

*The sequential pill.* Because of some complaints regarding the side effects of the combined pill, the sequential pills were developed. They amount to two different pills, one taken from day 5 through day 19 and the other from day 20 through day 24. (The days differ for different brands.) The pills taken the first 15 days contain estrogen only; the pills taken the last 5 days contain both estrogen and progestin (like the combined pill). The sequential pills are packaged so that the pills are easily taken in the right order. The action of both pills is similar. The effectiveness of the sequential pill is less than that of the combined pill. Of one hundred women taking the sequential pill for one year, one or two are apt to become pregnant.

*The "minipill."* A pill containing about one-fourth the progestin dosage of the standard pills and no estrogen is now available. Women using it take it every day of the year. Rather than inhibiting ovulation, the minipill is thought to reduce sperm motility—the sperm do not reach the egg. Its effectiveness appears to be about one pregnancy per one hundred women using it for one year.

Depending on the brand used, there are minor variations in the make-up and number of pills taken. The major advantage of all pill methods is their effectivness and the ease of taking them. When a woman wants to become pregnant, she merely stops taking the pills, and she should become pregnant with at least the same likelihood as before taking the pills.

Other hormonal contraceptives are now under investigation. The "20-year" pill is implanted under the skin and gradually releases its contents. A woman wanting a child would have her physician remove the pill. The "morning-after" pill is taken on the day following sexual intercourse. In fact, it may be taken up to 6 days afterward and still prevent pregnancy, but it is not recommended for regular use because of more extreme side effects. The morning-after pill works by preventing the fertilized egg from being implanted in the wall of the uterus. Pills for men are being tested that would make conception impossible by preventing the development of sperm or making them incapable of uniting with the egg. Vaccination appears to be another possibility. The idea of making the woman immune to sperm by injecting her with antibodies that would attack and reject sperm is being investigated.

Periodically the matter of the pill undergoes sensational publicity such as from congressional hearings and exposés in women's magazines. The pill is not a cure-all. The pill does have some harmful side effects, effects which are unpredictable in some women. It should never be prescribed for women who already show certain danger signals such as persistent headaches, swelling of the legs, vein tenderness, and chest pains. Studies suggest that among women using oral contraceptives there are about 3 clotting deaths per 100,000 women per year. But placed in perspective, about 24 women per 100,000 die each year as the consequence of pregnancy. This is about eight times more than die from pill-caused clotting deaths.

There are some 30 preparations of oral contraceptives on the market. For each commercial product the chemical structure of the synthetic estrogens and progestins may differ, as does the estrogen/progestin ratio. Some physicians believe that these side effects are essentially eliminated if the correct type of pill is chosen. Under any circumstance, the proper prescription of the pill, as with any contraceptive method, requires a thorough discussion between the patient and her physician. The patient must be made aware of the risks, real or suspected, of hormonal contraceptives. In terms of effectiveness as a contraceptive, the pill is two to four times more effective than the IUD and ten to thirty times higher than the diaphragm. Along with other forms of fertility control, Dr. Alan F. Guttmacher (1970) places the pill in perspective when he says that "it is a prophylaxis against one of the gravest sociomedical illnesses—unwanted pregnancy."

### Sterilization

Sterilization, or surgery that prevents parenthood, is a method of birth control that is common in certain parts of the world. It is a permanent method of fertility control that is virtually 100 percent effective. A man or woman who has been properly sterilized can have children only if a second operation is successfully performed to undo the first.

Sterilization does not remove any of the sex organs or glands and has no effect upon sexual desire or performance. For a woman,

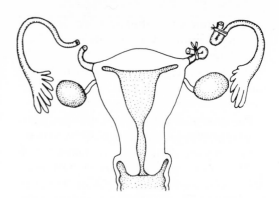

Tubal ligation, or sterilization by severing the fallopian tubes

the operation consists of cutting the two fallopian tubes and closing off the cut ends of the tubes. Once the tubes have been tied, the eggs can no longer reach the uterus. The procedure may be performed through an abdominal incision (commonly called a tubal ligation). Requiring several days of hospitalization, it is commonly performed shortly after childbirth. A more recent procedure is by laparoscopy, in which a tiny hole is made

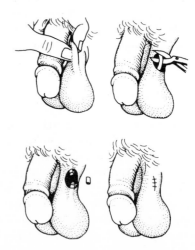

Vasectomy, or sterilization by severing the vas deferens

just under the navel, through which a slender instrument is inserted which clamps the fallopian tube, seals and cuts it. It may be performed in an out-patient department, the patient may go home the same day, and the procedure is relatively inexpensive.

For a man, the operation, called a vasectomy, consists of cutting and tying the vas deferens, the passages through which sperm travel from the testes to the genital passages. The man continues to produce semen as before; it is still ejaculated upon orgasm, but it contains no sperm. The sperm disintegrate and are absorbed by the blood vessels of the testes. The procedure requires only small cuts on both sides of the scrotum and can be safely performed in a physician's office.

Sterilization is legally permissible in every state of the union, as well as in many countries throughout the world. In a few states, medical reasons are required for the operation.

A disadvantage of sterilization is that the effects of the operation are commonly nonreversible. A second operation designed to undo the first fails in about half of all cases, with the techniques presently being used.

Sterilization is now being used in certain overpopulated countries of the world. Over 2 million men in India have been voluntarily sterilized. It is also being recommended in England and the United States. As a result of efforts to reduce misinformation and myths concerning the effects of a vasectomy, increasing numbers of couples are electing this method of contraception.

### Abortion

The removal of a growing embryo or fetus from the wall of the uterus to which it is attached is defined as an abortion. A natural abortion, commonly called a miscarriage, is the spontaneous termination of pregnancy by the body. It is believed that about one of every ten pregnancies ends in this manner. About 75 percent of these occur during the second and third months of pregnancy. Common causes are an abnormally developing fetus, abnormalities of the placenta, and maternal disease. An induced abortion is the expulsion of the embryo or fetus by artificial means. An induced abortion is legal or criminal depending on state laws.

Early in 1973, the U.S. Supreme Court voted to give every woman in the United States, regardless of existing state laws, the same right to an abortion during the first six months of pregnancy as she has to any other minor surgery. During the first three months of pregnancy the abortion decision must be left to the medical judgment of the pregnant woman's attending physician. After the first trimester, a state may regulate the abortion procedure in ways that are reasonably related to maternal health, for instance, by requiring hospitalization. But it is illegal to demand that a panel of physicians approve the abortion. Only after the fetus has developed enough to have a chance of survival on its own, usually during the seventh month, may a state regulate and even proscribe abortion except where it is necessary for the preservation or health of the mother.

The court has held that a woman's right to privacy overcomes any state interest in using abortion statutes (as some states have) to regulate sexual conduct, even though indirectly. It also holds that a fetus is not a person under the Constitution and thus has no legal right to life. Legal abortion during the first trimester is decidedly safer than childbirth. After the first trimester, the danger to the mother increases, hence the states' authority to protect the health of the mother. The United States has joined Japan, India, the Soviet Union, and the majority of Eastern European countries in making abortion freely available.

There are several common ways of aborting pregnancies. The most common is the classic D and C (dilatation and curettage) in which the cervix is dilated and the inside of the uterus is merely scraped clean. Up through the twelfth week, when performed by a physician under aseptic conditions, the D and C is a safe procedure. Another method which can be safely used before the twelfth week is the suction curettage. A machine which builds up a negative pressure sucks out the products of conception. As with the D and C, care must be taken not to perforate the uterus. From 12 to 17 weeks, a combined method is sometimes used, the suction curette being used to extract the products of conception after they have been broken up by a D and C. Another method which may be used up to 24 weeks of gestation is to introduce a hypertonic solution of saline or glucose into the uterine cavity. Not without risk to the mother, this should be performed only by a skilled physician. Improper administration can result in the rapid death of, or serious infection to, the woman. A physician may perform a curettage afterward to clean out the uterus. Occasionally, for a pregnancy of more than 12 weeks gestation, an abdominal procedure may be performed, perhaps with sterilization or hysterectomy. The physician may remove the uterus (hysterectomy) and/or tie off the fallopian tubes (tubal ligation).

Properly performed by a qualified physician in an aseptic setting, these methods may present little hazard to the woman, often less than allowing the pregnancy to continue on to full term. While some women do suffer from emotional problems following the abortion, other women do not. Most important is for the physician to make an individual determination and recommendation for each patient based on the factors in each case.

In countries where abortions are legally available to anyone wishing them, abortion is a common method of fertility control. In Japan, there are 46 abortions for every 100 pregnancies ending in childbirth; in Hungary, 132 abortions for every 100 pregnancies ending in childbirth.

In countries where abortions are legalized, there is very little danger since the procedure can be performed at the proper time in the ideal hospital setting. For example, in Hungary, the death rate from abortion is less than 6 per 100,000. The death rate in the United States from childbirth and its complications is almost four times as high; from removal of tonsils and adenoids it is more than three times as high. The procedure can be performed safely if performed early enough in the pregnancy. In Hungary, the death rate from abortion rises from about 6 per 100,000 when performed during the first 3 months to 300 per 100,000 when performed during the second 3 months of pregnancy, or is fifty times as high.

### Which Method to Choose

Fertility control is a highly individual matter which must rest upon a private decision between a man and a woman. It is plainly a matter of which method to choose, not whether or not to choose one. During a normal adult life, a woman may have four hundred chances to conceive. Such a woman could give birth to thirty or forty children. Few women would desire that many.

The choice of a method must be satisfactory to both partners. A choice ought to be made in terms of a couple's taste and preferences, their emotional dispositions, their physical requirements and any medical limitations, and their moral standards and religious attitudes. Methods ought to be discussed with a physician as part of any premarital counseling. Information may also be obtained from family planning clinics or from qualified agencies. (One such agency is Planned Parenthood Federation of America, 515 Madison Avenue, New York, New York 10022.) Ask for the address of your state or area organization. The address may also be obtained through a local telephone directory.

## INFERTILITY

For most couples, family planning means limiting the number of children they have, or at least spacing their arrival. The majority of young couples who desire children have little difficulty in producing them. Physicians estimate that at least 50 percent of all fertile couples can achieve pregnancy within 1 month of regular intercourse, and 75 percent are successful by the end of 6 months.

Yet for a significant minority, the problem is just the opposite. Some couples who practice no form of birth control would like to have children but have none at all. Other couples wish for more children than they have but are unable to have them. Out of every one hundred married couples, ten are unable to have any children at all and fifteen have fewer than they would like. This means that about 25 percent of the population are troubled with insufficient fertility.

There are two degrees of insufficient fertility. The total inability to produce children is termed sterility. A temporary inability to produce children is called infertility. A couple must consider themselves infertile until they can be shown to be sterile.

### Causes of Infertility

Childlessness has been looked upon in some places as a curse or a punishment, an object of scorn and ridicule. It is none of these. It may simply be the result of various physical and psychological conditions. It may be due to physical defects, emotional stress, a mistiming of ovulation, or a sperm allergy. It may be traceable to one partner or to both. For every one hundred cases of infertility, the wife is unable to conceive in fifty cases, the husband is unable to induce conception in thirty, and the problem is shared by both partners in twenty.

*The Husband.* In the male the problem is a failure to discharge enough active sperm to produce reasonable chances of fertilization. This difficulty has no relation to the male's masculinity, since the male hormones and the sperm are produced by different cells. A man may be sterile and still have normal sexual performance in all other respects.

Normal semen amounts to a minimum volume of 3 milliliters of ejaculate. (1 milliliter is approximately ¼ teaspoon.) There should be at least 60 million sperm per milliliter of semen, of which 60 percent must be normal sperm. (See figure showing normal and abnormal sperm.) 60 percent of the sperm should be motile 2 hours *after* ejaculation. If the sperm count falls below 10 million per milliliter or the percentage of normal sperm falls below 70 percent, the male is considered sterile.

Failure in sperm production may be due to poor health, inadequate nutrition, or emotional stress. Such conditions can often be corrected. Failure may also be due to birth defects, exposure to certain types of radiation, injury, or certain diseases. Some of these problems may be irreversible.

Techniques have been devised to improve the concentration of sperm. Some physicians advise the man to withdraw the penis after the first portions of ejaculated sperm have entered the vagina to prevent the first drops from being diluted. Portions of sperm can also be collected, combined, and artificially inseminated into the uterus of the wife.

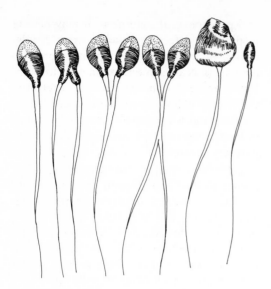

Various forms of human sperms: left, normal; others, abnormal. Sterility will result if the percentage of abnormal sperm reaches 25 to 30 percent of total sperm.

*The Wife.* The female reproductive system is not only more complicated anatomically than that of the male, it must also respond to the interaction of some critical hormones. Thus, the causes of infertility in the woman can be more extensive.

The first fact that must be known is whether a mature egg, which can be fertilized, is available each month. Basal body temperature readings and tissue examinations from the uterus can be used to help detect the course of ovulation. Depending on the cause, failure to ovulate may be treated surgically, hormonally, or by other medication. Some women ovulate after taking an oral contraceptive for several months and then stopping.

Other reasons for infertility in the woman might be an obstructed fallopian tube preventing the migration of the egg, uterine deformities which block passage of sperm, or vaginal fluids which kill the sperm. Also, the egg may be fertilized properly, but be

unable to make attachment to the uterine wall. This may be due to a hormonal imbalance that alters the nature of the endometrium. This condition can, however, be corrected.

*Emotional Factors.* In some underprivileged countries, diseased, half-starved humans existing in filthy conditions seem to have little trouble reproducing. Other women who are near physical collapse or who have undergone the psychological trauma of rape (and who would prefer not to be pregnant) bear children. Yet, strangely enough, the fertility of some couples desiring children seems to be upset by subtle emotional matters.

Some women have become pregnant after they have moved out of an annoying neighborhood or after they have taken leisurely vacations. Women who apparently could not conceive have become pregnant shortly after adopting a child.

With some, emotional tension may be the basis of the problem. Tension may prevent the release of the ripe egg or prevent its movement. It may interfere with the production of sperm. Low sperm counts have been revealed among male college students during examination periods, among airplane pilots during wartime combat, or in men who are in a state of nervous exhaustion due to overwork. Such sperm counts have changed when the emotional stress has been relieved. Some couples become fertile when they begin visiting a fertility clinic, but before they have actually received treatment.

*Timing of Intercourse.* To achieve pregnancy, it is important to have intercourse near the time of ovulation. Physicians frequently suggest methods of improving the chances of fertilization during this period; for example, the couple might refrain from intercourse in the few days preceding ovulation in order to conserve sperm, and then repeat intercourse in forty-eight hour intervals during the fertile period.

*Sperm Allergy.* Occasionally women are allergic to their husband's sperm. The woman develops antibodies that attack and reject the sperm, thus making fertilization almost impossible. Such immunities are sometimes known to wear off when the wife's body is not exposed to the sperm for a period of months. This type of infertility has been successfully treated in some cases by the man using a condom during every intercourse and preventing the sperm from entering the woman's body. The immunity may wear off and the allergy may disappear. The condom can then be eliminated and pregnancy may occur.

A couple ought to consult their family physician if they are unable to conceive after several months. In the event the physician feels his training is insufficient for the problem or is unable to find the cause, he may refer the patient or couple to a specialist or clinic. Medical schools often have fertility clinics. Help may also be obtained from a local Planned Parenthood Committee. (Another source is the American Fertility Society, 944 South 18th Street, Birmingham, Alabama 35205.)

### Artificial Insemination

Many couples, where one of the partners is sterile (either naturally or surgically) and who desire children, turn to artificial insemination. In this process sperm of the husband or of a nonhusband donor are mechanically introduced into the uterus of the wife at the time when conception is most likely to occur. When freshly donated sperm is used, pregnancies occur about 80 percent of the time. When the husband's sperm is used (where husband fertility is very low), pregnancy is successful in about 5 percent of the attempts.

Some physicians are now freezing sperm and storing it until needed. With frozen sperm, impregnation is successful in slightly over 50 percent of the cases. Repeated inseminations over several months are often necessary. Some men have requested prevasectomy storage of their sperm as insurance against unforeseen events. Although sperm stored for as long as ten years has produced live births, frozen sperm loses much of its effectiveness if stored for more than 16 months. Frozen sperm has several advantages. Not only is sperm available at all times when tests show that ovulation is occurring, but parents can come back and request specimens from the same donor. There is also less chance of the donor meeting the recipient.

Donor insemination, as nonhusband artificial insemination is sometimes called, may be looked upon as a type of semiadoption. There are often good reasons for requesting donor insemination over obtaining children through adoption. In the event the husband is sterile, the child will at least be partially like one of the parents. It will, of course, inherit some of the characteristics of the wife. The wife knows this is her baby physically, psychologically, and legally. The husband should look upon the child as his own child psychologically and legally.

The use of artificial insemination is slowly gaining acceptance. It requires a great deal of serious planning and discussion, between the prospective parents—to determine their emotional satisfaction with the process—and with the physician to determine the best method and to find an appropriate donor. Some couples have had more than one child by this technique.

### Adoption

Pregnancy for some couples wanting children is impossible or too dangerous for the mother.

351

These couples may still have the pleasure of raising a family through adoption. Adoption has many advantages. It provides a good home for the child; it does not contribute to population increase, and it guarantees the parents a healthy child of the desired sex.

The availability of children for adoption varies from area to area and from year to year, but there are fewer available infants for adoption each year. This is due to a variety of reasons, including more effective use of birth control by unmarried persons, more readily available abortions, more unmarried women choosing to keep and raise their children, and more couples choosing to adopt a child rather than contribute to the population problem.

However, certain types of children are still readily available for adoption; these include children who are beyond infancy, children of certain ethnic minorities, and children with physical or mental disabilities. Many couples have found the adoption of such children to be a very rewarding experience.

About half of all adoptions involve the children of blood relatives (as in cases where both parents are lost through death or desertion). Adopting a child who is a blood relative is a rather simple matter and can usually be handled by a family attorney. Adopting an unrelated child is handled either through a licensed agency or privately through direct arrangements with the child's family. The great majority of children adopted by non-relatives are the children of unwed mothers.

*Determination of Eligibility.* The operations of adoption agencies are controlled by law; consequently, these agencies usually provide the best protection for the child, the natural parents, and the adoptive parents. The major element in this protection is the determination of eligibility. Though the standards do vary from agency to agency, certain points are commonly found.

Agencies attempt to place children in homes where the atmosphere, attitudes, financial circumstances, living conditions, and health of the family are conducive to a satisfactory adjustment of the child. The age of the prospective parents, their religious and racial background (though these factors are less important now than in previous years), their obvious attitudes towards the idea of adoption and the child in particular, and the stability of the marriage of the prospective parents are easily discernible and valuable indices.

*Adoption Procedure.* Once the "match" between parents and child is made to the satisfaction of all parties concerned, the child enters the adoptive home, generally for a probationary period of one year. If the adoption proves suitable during this time, an adoptive decree will be issued for the child; a new birth certificate, giving him the family name of his new parents and their chosen first and middle names, will be drawn up. The original birth record is sealed by the court, never to be opened again except on court order. From this moment, the adopted child is treated as a natural child of the couple. He is entitled to matters of inheritance as is a natural child and is so treated by the courts.

## PREGNANCY AND CHILDBIRTH

Although many millions of sperm are deposited in the female genital tract, only one will penetrate the egg. This requires the efforts of many other sperm surrounding the egg. These sperm give off an enzyme which detaches a covering over the egg, the corona radiata, allowing one sperm to enter.

As soon as the sperm has penetrated the egg, the membrane covering the egg thickens and prevents the entry of any other sperm.

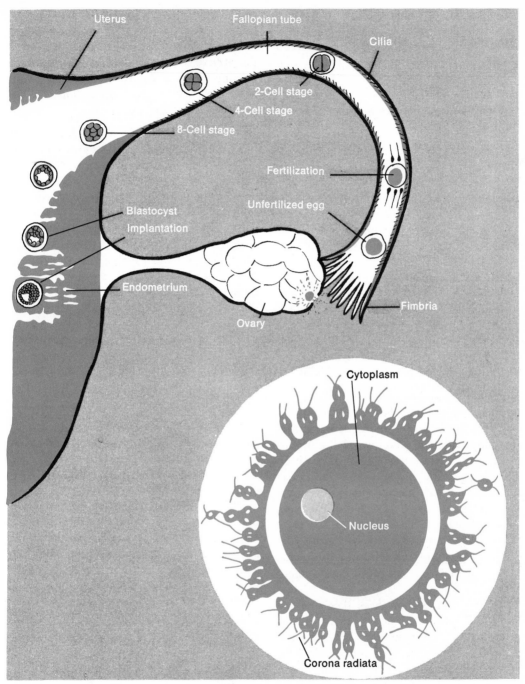

The human ovum (lower right) and its path during ovulation, fertilization, and finally implantation in the uterus.

Following entry, the nucleus in the head of the sperm fuses with the nucleus in the egg, and fertilization has occurred. The united cell is now referred to as a zygote. The woman is now said to be pregnant.

### Embryology (The Development of the Fertilized Cell)

The zygote immediately begins to divide. From a 1-celled zygote, it divides to form 2 cells, 4 cells, 8 cells, and so on. It is now called an embryo. By the end of the first week it is a hollow ball of many cells. As cell division speeds up, one side of the ball of cells forms a depression or indentation. This is the first indication that specialized cells, tissues, and organs will be appearing. A fold develops called the neural groove, later to become the nervous system. The groove becomes a tube, and the head end of the tube enlarges to become a beginning brain. Blood vessels develop and spread out and by the twelfth day the primitive beginnings of the head, heart, and limbs are evident.

*Implantation.* While this development is being initiated, the embryo is being carried down the fallopian tube toward the uterus. The embryo spends about three days within the fallopian tube. By the time it leaves the fallopian tube and enters the uterus, the mass of cells looks like a hollow ball, but is actually filled with fluid. Even though the cell mass consists of many cells by this time, the whole mass is no larger than the undivided zygote. (See figure on stages of development of zygote.)

For the next two or three days the cell mass, now called a blastocyst, floats around in the cavity of the uterus. Then, at a site chosen by chance, the mass attaches onto the endometrial lining of the uterus and begins to take root. The site of this attachment, or implantation, is usually some place in the upper half of the uterus. The blastocyst sinks in the endometrium which closes over it. Here the embryo continues to increase in size, soon bulging into the cavity of the uterus, still completely surrounded with endometrial tissue, now called decidua.

*Placenta Formation.* From the outer wall of the blastocyst, small fingerlike growths called chorionic villi now begin to project into the decidua. In the decidua between the blastocyst and the uterine wall, spaces filled with maternal blood are formed. This area of special tissue for the transfer of nutrients from the mother to the child and for the transfer of wastes from the child to the mother is called the placenta. Even though there is a very close relation between the villi of the embryo and the tissues of the mother in the placenta, there is never a direct connection between the two circulations. Blood does not cross directly from the mother to the embryo, and vice versa. The placenta actively transfers materials from the end of the fourth week after fertilization.

*Amniotic Fluid.* The embryo is attached to the placenta by the umbilical cord, and is surrounded by a double membrane which consists of the amnion and chorion. The space inside of these layers is often called the "bag of waters." The space is filled with amniotic fluid, which bathes the developing embryo. This fluid contains embryonic wastes which are exchanged with the mother's fluids. It also serves to give the embryo space in which to develop, protects it against injury, and keeps it at a constant temperature.

*Lunar Months of Pregnancy.* During the first 8 weeks of pregnancy, the developing child is called the embryo; the rest of the time, it is known as the fetus.

A full-term human pregnancy usually lasts

about 266 days from the time of conception, or about 280 days after the beginning of the last menstrual period (ovulation occurs about 14 days after the beginning of menstruation.) The events of pregnancy are commonly subdivided into lunar months; 280 days represents 10 lunar months, each 28 days or 4 weeks in length (although the true lunar month is 29½ days long). Thus a full-term pregnancy would be expected to last about 40 weeks.

According to the calendar, pregnancy lasts a little over 9 months. These 9 calendar months are commonly divided into three parts of three months each called trimesters. Each trimester is about 13 weeks. The chart on fetal development shows and describes the changes during each of the 10 lunar months of pregnancy (pp. 356–357).

### Diagnosis of Pregnancy

The determination of pregnancy can be based on symptoms a woman senses, signs the physician notes from physical examinations, and certain laboratory tests. The signs and symptoms of pregnancy are divided into three self-explanatory headings: presumptive, probable, and positive signs.

*Presumptive Signs.* Presumptive signs are the least definite evidence of pregnancy. Each of these symptoms which the woman can detect may also result from causes other than pregnancy.

The first symptom noticed is a missed menstrual period. One missed period is questionable evidence, but two missed periods is strong indication. The breasts may increase in size and firmness and be more sensitive. The nipples may become larger and darker. Nausea and vomiting ("morning sickness") may be associated with early pregnancy. The need to urinate more frequently is common to both early and late pregnancy. Pregnant women tend to fatigue more easily.

*Probable Signs.* The probable signs are discovered by the physician. They consist of: enlargement of the abdomen; changes in the shape, size, and consistency of the uterus; changes in the cervix; the detection of contractions of the uterus; and a positive hormonal test. Each one of these again might be caused by conditions other than pregnancy, thus should not be considered an absolute indication.

The hormonal tests call for some explanation. In the event of implantation, the chorion of the embryo gives off a hormone called chorionic gonadotropin. Carried by the bloodstream, some of it gets into the urine. Tests may detect the presence of the hormone in the urine about ten to fourteen days after the first missed menstruation or about the end of the first lunar month. There are several such tests for pregnancy.

*Immunological tests.* These are based on an antigen-antibody response. The hormones present in the urine sample serve as the antigen and will react with the prepared antibody being used in the test. Absence of agglutination is considered a positive test.

*Animal tests.* Various virgin female animals such as rats, frogs, rabbits, and mice may be used for such tests. Urine from the woman is injected into the animal. In the event she is pregnant, her hormone-laden urine will cause follicular development and ovulation in the female animal and show the presence of the corpus luteum.

*Hormone test.* In the event a woman has missed a menstruation, estrogen and progesterone hormones are given to her for two or three days. If she is not pregnant, a normal menstrual flow should occur within several

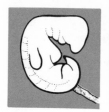 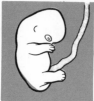 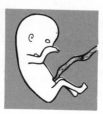 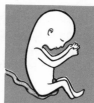 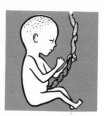

| FIRST LUNAR MONTH | SECOND LUNAR MONTH | THIRD LUNAR MONTH | FOURTH LUNAR MONTH | FIFTH LUNAR MONTH |
|---|---|---|---|---|
| Embryo about ¼ in. long; mouth and jaws present; eyes, ears, and nose forming; arms and legs budding out; heart beating and pumping blood through simple vessels; head very large in proportion to body | Embryo about 1 in. long; face human; eyes, ears, nose visible; thin skin forming; hands and feet forming; fetus begins slight movements; external genitalia beginning to form | Fetus 3 in. long, weight 1 ounce; teeth forming under gums; fingers and toes well formed and bear nails; eyes covered by closed lids; kidneys working; fetus starts swallowing amniotic fluid; sex distinguishable; responds to stimuli; fetus moves easily—not felt by mother | Fetus 6¼ in. long, weight 4 oz; fine hair on body; fetal skeleton visible on x-ray; mother may feel fetal movements; wall of uterus begins stretching | Fetus 9½ in. long, weight 11 oz; buds for permanent teeth begin to form; hair on the head; fetal movements strong; heartbeat perceptible with stethoscope; breasts stop enlarging; uterus as high as navel |

days. In the nonpregnant woman, the hormones quickly build up the uterus lining; then with their discontinuance this lining is shed in bleeding. In the event she is pregnant, no unusual bleeding will occur.

Once more, none of these hormonal tests provides positive proof of pregnancy. Many obstetricians use them with reservations.

*Positive Signs.* There are three positive signs of pregnancy. All three arise from the fetus: fetal heartbeat, perception of active movements of the fetus, and ability to see the fetal skeleton by x-ray. Hearing and counting the fetal heartbeat is unmistakable evidence of pregnancy. The pulse rate will be about twice as fast as the mother's pulse. Fetal movements are commonly felt after the fifth month of pregnancy by placing the hand over the abdomen. The fetal skeletal outline will be visible sometime after the fourteenth week of pregnancy. X-ray is especially useful with obese women in order to distinguish between a tumor or a normal pregnancy.

### Care of the Pregnant Mother

The care of the mother from conception to the beginning of childbirth is called prenatal

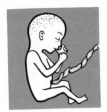 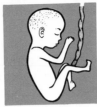 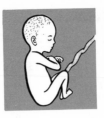 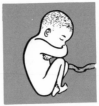 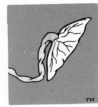

| SIXTH LUNAR MONTH | SEVENTH LUNAR MONTH | EIGHTH LUNAR MONTH | NINTH LUNAR MONTH | PLACENTA |
|---|---|---|---|---|
| Fetus 12 in. long, weight 1½ lb; skin very wrinkled, fat forming underneath; growth now more rapid at head end; eyebrows and eyelashes forming; eyelids reopened; fetus sucks thumb, has hiccups, rolls freely in amniotic fluid | Fetus 14 in. long, weight 2½ lb; skin reddish; thin and scrawny; organs immature, but chance of survival if born | Fetus 16 in. long, weight 3½ lb; skin wrinkled; hair on head abundant; good chance of survival if born | Fetus 18 in. long, weight 6 lb or more; more fat beneath skin makes it plumper, less wrinkled; chances of survival excellent; tip of uterus near breastbone<br><br>Term—fetus 20 in. long, weight 7¼ lb or more; skin smooth | Placenta—1 to 2 in. thick, 6 to 9 in. diameter at birth. Serves two purposes: (1) anchors fetus to the interior of the uterus through the gestation period; (2) includes a complex web of blood vessels through which nutrients pass from the mother to the developing fetus. Also called the afterbirth, and is expelled from the uterus as the final step of a normal birth. |

care. This care is most important in order to ensure the good health of both the mother and the child. Unfortunately, many women are not able to obtain this care. It has been estimated, for instance, that one-third to one-half of the women delivering children in major city public (tax-supported) hospitals see a doctor for the first time when they are in labor.

Due to the demands a pregnancy places on the body of the mother, a disorder or disease that might normally have little effect on her can turn into a major complication. A condition affecting the mother can have a similar effect on the fetus. Careful medical supervision during this time can avert many damaging conditions.

When a woman suspects that she is pregnant, she should have a complete physical examination, including blood tests and pelvic examination. Follow-up examinations should be made every four weeks until the seventh calendar month of pregnancy; then every two weeks, or more frequently as indiciated, until the final month; then once a week until labor begins.

Certain conditions that ought to be watched for closely in case the woman is pregnant include heart disease, diabetes, syphilis, gonorrhea, and acute infectious diseases.

Two particular conditions are also worth serious attention. Toxemias are a group of body poisonings that may occur during the last trimester of pregnancy. They can cause serious complications, even death, to both the mother and the fetus. The conditions are all characterized by a swelling of the body, particularly the feet or ankles; increased blood pressure; albumin in the urine (albuminuria); and a more-than-normal increase in body weight. Treatment by a physician may include a low-salt diet, complete bed rest, drugs to quiet the mother and to reduce swelling, and prescribed amounts of water.

About 85 percent of all pregnant women experience a feeling of nausea or "morning sickness" during the first three months of pregnancy. Experienced on arising in the morning, it may be accompanied by vomiting.

If the vomiting does not disappear during the day, it is known as pernicious vomiting. It may become so severe that it may interfere with sound nutrition, leading to dehydration and starvation. A physician can normally control this condition by the use of indicated foods and drugs. When treated, the mother usually recovers quickly.

### Diet

The pregnant mother must remember that she is eating both for herself and for her developing child. Not only does proper nutrition help maintain maternal health, it also reduces the chances of complications. Proper foods are of importance in the development of the fetal teeth, bones, and other tissues.

As pregnancy advances, the importance of certain foods changes. The intake of protein, minerals, and vitamins must be increased far more than that of calories. Many women have difficulty in increasing their intake of certain kinds of foods, yet limiting calorie increase to only 200 per day. It may be shocking for the mother to discover that not all her weight gain during pregnancy disappears at childbirth. The amount she will be allowed to gain will depend upon her weight at the beginning of pregnancy. If her weight is ideal at that time, she should gain from 20 to 24 pounds.

It becomes very easy for a woman to gain more weight than she should during this time. One study showed an average weight gain at the end of pregnancy to be:

| Baby | 7¼ pounds |
|---|---|
| Placenta | 1 pound |
| Amniotic fluid | 1½ pounds |
| Uterine muscle | 2 . pounds |
| Breasts | 2-3 pounds |
| Water storage | 5 pounds |
| Protein storage | 4 pounds |

Only about 11 pounds of this is lost with delivery. Some weight is lost within the next several weeks. Any excess weight will likely remain permanently.

### Childbirth

*Fetal Position.* As shown in the figures here, by the end of pregnancy the upper point of the uterus has pushed up almost to the breastbone of the mother. As a rule, in the later months of pregnancy, the fetus forms a mass roughly similar to the shape of the uterine cavity, folded upon itself so that the chin is almost in contact with the chest, the thighs bent over its abdomen, the legs bent at the knees, and the arms either crossed over the chest or parallel to the sides.

Over 99 percent of the time the long axis of the fetus is parallel to the long axis of the mother; in less than 1 percent it is transverse, that is, at right angles (this is a serious obstetric complication).

The lowest part of the fetal body or that part first seen in delivery is called the presenting part. The presentation is named according to the presenting part. When the head is lowermost it is a cephalic presentation; when the buttocks are lowermost it is a breech presentation. If the fetus is transverse it may make a shoulder presentation. Almost all babies are born with the back of the head (the vertex) appearing first.

*Estimated Date of Delivery.* A customary way of estimating the expected day of delivery is to count back three months from the first day of the last menstrual period and add seven days (Naegele's rule). For example, if a woman's last menstrual period began on June 10th, the expected day of delivery would be March 17th. Few mothers deliver on the expected day, but will commonly deviate only two weeks on either side.

*False Labor.* False labor contractions may occur as early as three or four weeks before the termination of pregnancy. They are nothing more than an exaggeration of the irregular uterine contractions that occur through the entire period of pregnancy.

There are ways of distinguishing them from true labor. They occur chiefly in the groin rather than in the top region of the uterus. Their duration is short and they are rarely intensified by walking about (walking may even relieve them). They do not increase progressively in intensity, duration, and frequency. True labor contractions cause a dilation (expansion) of the cervix of the uterus within a few hours, whereas false labor does not.

*Labor.* Labor is the process by which the products of conception are expelled by the mother (also commonly called childbirth, travail, or parturition). The word delivery refers to the actual birth of the baby. This

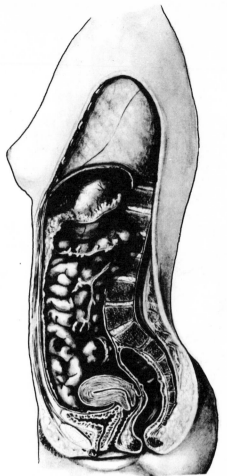

The three illustrations appearing here and on the next page are cut-away views of the way in which a woman's body changes during pregnancy.

is expected to occur at term, or the end of the fortieth week.

Labor is conveniently divided into three stages: (1) preparatory state, (2) birth of the baby, (3) and delivery of the afterbirth.

*Preparatory stage.* This period starts with the beginning of labor contractions and lasts until the cervix of the uterus is fully dilated and ready for the passage of the child. The

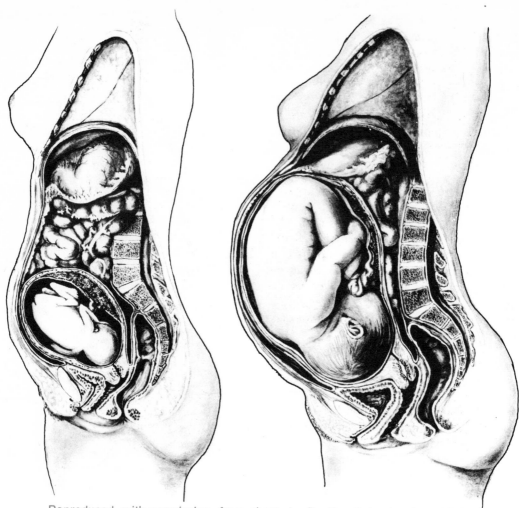

Reproduced, with permission, from charts by Dr. Eva Schuchardt, published and copyrighted by Maternity Center Association, New York.

initial contractions are short, mild, and separated by intervals of 10 to 20 minutes. The woman may walk around to remain comfortable between contractions. The discomfort usually starts in the small of the back and then sweeps around to the front of the abdomen. As labor progresses the contractions become more frequent (every 3 to 5 minutes), become more intense, and last longer. The contractions preceding full dilation may be quite painful. The average duration of the first stage of labor is about 12 hours for the first child and about 8 hours for children born subsequently.

*Delivery of the child.* Delivery starts with the full opening of the cervix and ends with the completed birth of the child. Contractions are severe and may last 50 to 100 seconds, occurring at intervals of 2 or 3 minutes. The

## BIRTH OF A BABY

Courtesy of the Cleveland Health Museum and Education Center.

pressure of the contractions will usually cause the rupture of the amniotic sac during the early part of this stage (but also sometimes before or during the first stage). During the contractions the mother strains and bears down strongly.

When the cervix is open, the child begins to move down into the vagina. Each labor contraction moves the head down farther. With the cessation of each contraction, the head recedes somewhat. Just before the head emerges, it rotates to the side to pass the front part of the pelvic bone. With the next few contractions the neck and shoulders emerge. The body of the child is then quickly expelled. Immediately afterward the rest of the amniotic fluid gushes out. As soon as the child has emerged, the physician ties off the umbilical cord several inches from the navel. Immediately after birth he assists the child to begin breathing. The child usually begins breathing within one minute and follows this with a strong cry.

The average length of the second stage is 50 minutes in the first delivery and 20 minutes in later ones.

*Delivery of the afterbirth.* Contractions stop for a few moments following passage of the child and then begin again at regular intervals until the placenta is separated and expelled. Placental separation lasts about 2 to 3 minutes. Its expulsion from the uterus will take 5 to 6 additional minutes.

*Reducing the Pain of Delivery.* Pain is normally involved in the delivery of a child. The amount of this discomfort can be reduced by preparing the mother. This preparation should include an understanding of the physical and emotional aspects of delivery. Learning controlled relaxation and breathing before delivery can reduce muscle spasms during labor. Such natural methods to reduce childbirth discomfort are referred to as natural childbirth.

Drugs are commonly used if the pain becomes too severe. Some reduce the pain but allow the mother to remain conscious; others act only on specific parts of the body; some cause her to lose consciousness. Drugs may be injected into the spinal cord to deaden nerves coming from the uterus, but not affect her consciousness. The drugs used depend upon the wishes of the mother and the choice of the physician.

With mothers who are receptive to it, hypnosis has been effective in allowing labor with little or no drugs. Although recognized by the American Medical Association, it has limited use. It requires time and patient response.

*Handling the Newborn.* The completed delivery of the child is the official time of birth. As soon as the baby is delivered, it is grasped by the feet and held head down to drain fluids from the nose and mouth. The umbilical cord is clamped and cut (within a few days the cord drops off). The baby must now breathe almost immediately, in order to obtain his own oxygen. Some cry and take their first breath almost as soon as they are born; in most cases breathing starts within one minute. A strong cry indicates that the respiratory system is functioning well. In case of any breathing difficulty, resuscitation must be applied immediately to prevent asphyxiation (suffocation). Delay in breathing can cause damage to the brain cells or the death of the infant.

The child is quickly checked for normal heartbeat, regular breathing, good movement of arms and legs, nervous reflex, and pink color. The infant's eyes are treated with a germicide to prevent a possibility of gonorrheal infection, or ophthalmia neonatorum (this is required by law in most states). The physician inspects the infant for any apparent abnormalities, such as birthmarks, clubfeet, or improperly formed body openings. He must also decide whether the infant needs incubator care or not.

To prevent confusing it with other babies in the nursery, the infant must be properly identified before he leaves the delivery room. Identification bands with numbers are commonly fastened to both the baby (wrist and/ or ankle) and the mother. Some hospitals also take inked footprints. This can serve as positive identification.

*Observation of the Mother.* The mother is now ready to be moved from the delivery room. She will need close observation for the next few hours to prevent any complications that may arise following delivery. She is exhausted and cold and will need to be kept warm. She should see her husband as soon as possible after leaving the delivery room for his reassurance. To insure rest and relaxation, she may need to be given a sedative.

### Complications of Delivery

*Premature Birth.* Occasionally a pregnancy ends before the fetus is mature. Whether or not the fetus survives will depend on what point during the pregnancy the termination occurs, the causes, and the conditions of the termination.

By definition, a premature infant is one which is born so early during the course of pregnancy that its organs have not reached full development. As a result, its chance of survival is poorer than that of a full-term infant. The most accurate rule used to measure maturity is weight. A premature infant is one whose weight is 5½ pounds or less at delivery.

The less an infant weighs at birth, the less its chances of survival. The survival chance of a fetus at birth is often classified according to the following scale:

| | |
|---|---|
| 1 lb 1 oz or less | no chance of survival |
| 1 lb 2 oz to 2 lb 2 oz | extremely poor chance of survival |
| 2 lb 3 oz to 5 lb 8 oz | chances of survival range from poor to good according to weight |
| 5 lb 9 oz or more | excellent chance of survival |

In terms of age of the fetus, the fetus may weigh 1 pound, 1 ounce during the sixth lunar month (22 weeks), or 2 pounds, 3 ounces at the end of the twenty-eighth week.

As many as half of all premature births are without explanation. However, suspected maternal causes include high blood pressure, placental problems, and untreated syphilis. Prematurity is the leading cause of infant mortality (death between the time of birth and the first year of age). The death of the infant may often be caused by respiratory difficulties or infections of various kinds.

*Forceps Delivery.* An obstetric forceps is an instrument used for the extraction of the child when it presents its head. It is used when passage is slowed and there may be danger to the mother and/or the fetus. The forceps is a curved instrument which fits around the head of the fetus. The physician applies a gentle pull and rotates the head. Reasons for its use would include an abnormal fetal heartbeat, separation of the placenta from the uterus, or a shortage of oxygen supply to the fetus.

*Cesarean Section.* The delivery of the fetus through an incision in the wall of the abdomen and uterus is a cesarean section.

About half of all cesarean sections are performed on women bearing their first child. The most frequent indication for cesarean section for a first delivery would be a space limitation—too large child for the birth canal, a birth canal tumor, or pelvic contractions. Other reasons might be a breech presentation, maternal diabetes, placental, or umbilical cord complications. It might also be done in an attempt to save the fetus in the event a mother late in pregnancy dies from other causes.

The other half of all cesarean sections are performed on women who have had cesarean sections before. In such cases the concern is over the rupture of the scar, especially during labor. Although women who have experienced a previous cesarean section may give birth to a fetus through natural labor, more commonly subsequent deliveries would also be by cesarean section. Accordingly, how often a mother could deliver in this manner would depend upon the counsel of her physician. Most commonly a mother is counselled to limit her children to two or three, although some women have had more cesarean sections.

Commonly, a physician will set a definite date for performing the operation if he can estimate the maturity of the fetus with confidence. Otherwise, he may wait until the patient goes into labor. In any event, the physician may not want to perform a section more than ten days before the calculated date of the delivery.

*Multiple Pregnancies.* A multiple pregnancy is one in which the uterus contains two or more embryos. Twins occur in about 1 out of every 86 pregnancies, and triplets in about 1 out of every 7000 births. Twins occur more commonly among blacks than among whites.

Twins may result from the fertilization of either two separate eggs or a single egg. Twins developing from two separate eggs are called fraternal twins. Since they are from two separate eggs, fertilized by two separate sperms, they are the same as two different individuals born of the same parents, but at different times.

In about one out of every three cases of twins, one mature egg, fertilized by a single sperm, completely divides into two halves. Since both developing embryos are from the same egg and are fertilized by the same sperm, they are both alike genetically or identical.

Triplets may arise from one, two, or three eggs. If from one egg, the egg has completely divided into three parts, in which case the triplets are identical. If from two eggs, one of the eggs has divided into two halves, two of the triplets are identical and one not. The same would hold true for quadruplets, quintuplets, or other kinds of multiple pregnancies. In one case, the Dionne quintuplets, it is believed that all five were from a single egg.

Current treatment of sterility due to lack of ovulation with human gonadotropins has not only successfully induced ovulation, but has also produced multiple eggs, often two or three. The common result has been multiple pregnancies. Efforts are being made to reduce this side effect from the use of these hormones.

*Extrauterine Pregnancies.* Some pregnancies are located outside the uterus. Almost all of these occur in the fallopian tubes. This type of pregnancy is believed to be caused by slowed movement of the egg down the tube and by increased receptivity of the tube to the egg. Regardless of the place the egg lodges, the fetus usually aborts. The mother may feel severe abdominal pains and, if hemorrhaging occurs, may show vaginal bleeding. In any event, the affected tube must be removed. This does not preclude later pregnancies, since another fallopian tube is still available for egg transport.

*Induction of Labor.* Where a pregnancy has developed medical complications, it may be necessary to terminate the pregnancy artificially in order to save the life of the fetus, the mother, or both. In a few cases a physician may decide to terminate the pregnancy for reasons of convenience—a mother who has had a history of rapid deliveries and who might not make it to the hospital in time or who lives a great distance from a hospital. The timing and technique used to induce labor may present hazards to both the fetus and mother and must be decided upon only by a qualified physician.

### Changes in the Mother after Delivery

By the end of the first week after delivery, the tissues of the vagina and uterus have greatly contracted. Within six weeks, the

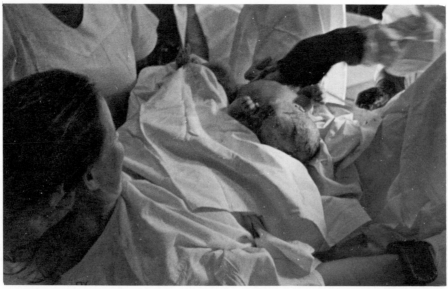

Rondal Partridge, BBM

uterus is virtually back to normal. The abdominal wall ought to be back to original shape and firmness within two to three months.

*Loss of Weight.* With delivery a weight loss of around 11 pounds occurs. Within the next several weeks the mother should lose an additional 4½ to 5½ pounds. Unless she has gained excessively during pregnancy, she should return to her nonpregnant weight within six to eight weeks.

*Menstruation.* Women who do not nurse their babies usually menstruate within eight weeks after delivery. With those who do nurse them, menstruation is often delayed until the fifth or sixth month, although it may vary from two to eighteen months. It may return before or after milk production by the breasts is ended. The first menstrual cycles may be irregular. Although ovulation is normally suspended while milk is produced, a nursing mother may become pregnant even though she has not yet menstruated since delivery.

*Breasts.* Breasts begin enlarging early in pregnancy, during which time they may produce small amounts of colostrum, a yellowish fluid. On about the third day after delivery, the breasts become engorged with milk. At first they may feel uncomfortable, but within several days these feelings disappear as production becomes regulated. Frequent and complete emptying of the breasts stimulates production. If the baby cannot empty the breasts in the early days of nursing, it is sometimes necessary to empty the breasts artificially. The length of time a mother breastfeeds her child will vary. Discontinuing of nursing should be a gradual process allowing milk production to decrease.

A mother may choose not to nurse her baby. Milk production can be suppressed by stopping the production of milk-producing hormones. Failure to remove accumulated milk from the breasts will also inhibit further milk production. However, the breasts will become engorged with milk in the meantime and this may cause some discomfort for several days.

## THE SEX EDUCATION OF CHILDREN

Sex education is often one of the worst-handled duties of parenthood. The subject may be avoided entirely or handled on a "too little and too late" basis. Many children get most of their sex education from their friends, who are typically poor sources of information, since their own sex education has been just as poorly handled. Often many serious misconceptions are picked up from misinformed friends.

Even parents who have handled other phases of parenthood very well often fail in the area of sex education. The parents who have the most difficulty in sex education are those who, as a result of their own poor sex education, hold negative attitudes toward sex, feel uncomfortable about their own sexuality, or fear that the information will encourage further curiosity and experimentation. Out of embarrassment or a feeling that sex is "dirty," these parents delay giving factual information to their children. The questions of the child are either dodged with a hasty change of subject or else answered with outright lies or with a stern moralistic lecture ("nice girls don't ask questions like that").

Successful sex education of children (whether by parents or by school teachers) requires that the instructor have correct factual knowledge about sex as well as positive, healthy attitudes toward sex. Sex education can be considered successful only if both correct facts and positive attitudes are learned by the child. The parent who feels uncomfortable about sex education should start by examining his own knowledge and attitudes about sex.

A detailed explanation of sexual anatomy and physiology without reference to sexual attitudes and sexual behavior is not complete sex education. Nor is the negative approach—sitting a child down and telling him all the things he must not do, accompanied by threats of retaliation if he does. But all too often, sex education takes one of these forms.

### How Much, How Soon?

Parents (and even schools) are often in a quandary as to how much about sex should be taught to a child of a given age. Sex education should not be tied to any particular schedule because growth patterns vary from child to child and there can be several years difference in the emotional maturity of two children of the same age. But there are some guidelines to follow.

The first is to provide the child with an honest answer for any questions he asks at the time the question is asked. The answer should not be postponed, for several reasons. The child is likely to detect a parent's feeling of embarrassment or uncertainty about sex if his questions go repeatedly unanswered. An opportunity to reveal a positive attitude toward sex will be lost. The child should never be given a false answer. He will soon realize its dishonesty and turn to another source, such as his friends, for sexual information which, quite often, will be wrong. Any reluctance of the parents to discuss sex honestly can only create doubts about sex in the mind of the child and will close the door to open and honest discussions of sexual problems in the coming adolescent years.

Another guideline is to be sure the child has necessary information before he will need it. For example, a girl should know the facts regarding menstruation and breast development in advance of the actual events so that she will not be frightened or embarrassed when they occur, which may be as early as age ten. A boy should similarly know about erection, seminal emission, masturbation, and ejaculation by age ten, to prevent his feeling frightened or guilty at the time they occur.

When discussing sex with children, it is best to concentrate on human sex, which is where the child's interest really lies, rather than dwelling on sex in various plants and animals ("the birds and bees") in which he is only moderately interested. Of course, animals can be drawn upon occasionally for purposes of illustration and comparison, such as in egg production and nursing. Similarly, when animals are observed mating, giving birth, or nursing their young, it is useful to tell the young child in frank and honest terms just what is happening, pointing out similarities to and differences from human reproduction, and honestly answering all questions raised by the child.

There are many intangibles in sex education. Attitude development, for example, is influenced every day as the child detects his parents' attitudes toward sex, not just in "facts of life" talks. Even little things like the inflection given to certain words will betray the parents' true feelings. The child acquires his concepts of masculinity and femininity largely through the daily observation of the roles taken by his parents.

### Some Specific Considerations

*Nudity in the Home.* Parents often wonder to what extent their child should see them or his brothers or sisters in the nude. Certainly, an important part of the early sex education of any child is that realization that boys and men are different from girls and women and that this difference is perfectly natural.

Home nudity among young children and their parents can be quite harmless, and even useful, if neither the parent nor child is embarrassed by nudity and the nudity is in a normal context such as bathing or dressing. Parents should never flaunt their nudity before their children.

Older children and adolescents are likely to be self-conscious about their developing bodies and will probably wish privacy. Their wishes for privacy should be respected by their parents as well as their brothers and sisters.

*Proper Terminology.* Many parents are reluctant to teach a child the proper words for sexual parts and functions. This may reflect the embarrassment of the parent or perhaps even his doubt about what the proper word is. Another problem is that some of the terms are difficult for the very young child to pronounce.

The best policy is to teach the proper word as soon as the child can pronounce it. For example, the mother trying to toilet train her 2-year-old need not try to teach him to say *urinate,* but when he reaches an age where he can pronounce the word, it should be taught and used.

*Masturbation.* Another problem topic for many parents is masturbation. The parents may carry residual fears and guilt about masturbation as a result of the way their own parents cautioned or threatened them about masturbation. It is only in recent years that masturbation has been recognized as perfectly harmless and a normal part of both male and female sexuality. Parents should accept masturbation as a harmless way of relieving the powerful sexual tensions of adolescence. Threats should never be made nor fear or guilt created as a result of adolescent masturbation.

*Nonmarital Sex.* Parents should frankly and calmly discuss nonmarital sexual relationships with their early adolescents. Too often, the only real discussion comes after a 15-year-old daughter is already pregnant. Rather than centering around threats and accusations, the discussion of nonmarital sex should rationally discuss the issues mentioned at the beginning of this section.

*Contraception.* An often neglected topic in sex education is fertility control. Some parents are actually afraid that a knowledge of contraception will encourage nonmarital intercourse by their adolescents. But studies have shown that this is not the case. In fact, many adolescent sexual relationships include absolutely no precautions against pregnancy. Knowledge of contraception is seldom, if ever, the deciding influence in determining whether or not a teen-age couple engages in intercourse. But it is certainly desirable that those adolescents who do engage in intercourse make use of an effective contraceptive method.

Even more important than teaching the technique of contraception is teaching why nonmarital pregnancy is undesirable, why pregnancy should be delayed in early marriage, why children should be spaced, and why the total number of children a couple produces should be limited.

*Venereal Disease.* Children should be given a thorough and factual knowledge of venereal diseases, not as a scare tactic to prevent nonmarital intercourse, but as a protection against several serious diseases which are now in an epidemic state among adolescents.

Syphilis and gonorrhea should be stressed—their early symptoms, and what to do in case these symptoms appear. The adolescent must feel free to seek treatment for the venereal diseases. Delayed treatment may result in permanent damage.

*Homosexuality.* Parents should expect questions from their children regarding homosexuality and should be ready to give honest answers. Homosexuality is and will continue to be prominently featured in literature, theater, television, and popular music. Many adolescents pass through a stage where homosexual attractions are felt. This may create fear or guilt which, when combined with a lack of understanding from parents, may lead to the adoption of homosexuality as a way of life.

# FOR FURTHER READING

Gebhard, Paul, et al., *Sex Offenders,* New York: Harper & Row, 1965. *A major contribution to the recent general literature on sexual deviancy.*

Gillette, Paul, *The Pill and Other Birth Control Methods.* New York: Bantam, 1970. *Explains the choices available to a woman who wants to control the number of children she would like to have.*

Guttmacher, A.F., *et al., Complete Book of Birth Control.* New York: Ballantine Books, 1970. *Written by one of America's foremost advocates of informed family planning; one of the best books available on the subject.*

Hamilton, Eleanor, *Sex Before Marriage.* New York: Bantam Books, 1970. *Comments on the implications of sex before marriage; a good book to read for knowledgeable decision making on an important personal topic.*

Havemann, Ernest, and Editors of Time-Life Books, *Birth Control.* New York: Time, 1967. *An explicit word and picture guide to conception, fertility problems, and the choices of methods of birth control.*

Kinsey, Alfred C., et al., *Sexual Behavior in the Human Male,* 1948; *Sexual Behavior in the Human Female,* 1953; Philadelphia: Saunders. *Pioneering and, at the time, controversial studies.*

Masters, William H., and Virginia E. Johnson, *Human Sexual Response.* Boston: Little, Brown, 1966. *A pioneering physiological study of male and female sexual response.*

Masters, William H., and Virginia E. Johnson, *Human Sexual Inadequacy.* Boston: Little, Brown, 1970. *Descriptions of clinical procedures developed by the authors for the medical treatment of problems of sexual inadequacy.*

Mohr, J. W., et al., *Pedophilia and Exhibitionism,* Boston: Little, Brown. *Applies detailed methods of testing and evaluation to two specific areas of sexual deviance research.*

Neubardt, Selig, *A Concept of Contraception.* New York: Trident Press, 1967. *A practical, nontechnical description of the available contraceptive techniques; mixes humor with important clinical observations.*

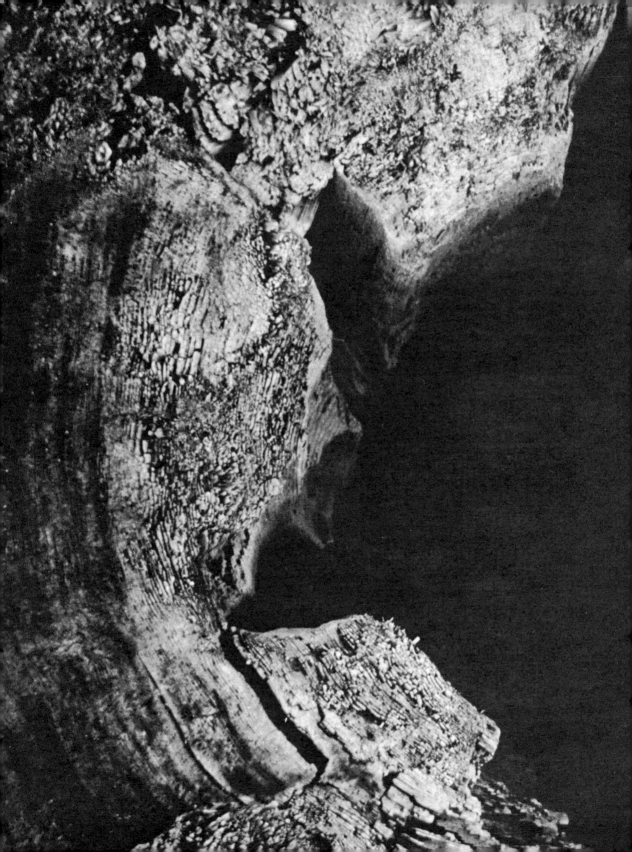

# 6
## Disease

# 17  The Communicable Diseases

Theories of Communicable Diseases • Stages of Communicable Diseases • Protection Against Communicable Diseases • The Major Communicable Diseases • The Venereal Diseases • Prevention of Venereal Diseases • Other Infections of the Reproductive and Urinary Organs

# 18  The Noncommunicable Diseases

Cancer • Other Major Noncommunicable Diseases • Heart and Artery Diseases

# 17
# The
# Communicable
# Diseases

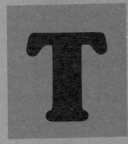

The word disease has a very broad meaning, being properly applied to any process in which the physical or mental health is impaired. Within this framework would fall such diverse conditions as nutritional deficiencies, emotional problems, drug or alcohol dependence, allergies, noncommunicable degenerative conditions, and the communicable diseases. Throughout most of the history of man, the communicable diseases have been the principle limiting factor in life expectancy. Malaria, tuberculosis, pneumonia, smallpox, yellow fever, plague, cholera, and a host of other infectious conditions for centuries held the life expectancy to only 30 or 40 years.

In recent years, however, the communicable diseases have been largely controlled in many parts of the world, increasing life expectancies in those regions by 30 years or more. As a result, in the developed countries of the world, the noncommunicable degenerative diseases have emerged as the principle causes of death. Any further increase in life expectancy must now come from control of degenerative circulatory conditions, cancers, and other degenerative diseases.

Yet the communicable diseases still lurk in the background as potential killers of vast numbers of people. The germs that cause these diseases have not been eliminated from the face of the earth; they have only been controlled. Any of them could reemerge if sanitation, immunization, or other control measures were neglected. Also a constant threat is the development of a new disease or more resistant strain of an existing disease through mutation of its germ. Still another threat to our control of communicable diseases is the current explosive growth in world population, which will make adequate sanitation difficult or even impossible to maintain, allowing many of the presently controlled diseases to reemerge.

## THEORIES OF COMMUNICABLE DISEASES

Communicable diseases are diseases which are transmitted by living organisms or their metabolic products. Other terms used to describe this class of diseases are *contagious* and *infectious*. Communicable diseases have a unique place in human history. They have been responsible for more suffering, death, and destruction than all the wars which have ever been fought by man. For many centuries, they were the primary natural population control device of several regions, and despite the great advances medicine has made against them during the past century, some diseases still have this dubious distinction in certain areas of the world.

The awesome power of disease, such as the bubonic plague, cholera, and malaria, to debilitate their victims and seriously interrupt the normal functioning of entire nations kept understanding of the causes and control of these diseases inextricably tied up with myth and superstition. It appeared that only supernatural forces and demonic powers could cause such misery. The progress against these diseases made by European and American bacteriologists, chemists, and physicians during the eighteenth and nineteenth centuries seemed almost anticlimactic. It was based on the theory that minute, invisible life forms—pathogens—were responsible for the transmission of these diseases. The obvious corollary of this theory is that the cure and treatment of such conditions as smallpox, tuberculosis, and yellow fever relates directly to the control of these organisms.

### Pathogens

The first step in understanding communicable diseases is to gain some familiarity with pathogens and their role in the causation of these diseases. A disease is "caught" when a pathogen invades the body. The disease that follows is caused by some aspect of the parasitic life of the pathogen. (See table on the major pathogen groups.)

Pathogens cause disease in a variety of ways; identification of a particular organism as the causative agent of a disease does not necessarily explain which of these modes is involved. Many pathogenic bacteria, fungi, and protozoa release enzymes which destroy and digest the surrounding human tissues, making the products of their digestion available as food for the pathogens. Other pathogens, particularly bacteria, release powerful toxins (poisons), some of which destroy cells near the site of the infection and some of which are carried by the blood to work in other parts of the body, often on the nervous system, heart muscle, liver, or other organs. Some of the bacterial toxins are among the most poisonous substances known to man.

Pathogenic viruses produce disease in an entirely different manner. When a virus enters a host cell, such as a human cell, the genetic material of the virus takes over the control of the host cell. The virus genes direct the protein synthesizing mechanism of the cell to produce the protein needed for the reproduction of the virus, while neglecting to produce the proteins needed by the cell itself. This disruption of cell function leads to the symptoms of many virus diseases. After several hundred virus particles have been produced, they leave the host cell to infect other cells. Some viruses kill the host cell as they burst out while other viruses leave the host cell capable of recovery.

### Vectors

The transmission of many diseases from an infected person or other reservoir of pathogens to a healthy person requires a *vector*. In its more general sense the word vector means a carrier. In reference to diseases it usually applies to an arthropod (insect, tick, mite, etc.) that carries the pathogen. The arthropod may or may not suffer from the disease it carries. In most cases it is the bite

# MAJOR PATHOGEN GROUPS

| ILLUSTRATIVE PLATE | GROUP AND SIZE SCALE | DESCRIPTION | DISEASES CAUSED | MODE OF ACTION |
|---|---|---|---|---|
| | Viruses (10 to 250 nanometers) | Minute, submicroscopic particles composed of nucleic acids and protein; intracellular parasites | Rabies, polio, yellow fever; colds, influenza | Disrupt protein synthesis of cells, sometimes kill cells |
| | Rickettsia (less than one micrometer) | Small bacteria always associated with insects and other arthropods | Typhus fever; Rocky Mountain spotted fever; Q-fever | Interfere with metabolism of host cells, all are intracellular parasites |
| | Bacteria (1 to 10 micrometers) | Single-celled, plantlike; abundant in the biosphere; secrete disease-causing toxins; are commonly found in rod, spiral, or spherical shape | Tuberculosis, syphilis, pneumonia, scarlet fever, boils, meningitis | Produce toxins and enzymes that destroy cells or interfere with their function |
| | Fungi (A few micrometers to several inches) | Single-celled or multi-celled plantlike organisms; consist of thread-like fibers and reproductive spores | Athlete's foot, most commonly diseases of the skin, hair and nails, and lungs | Release enzymes that digest cells |
| | Protozoa (A few to 250 micrometers) | Microscopic animals; each is single-celled | Malaria, amebic dysentery, and African sleeping sickness | Release enzymes and toxins that destroy cells or interfere with their functions |
| | Parasitic Worms (1/32 inch to 20 or 30 feet) | Multicellular animals; common types are round or flat | Pinworm, trichinosis, tapeworms | Release toxins; compete for foods; block digestive tract and blood and lymph vessels |

A nanometer is one billionth of a meter; a micrometer is one millionth of a meter; a meter is 39.37 inches.

of the vector which transmits the pathogens, but some pathogens are transmitted through the feces of the vector or are carried on the feet or body of the vector.

Mosquitoes are among the most important vectors of disease, transmitting malaria, yellow fever, encephalitis, filariasis, dengue fever, and other diseases. The piercing mouthparts of the female mosquito contain two ducts, one for sucking blood and one for injecting saliva. The saliva of a mosquito contains an anticoagulant to prevent clotting of blood and is always injected into the man or other animal being bitten before any blood is drawn out. This makes the mosquito an efficient vector of disease. (The male mosquito never bites, feeding on nectar of plants.)

Other important vectors include ticks, mites, fleas, lice, flies, kissing bugs *(Triatoma),* and other arthropods. Each transmits specific diseases in specific ways. The pathogen-vector relationship is generally quite specific. For example, each of the diseases mentioned as being transmitted by mosquitoes is carried by only certain specific mosquitoes.

A worldwide conflict is developing between public health workers, on the one hand, who have sought to control vectors, especially mosquitoes, through the application of insecticides and elimination of breeding areas by draining swamps; and environmentalists, on the other hand, who feel that these measures are ecologically unwise. The outcome of this controversy may determine whether vast areas of the earth's surface are suitable for human habitation.

## STAGES OF COMMUNICABLE DISEASES

Most communicable diseases progress through several definite stages. The identification of these stages in particular cases is of great importance for three major reasons:

(1) some diseases involve stages during which no obvious symptoms are present, but the patient is still clinically in danger; (2) contagion control requires that those stages during which the disease can be transmitted be clearly identified; (3) the possibilities of isolation and immunization frequently relate to the progress of the disease.

### Transmission and Infection

Transmission is the process whereby a disease is "caught." In this process the pathogen is carried in some way from its source and enters the body in an area where it can cause infection. Infection is the process establishing a pathogen as a parasite in the body. Transmission and infection require the following:

1. *Pathogen.* The pathogen, as discussed earlier, may be one of a number of viruses, rickettsia, bacteria, fungi, protozoa, or parasitic worms.

2. *Source.* The source, also called the reservoir, may be human or animal, soil, water, food, or an object that will allow the pathogen to survive.

3. *Method of transmission.* Pathogens are often passed from person to person or animal to person by direct or indirect contact. Transmission by direct contact can occur as a result of touching, kissing, or other close personal contacts. Indirect transmission takes place when pathogens are released during coughing, breathing, or talking. Transmission also can take place when contaminated food or water is taken into the body.

4. *Portal of entry.* The pathogen must get into the body. This occurs as the result of a vector bite, a wound, or entry through body openings such as the nose, mouth, eyes, genital openings, and skin and mucous membranes.

5. *Susceptible host.* A susceptible host is an individual who is unable to resist the pathogen and its effects.

Should all five links in the cycle be present,

then infection will occur and the cycle may begin again. If any link in the cycle is broken, however, the disease will be prevented.

### Incubation Period

Once a communicable disease has been caught, it progresses through an incubation period, the interval between the time of infection and the appearance of the first symptoms. During this time, the pathogen multiplies in numbers until it is abundant enough to overcome the body's defenses and produce its disease.

The incubation period may be as short as a few hours or as long as several months or years, depending on the disease. Most diseases have an incubation period of a few days to a few weeks. Generally, diseases are not contagious during the early part of the incubation period, but they do become highly contagious at the end of the period, just before the symptoms appear.

### Prodromal Period

The prodromal period is the time during which vague, nonspecific symptoms of a disease appear. This period lasts from a few hours to several days and is characterized by fever, headache, and various aches and pains. Many diseases are highly contagious during this period.

### Typical Illness Period

After the prodromal period a group of specific symptoms will appear. This is the typical illness period during which a recognizable disease is present. The term syndrome often is used to indicate a group of symptoms characteristic of a given disease.

### Recovery Stage

The recovery stage begins when the body defenses start to overpower the pathogens and the symptoms disappear. It is important to remember that the pathogens are still present in the body during the recovery or convalescence stage. If a convalescent person resumes full activity too soon, his body defenses will be weakened, and he will have a relapse (return of the symptoms of the disease.) As is indicated in the figure showing the stages of communicable disease, there are degrees of recovery, each of which has long-range significance both to the future health of the patient and to contagion of the disease.

## PROTECTION AGAINST COMMUNICABLE DISEASES

Not too many years ago, little could be done to control the spread and effects of communicable diseases. As we have seen, this was partly due to the lack of knowledge about pathogens and how they cause disease. Another factor, however, was the need for collective (public) responsibility. Many protections against diseases are impossible or extremely difficult for the individual to carry out on his own. The responsibility for these protections, therefore, has been assumed by modern public health agencies.

The major emphasis in public health is on prevention. This is reflected in such functions as immunization, the inspection of such reservoirs of pathogens as food, water, air, and insect vector sources, and the discovery and isolation of carriers. Public health agencies have increasingly also served an educational function—alerting the public to the symptoms of common and dangerous diseases, and encouraging anyone suspected of being ill to receive treatment; in many cases, the government will provide treatment free of charge to those who cannot afford to pay.

Though it is becoming less common, public health agencies occasionally deal with the consequences of widespread epidemics. The

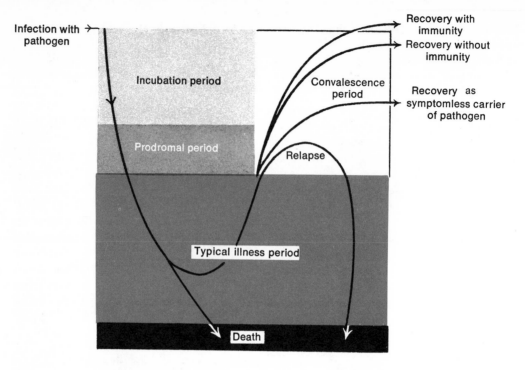

Infection with pathogen →

Incubation period

Prodromal period

Typical illness period

Relapse

Convalescence period

Recovery with immunity

Recovery without immunity

Recovery as symptomless carrier of pathogen

Death

The stages of a communicable disease from infection to death or recovery.

"flu" epidemics of recent years have mobilized the facilities of health agencies across the country. The control of carriers of smallpox is a continuing function, whose importance is dramatized by the constant possibility that a widespread epidemic of this disease could sweep the country within days of a break in this protection.

To a certain extent, the success or failure of public health facilities to control communicable disease hinges on the degree to which the individual's natural body defenses can be activated.

The human body has a great ability to resist disease. We are constantly being exposed to germs. Most of the time we completely resist these germs, and no infection occurs. When infection does take place, re-covery is often possible through the body's own unassisted defenses. Some of these natural defenses are:

*Skin and mucous membranes.* The unbroken skin or mucous membrane keeps out most pathogens, even though a few can penetrate healthy skin.

*Tears.* Tears, constantly flowing over the surface of the eyes, contain a substance (lysozyme) that inhibits bacteria. Without this substance, the eyes would have many more infections than they do.

*Cilia lining the respiratory system.* The ducts of the respiratory system have an inner lining of cilia. These are millions of microscopic hairs that pick up inhaled bacteria, dust, and foreign matter on a thin layer of mucus. The cilia wave in such a manner that the foreign matter is carried up to the throat and swallowed. This action helps keep the lungs free of infection. In the heavy smoker these cilia completely disappear. The smoker then must cough frequently to clear foreign matter from the lungs. Years of coughing may lead to emphysema, a serious condition in which the air sacs of the lungs break down.

*White blood cells.* The white blood cells, or leucocytes, are able to surround bacteria and digest them.This action is very important in overcoming infections reached by the bloodstream.

*Interferon.* Virus-infected cells release a chemical called interferon. Because this chemical protects other cells from invasion by viruses, it is thought to be important in our recovery from virus diseases.

*Antibodies.* The invasion of the body by pathogens or certain other foreign substances stimulates the production of antibodies. Antibodies are proteins that destroy the foreign substances that stimulated their production, the *antigens.* Thus, antibodies are very specific in their action. Antibodies are the basis of immunity.

The antigen—antibody—immunity relationship is the basis of a man-made method of disease prevention, immunization. Through immunization, a person can develop immunity to a disease without having to suffer from the disease first. There are two basic methods of immunization. Active immunity is obtained by injecting or otherwise exposing a person to an antigen, which causes the person to produce his own antibodies. The resulting immunity is usually long lasting; that is, it is effective for several years or even for a lifetime. Passive immunity is obtained by injecting a person with antibod-

ies extracted from the blood of an animal or from another person. Passive immunity is instant immunity, but it has a short duration. The injected antibodies break down in a few weeks without stimulating the person to produce antibodies of his own. Only his exposure to antigens can give him long-term protection.

A special type of passive immunity is congenital immunity. During pregnancy, antibodies pass across the placenta from the body of the mother into the blood of the child. These antibodies give the newborn child an immunity to many common diseases. But since this is passive immunity, it lasts only for several months. The proper protection of an infant requires a series of injections given at regular intervals during the first few years of his life. It is the responsibility of parents to see that their child receives these immunizations. The first injections are usually given when the infant is about two months old. Every child born in the United States should be immunized against seven diseases: diphtheria, tetanus, whooping cough, polio, measles, German measles, and mumps. (See table on typical immunization schedule.) It should be remembered that continued protection against diphtheria and tetanus requires booster immunizations every ten years throughout adult life.

Immunizations against several other common diseases are still being developed, and may eventually become part of the standard immunization series. In addition, immunizations against many other diseases are already available for use in special cases, such as before travel into foreign countries.

### Treating Communicable Diseases with Drugs

The use of drugs to treat diseases is called chemotherapy. In general, the drugs devel-

## TYPICAL IMMUNIZATION SCHEDULE

| AGE | PREPARATION |
|---|---|
| 2 months | DPT (diphtheria, whooping cough, tetanus) |
| | Trivalent OPV (oral polio vaccine containing types I, II, and III) |
| 3 months | DPT |
| 4 months | DPT |
| | Trivalent OPV |
| 12 months | Live measles vaccine[a] |
| 12 months to puberty | German measles vaccine[a] |
| | Mumps vaccine[a] |
| 15 months | DPT |
| | Trivalent OPV |
| Before school entrance | DPT |
| | Trivalent OPV |
| 15 years | Td (adult type tetanus and diphtheria booster) |
| Over 15 years | Td boosters every 10 years for life |

[a]Measles, German measles, and mumps vaccines may be combined into a single trivalent vaccine.

NOTE: This schedule is recommended as a flexible guide which may be modified within limits to meet the needs of the individual patient or physician.

SOURCE: *Public Health Service Advisory Committee on Immunization Practices*, 1972 Recommendations, National Communicable Disease Center Morbidity and Mortality report, Vol. 21, No. 25, June 24, 1972.

oped so far have had the greatest successes against bacterial diseases, moderate success against protozoan, fungal, and parasitic worm diseases, and little or no effect on the viral diseases. A few antiviral drugs have been developed, however, and there is good probability that others will follow.

The discovery of sulfa drugs (sulfonamides) in 1935 was the first major step toward the control of bacterial infection. Sulfa drugs prevent the multiplication of bacteria by interfering with the bacterial metabolism. When a person takes sulfa drugs, he must drink plenty of fluids; otherwise, the drugs might crystallize in his kidneys and cause damage.

Antibiotics are substances that are produced by soil-inhabiting microorganisms in order to inhibit the growth of competing soil organisms. Antibiotics are made for drug use by growing the organisms that produce them in large vats. The liquid growth of these organisms is released from the vats; from this liquid, antibiotics are extracted and then purified. Most antibiotics are given by injection, but some are effective if taken by mouth.

Antibiotics are generally effective only against bacteria; they have no effect on viruses. Antibiotics cannot cure a cold, influenza, measles, mumps, or other common viral diseases.

When a person is taking drugs, he should follow these precautions:

1. Follow instructions exactly.

2. Use a drug only for the illness for which it was prescribed. Do not keep leftover drugs for future use. Many drugs break down in storage and may become worthless or even harmful.

3. Avoid borrowing or lending prescriptions. Entirely different diseases may have very similar symptoms, and a borrowed prescription may be very dangerous. (It is also illegal to possess a prescription drug without having a prescription.)

4. Keep all drugs out of the reach of children.

5. Avoid unnecessary use of antibiotics. The indiscriminate use of antibiotics has two undesirable effects. First, it can cause the development of allergic reactions to the antibiotic, which can later be serious or even fatal. Second, it speeds the development of drug-resistant strains of bacteria. Such bacteria have already become a critical problem in public health, since by definition, they are not susceptible to man's major weapon against disease.

## THE MAJOR COMMUNICABLE DISEASES

The major communicable diseases include several diseases commonly called "childhood" diseases because the greatest number of cases are in the age group of one to fifteen years. Since these diseases usually confer lifelong immunity, repeated infection is not common. It is not unusual, however, for a person to escape infection during childhood and then catch one of these diseases as an adult. Frequently, the consequences of an adult case of a "childhood" disease can be more serious than that occurring in earlier years.

In addition, the common diseases include the common cold and influenza, neither of which confer any long-term immunity; thus, they can be contracted many times. (See table of major communicable diseases.)

## THE VENEREAL DISEASES

Venereal diseases are communicable illnesses which are transmitted primarily through sexual intercourse; "venereal" is derived from Venus, the Roman goddess of love. They have been set apart from the other communicable diseases because of their tremendous importance in the United States today. There are more cases of venereal disease occurring in the United States today than all of the cases of the other communicable diseases put together (excepting the common cold).

Venereal diseases occupy an anomalous position in our country today. They are readily preventable (not by immunization, but by proper hygiene methods), easily treatable, and extremely dangerous if not promptly diagnosed and medicated. Yet, they are in an epidemic state in our country on the basis of the reported cases, which we may assume are only a portion of the total number of cases occurring each year. Despite the serious consequences of these diseases, many people will not or cannot seek treatment which is available through most public health agencies and all physicians.

Part of the problem is the moral stigma attached to venereal disease. Many people will ignore painful and alarming symptoms rather than undergo treatment. Perhaps the more important side of the issue is the one of education; education about venereal dis-

| NAME OF DISEASE | CAUSED BY | USUAL AGE INFECTED | MODE OF TRANSMISSION | INCUBATION PERIOD | EARLY SIGNS | LENGTH OF DISEASE |
|---|---|---|---|---|---|---|
| Common Cold | Over 50 types of viruses | Any age | Direct or indirect contact with nose or throat discharges (cough or sneeze) of infected person | 12 to 72 hours, usually 24 hours | Sore throat, running nose, chills, aches; classical prodromal period | 2 to 7 days |
| Influenza or "flu" | Many strains of viruses that fall into three types, A, B, and C. New strains always developing. | Any age | Direct or indirect contact with nose or throat discharges (cough or sneeze) of infected person | Quite short, usually 24 to 72 hours | Very rapid onset of fever, chills, headache, muscular aches, and severe coughing | 1 to 3 days |
| Chickenpox | Varicella virus. Same virus causes herpes zoster (shingles) in adults | Childhood disease, 2 to 8 years | Direct or indirect contact with discharges from skin or nose or throat lesions of infected persons. Virus may also be airborne | 10 to 21 days, usually 14 to 16 days | Slight fever, skin eruptions (lesions) | 9 to 14 days |
| Poliomyelitis "polio" | Three types of polio viruses | Any age, most common among children (called childhood disease) | Direct contact or close association with infected person. Indirectly by fecal contamination or nose or throat discharge of an infected person | 3 to 28 days, usually 7 to 12 days | Fever, headache, sore throat, nausea, muscle pain, and general weakness | Highly variable—up to several months |

ease is potentially the most effective "medicine" against it.

Five venereal diseases are recognized in the United States—gonorrhea, syphilis, chancroid, granuloma inguinale, and lymphogranuloma venereum—the first two being by far the most prevalent. Any one of these diseases, however, can be very serious.

It is impossible to give exact figures on the amount of venereal disease in the United States because of the previously mentioned problems of reporting and detection. The

| CONTAGIOUS PERIOD | PERMANENT AFTEREFFECTS | IMMUNITY | PREVENTION | ADDITIONAL INFORMATION |
|---|---|---|---|---|
| From 24 hours before onset of symptoms until 3 to 5 days after | None | Little or none | Avoid infected persons | Very serious side effects may result from the improper care of colds. When a high fever accompanies cold symptoms, a secondary infection is present and a physician should be consulted |
| One day before onset until 4 days after | Rare, but predisposes elderly or weakened persons to pneumonia. The general death rate goes up during flu epidemics. | Infection produces immunity of unknown duration to the type of virus infecting you; but not necessarily to other influenza viruses. | Annual immunization with vaccine based upon prevailing strains of virus | True influenza is an infection of respiratory tract. Many other types of viral, or even bacterial, infections are commonly, though incorrectly, called "flu." |
| From 1 day before eruption of lesions until 6 days afterward | Very rare; deaths from encephalitis or pneumonia do occur | One attack confers long immunity | No effective prevention has yet been developed | The same virus, when contracted by adults who have not had chickenpox, sometimes causes an infection of the nervous system called shingles—a painful inflammation of the skin is produced. |
| Maximum period from 1 week before symptoms to 3 months after onset of symptoms; usually from 3 days before to 10 days after onset | Two to 10% fatality rate in paralytic cases; or paralysis may be permanent | Most cases are nonparalytic and result in immunity to the specific type of virus responsible, but not to the other two types. | Oral polio vaccine (OPV) currently given in a mixed form containing all three types of weakened polio viruses; called trivalent OPV; should be taken 4 times during childhood for lifetime immunity | Polio is completely preventable by proper immunization. However, cases continue to occur in the United States among people who have had only partial immunization or whose parents were not interested enough in their welfare to even have them immunized. |

number of new cases of gonorrhea is estimated at over two and one half million each year. Syphilis is estimated at 75,000 to 100,000 new cases per year.

There has been a great increase in venereal disease during the past ten years. The majority of this increase has been in the young population. Over half of all venereal disease cases today are among persons under twenty-five years of age. People who have a multitude of casual sexual partners are likely to be infected. Anyone having sexual contact

| NAME OF DISEASE | CAUSED BY | USUAL AGE INFECTED | MODE OF TRANSMISSION | INCUBATION PERIOD | EARLY SIGNS | LENGTH OF DISEASE |
|---|---|---|---|---|---|---|
| Smallpox | *Variola* or Smallpox *virus* | Any age | Direct or indirect contact with throat or skin discharges of lesions of infected persons; airborne transmission of virus over a short distance | 7 to 16 days | High fever, headache, prostration, skin eruption | 1 to 7 weeks |
| Measles "red measles" (Rubeola) | *Rubeola virus* | Childhood disease, 2 to 8 years | Direct or indirect contact with nose or throat discharge of infected person; also airborne | 7 to 14 days, usually 10 to 12 days | Gradually increasing fever, cold symptoms, severe cough, conjunctivitis, running nose; rash appears on third or fourth day | 6 to 12 days |
| German Measles "three-day measles" (Rubella) | *Rubella virus* | Childhood disease, 2 to 15 years | Direct or indirect contact with nose or throat discharge of infected person; also airborne | 10 to 28 days, usually 14 to 21 days | Slight fever, swelling of lymph glands, rash | 1 to 4 days |
| Diphtheria | *Corynebacterium diphtheriae,* the diphtheria bacillus | Childhood disease; under 15 years of age | Contact with nose or throat discharges of a patient or carrier | 1 to 6 days | Sore throat, mild fever, running nose | Highly variable; possibly several weeks |
| Whooping Cough (Pertussis) | *Bordetella (Hemophilus) pertussis,* the pertussis bacillus | Childhood disease, birth to 10 years | Direct or indirect contact with nose or throat discharges of infected person | 5 to 16 days, usually 7 to 10 days | Gradually increasing *dry* cough | 2 to 10 weeks, usually 4 to 6 weeks |

with them takes a great risk of catching a venereal disease.

Like all infectious diseases, venereal diseases are the result of infection of the body by germs. The germs causing these diseases enter the body through the mucous membranes and the skin. They are among the more delicate germs, sensitive to chilling and drying. The most ideal means of transmitting them is through sexual contact or other close bodily contact.

### *Gonorrhea*

Gonorrhea is the most common venereal disease in the United States today. It is caused by a bacterium commonly called the

| CONTAGIOUS PERIOD | PERMANENT AFTEREFFECTS | IMMUNITY | PREVENTION | ADDITIONAL INFORMATION |
|---|---|---|---|---|
| From 4 to 5 days before rash appears until rash disappears | From 1 to 40% of cases die; blindness, brain damage, scars | Second attacks are very rare | Vaccination when traveling outside the U.S. | Smallpox is caused by a highly contagious virus that is very easily transmitted. A few isolated cases do occur in improperly immunized individuals outside of the U.S. Only required vaccination for entry into the United States |
| From 4 days before until 5 days after rash appears | Occasional death or brain damage due to encephalitis | Congenital immunity lasts a few months. The disease usually confers permanent immunity. | Immunization with live measles vaccine | A single injection gives an active immunity against measles for life. Some states require immunization before registering for school. This disease can cause death and disability. All children should be immunized. |
| From 1 week before until end of rash | Rare, except to fetus of an infected expectant mother | One attack usually confers permanent immunity | Immunization with German measles vaccine | There is a high chance of permanent damage to the fetus of a woman who is in the first six months of pregnancy when contracting German measles. This vaccine should not be given to a pregnant woman or one who may become pregnant within two months after the shot. All girls should be immunized before their first menstrual flow. |
| Variable; usually from 3 days before until 10 days after onset of symptoms | Five to 10% of cases die; toxin may permanently damage heart or nervous system | Congenital immunity lasts for several months. The actual disease usually confers a lasting immunity | Immunization with DPT shots | Diphtheria bacteria release a toxin which, when carried by the blood, has serious destructive effects on many parts of the body. |
| Variable; usually first two weeks | In infants, death or brain damage | No congenital immunity; second attacks rarely occur | Immunization with DPT shots. | In the United States today, whooping cough occurs mainly among young children from low-income families where proper immunization practices are not always followed. It is very dangerous to young children, especially those under six months of age. |

gonococcus. Slang names for the disease include "the clap," "a dose," "morning drop," "g.c.," and "strain."

Gonorrhea is usually limited to a local infection of the lining membranes of the reproductive system. Unlike syphilis, it does not usually enter the bloodstream to be carried to other parts of the body. The first symptoms of gonorrhea usually occur about three to five days after exposure, but the incubation period may be from two to ten days. Gonorrhea begins as an acute disease and then progresses into a chronic condition.

Male gonorrhea starts as an infection in the inner lining of the urethra. This infection causes the first symptoms of male gonor-

| NAME OF DISEASE | CAUSED BY | USUAL AGE INFECTED | MODE OF TRANSMISSION | INCUBATION PERIOD | EARLY SIGNS | LENGTH OF DISEASE |
|---|---|---|---|---|---|---|
| Tetanus "Lock jaw" | *Clostridium tetani,* the tetanus bacillus | Any age | Tetanus spores in dust or dirt infect the body through an open wound or cut | Commonly 4 days to 3 weeks | Painful contractions of the body's muscles | Variable; several weeks |
| Mumps | Mumps virus | Childhood disease, 2 to 14 years | Direct or indirect contact with nose or throat discharge of infected person | 12 to 28 days, usually 16 to 20 days | Fever, swelling of salivary gland | 4 to 10 days |
| Tuberculosis | *Mycobacterium tuberculosis,* the tubercle bacillus | Any age | Contact with patients, indirect contact through contaminated articles, unpasteurized milk; bacillus may be airborne | 4 to 6 weeks | None (may go undetected for long period of time) | Indefinite |
| Infectious Hepatitis | A virus infection of the liver | Any age | Contact with feces, urine, blood, and probably nose and throat discharges of infected persons | 2 to 7 weeks, commonly 3 to 4 weeks | Fever, mild headache, chills, fatigue and jaundice | Variable; often 2 to 4 weeks |
| Infectious Mononucleosis | A virus infection centered in the lymph nodes | Can be a childhood disease; 2 to 20 years of age | Unknown—believed to be direct contact with nose or throat discharges of infected persons; some implication of cats as a reservoir | 2 to 6 weeks | Fever, sore throat, fatigue, enlarged lymph nodes | Variable; 1 week to several months |

rhea—burning or stinging urination and a discharge of pus from the penis. These symptoms usually begin three to five days after exposure to the disease in about 80 percent of infected males. The other 20 percent show no outward symptoms. If treatment is promptly given at this stage, no permanent damage will take place. But if the disease is not promptly treated, the infection will work further up the male reproductive system. Scar tissue may form inside the delicate structures of the testes and the small tubes that carry the sperm. The result may be permanent sterility; gonorrhea is one of the major causes of sterility in males today.

Female gonorrhea usually starts as an in-

| CONTAGIOUS PERIOD | PERMANENT AFTEREFFECTS | IMMUNITY | PREVENTION | ADDITIONAL INFORMATION |
|---|---|---|---|---|
| Not contagious from human to human | Fatality rate about 50% of cases; usually no permanent damage to someone who recovers | Second attacks are known to occur. | Immunization with DPT shots | When tetanus infection occurs, the toxin released by the bacteria is picked up by the blood and acts upon the central nervous system. The muscles contract fully, become rigid, and convulsions occur. Death is usually because of failure of the muscles needed for breathing. |
| Seven days before swelling until end of swelling. | Very rare; brain damage, atrophy of one testis in some older males or ovarian involvement in some females | The disease usually confers life-long immunity. | Immunization with live mumps virus vaccine | An effective vaccine is available and should be given to all children over one year of age and to any adult who has never had mumps. After puberty there is a chance (25%) that one testis of an infected male may degenerate. In mature females ovarian degeneration may occur. |
| As long as disease is active | Death; destruction of lungs, bones, kidneys and skin | Immunity conferred by healed infection is very limited. | Avoidance of crowding, proper nutrition, chest x-ray, skin test, BCG vaccine for high-risk individuals | Tuberculosis is a disease of poor health conditions, poverty, and crowding. Adequate health conditions can overcome it. |
| Unknown; believed to be from 1 week before onset until 1 week after | Rarely death or permanent liver damage | Second attacks are rare. | None | This disease is more severe in adults than in children. It is often transmitted through traces of blood remaining in or on an injection needle, through blood transfusions, or by shared needles when abusing drugs. |
| Probably from several days before symptoms until end of sore throat | None | Infection with or without symptoms is believed to confer lasting immunity. | None | This disease is most severe among young adults. It is rarely fatal but a period of general weakness may last for several months. |

ᵃFor a more complete listing of the communicable diseases see: K. L. Jones, L. W. Shainberg, and C. O. Byer, *Health Science*, New York, Harper & Row, 1974.

fection in the inner lining of the vagina and in or on the cervix of the uterus. This infection is usually painless. Its only symptom, a slight discharge of pus from the vagina, is so mild that it often goes unnoticed. For this reason, females seldom seek prompt treatment for gonorrhea. Because they may remain highly infectious for many months, promiscuous females are believed to be the main sources of gonorrhea outbreaks. Fully 80 percent of females (some authorities say 90 percent) are truly asymptomatic. They show no outward symptoms of their infection. Prompt treatment is seldom received unless they are warned of their infection by a sex partner or the public health department. It is these symptomless females that provide the *reservoir of infection* that makes gonorrhea so common today.

Eventually, untreated gonorrhea may progress up through the female reproductive system to the fallopian tubes. As in the male, scar tissue forms. This may result in permanent sterility if the eggs can no longer travel down the tubes.

The eyes can be severely infected or permanently blinded by the effects of the gonococcus. Persons having gonorrhea of the reproductive system must be very careful to avoid infecting the eyes. They must thoroughly wash their hands with ordinary soap after they have had contact with the infected sexual organs.

A newborn infant may also be blinded by gonococcus. If the mother is infected at the time of the child's birth, the bacteria may get into the child's eyes as he passes through the vagina. To prevent possible gonorrhea blindness, it has been a standard practice in hospitals throughout the United States for many years to place drops of silver nitrate or an antibiotic into the eyes of the newborn to kill any gonorrhea germs that might be present. All infants are routinely treated in this manner.

There is no blood test available for the detection of gonorrhea, though one which shows promise is being tested. The disease is diagnosed when the gonococcus is found in a stained microscope slide made of the pus discharge from the urethra of the male or the vagina of the female. Even this test is not highly reliable. It works only in about 75 percent of male cases and 25 percent of female cases. The infected female is usually found only after being named as a sexual contact by one or more infected males.

The gonococcus has a long history of developing resistance to everything that has been used for its treatment. Drugs that were miraculous when first used have gradually lost their effectiveness. Some of these drugs have been plain sea water, potassium salts, silver compounds, sulfa drugs, and penicillin. Although penicillin is still the drug most commonly used against gonorrhea, treatment now requires a much larger dose than when the drug was first available. If penicillin eventually is of no further value, there are, fortunately, other drugs that can be used. Penicillin has remained the drug of choice because of fewer undesirable side effects than many other antibiotics.

It must be emphasized that there is no effective home remedy for gonorrhea. Nothing can be mixed up or bought without prescription or by mail that will cure this or any other venereal disease. The infected person must see a private physician or his local public health department for effective treatment. Untreated gonorrhea may enter the bloodstream, leading to infections in other parts of the body. Among the more important of these are arthritis (infection of the joints) and endocarditis (infection of the inner lining and valves of the heart). Permanent damage such as sterility can also occur.

In addition, there is no vaccine that will prevent gonorrhea. Similarly, no natural immunity results from a case of the disease. After antibiotic treatment wears off in a few days, reinfection can occur.

### Syphilis

Syphilis is the most serious and the second most prevalent veneral disease. Slang names for syphilis include "siff," "pox," "lues," and "bad blood." Syphilis is entirely different from gonorrhea. Gonorrhea is normally a local surface infection, but syphilis is always a systemic infection, spread throughout the body. Their only similarity is that both are transmitted by sexual intercourse.

The organism causing syphilis is a spiral bacterium called *Treponema pallidum;* it is very frail and cannot survive drying or chilling. It is killed within a few seconds after its exposure to air. Since the germ is so easily killed by air, it is easy to see why transmission requires intimate bodily contact. The germ requires warm, moist skin or mucous membrane surfaces for its penetration into the body. After the pathogen burrows through the skin or mucous membrane (which it does very quickly) and enters the blood, it can be readily carried throughout the body. Because its symptoms are so varied that they can resemble any one of many other diseases, syphilis has been called the "great imitator." It progresses through definite stages, which are explained in the following pages.

*Primary Syphilis.* After infection with syphilis, there may be a symptomless incubation period of ten to ninety days, although the usual period is three to four weeks. During this time the bacteria multiply in the body.

The first symptom that appears is the primary lesion or chancre (pronounced "shanker"). This is a sore that appears at the exact spot where infection took place. The chancre is swarming with bacteria and any contact with it is likely to result in a syphilitic infection.

The chancre may range in size from very small up to about the size of a dime. It's color ranges from pink to red, and it is raised, firm, and not usually painful. It is usually on or near the sex organs (often within the vagina), but it may occur *anywhere* on the body.

Even if primary syphilis is not treated (which it definitely should be), the chancre will disappear spontaneously in two or three weeks. But this disappearance of the chancre does not mean that the disease is cured. It is just progressing to the next stage. At about the time the chancre disappears, blood tests for syphilis become positive.

*Secondary Syphilis.* In secondary syphilis, the true systemic nature of syphilis becomes obvious. Symptoms may appear throughout the body, starting one to six months after the appearance of the chancre, though in many cases this stage is skipped over. The most common symptom of secondary syphilis is a rash that does not itch. This rash is quite variable in appearance; it may cover the entire body or any part of it. Large, moist sores may develop on or around the sex organs or in the mouth. Other symptoms include sore throats, headaches, slight fevers, red eyes, pain in the joints, and patches of hair that fall out. When a person has these symptoms and thinks he may have been exposed to syphilis he should explain this fact to a physician. Because syphilis can easily be mistaken for one of many other diseases, it is difficult to diagnose. Without an accurate diagnosis, it may not be properly treated. Syphilis at this secondary stage is best diagnosed by means of specific blood tests for the disease.

*Latent Syphilis.* Latent syphilis begins when the symptoms of secondary syphilis disappear. It may last for only a few months or for a lifetime. The average length of latent syphilis is five to ten years. During this time there are absolutely no outward symptoms of the disease. The only way latent syphilis can be detected is through a blood test. Throughout the period of latent syphilis, the germs remain alive in the body but are temporarily held in check by the body defenses.

For its first two years, latent syphilis is called early latent syphilis. During this time the symptoms of secondary syphilis may reappear from time to time. During these periods of returned symptoms, the disease can be transmitted.

The remainder of the latent period is called late latent syphilis. This may last from a few months to many years. There are never any symptoms of late latent syphilis; the major danger during this period is transmission by a pregnant infected mother to her fetus.

*Late Syphilis.* The latent period ends and late syphilis begins when the pathogens make their final destructive attack. In this period the vital organs of the body are violently attacked and permanently damaged. The end result is disability or death.

The most serious damage is to the circulatory and nervous systems. The heart and blood vessels may be severely weakened. Damage to the optic nerves may cause blindness. A general paralysis called paresis may result from damage to other parts of the nervous system. Mental changes might result from generalized brain damage.

Each year, more than 3000 people in the United States die from syphilis, and thousands more must be committed to mental institutions because of permanent syphilitic brain damage.

Late syphilis can still be cured (though with difficulty), but any damage it has produced is permanent damage. For this reason it is important that syphilis be diagnosed and treated in early stages.

### Congenital Syphilis

Syphilis in a pregnant woman presents a very great hazard to the unborn child. The spirochetes pass across the placenta into the blood of the child during the last half of the pregnancy. If a woman is syphilitic at the time of conception or contracts syphilis during pregnancy, the child might be the victim of congenital syphilis. A severe infection might cause a stillbirth.

There may be various visible symptoms of late congenital syphilis, some of which may not appear until late childhood or adolescence. One such late symptom is a clouding of the corneas of the eyes which can lead to blindness. Another symptom of late congenital syphilis is a characteristic abnormality of the permanent teeth—widely spaced and notched.

Congenital syphilis can be prevented by giving the pregnant woman a blood test for syphilis early in the pregnancy and again in the seventh month. If syphilis is found and treated early, the child will not be infected. If treatment is given later, after the child has been infected, the treatment will reach and cure the child as well as the mother.

Any person who has reason to suspect that he might have syphilis should see his private physician or the public health department immediately. He should not let fear or embarrassment prevent him from seeking help. The physician regards syphilis only as a dangerous disease that requires immediate treatment—not as evidence of a sin or crime that requires punishment. The sooner a venereal disease is treated, the easier will be its treatment and the lower the chances of dangerous permanent effects.

Syphilis is commonly confirmed by one of two means. Primary or secondary syphilis can be diagnosed by the presence of spirochetes in the fluid oozing from the chancre or other sores. It is easy to see these organisms under the microscope using special illumination techniques.

The other common way of diagnosing syphilis is with one of several available blood tests. These tests become positive about the time the chancre disappears and remain positive until the syphilis is successfully treated and often for some time thereafter. Blood tests are the only way to detect latent syphilis.

Penicillin or other antibiotics are used in treatment. Proper treatment will completely cure the disease. There is no home remedy, mail-order cure, or nonprescription drugstore product that will cure syphilis. It must have professional treatment.

Although no effective vaccine against

syphilis has yet been developed, an immunity occasionally develops in a person who has had the disease for several years before treatment. When syphilis is treated promptly, as it should be, no immunity will develop, and reinfection can soon take place. However, it would be very foolish to purposely delay treatment of syphilis on the chance that an immunity might result, because the permanent effects of the late stages of the disease might occur first.

## PREVENTION OF VENEREAL DISEASES

So far, our discussion of venereal diseases has revolved around recognizing their symptoms and the importance of obtaining prompt treatment if infection occurs. From both the personal health and public health standpoints, it is much more desirable to prevent any disease than to treat it. The prevention of the venereal diseases requires action by both the individual and public health personnel.

### Personal Prevention

As with most other diseases, the ultimate responsibility for the prevention of venereal diseases lies with individuals. The most important personal preventative measure is the avoidance of any sexual contact with anyone who is likely to be infected with a venereal disease. With today's high incidence of venereal diseases, that would include anyone who has sexual contact with a variety of partners or who has sexual contact with one sexual partner who in turn has a variety of sexual partners. Remember that venereal diseases can be transmitted through either heterosexual or homosexual contact and through either genital-genital, oral-genital, anal-genital sex, or even through certain "petting" practices.

Once again, the prime mechanism of prevention of the venereal diseases is selective sexual behavior. Unfortunately, for the public as a whole this has failed because it has never been widely practiced. The current VD epidemic is glaring evidence of this failure. Thus, for the person who chooses to be somewhat less discriminate in his choice of sexual partners, it becomes important to make maximum use of other personal preventive (prophylactic) methods to reduce the chances of infection. Note that we use the word reduce rather than eliminate, since even the best of the currently available prophylactic methods are far from certain in their action.

The single most important personal preventive method is probably the liberal use of soap and water immediately after sexual contact. The pathogens of the venereal diseases that enter the body through the skin can often be killed or removed in this manner. The three less common venereal diseases, chancroid, lymphogranuloma venereum, and granuloma inguinale can be almost entirely eliminated by this simple technique.

Urination by a male immediately after sexual contact may help reduce the chance of his infection with gonorrhea, as may prompt douching by a female. It should be pointed out that douching is not effective as a birth control measure and will reduce the contraceptive effectiveness of foams, jellies, and the diaphragm and jelly. In addition, frequent douching often results in vaginal irritations and infections. Douching should be reserved for venereal disease prevention or for special situations upon the recommendation of a physician.

The use of a condom (rubber) over the penis of the male will help prevent the transmission of VD, especially gonorrhea, in either direction—from male to female or from female to male. To be effective, the rubber must be applied onto the erect penis at the very start of any sexual activity, before any sexual contact is made. Also, care must be taken to prevent contamination of the condom from the fingers. Even though a condom is used, it is still important to wash with soap and water immediately after contact because the condom covers only the penis and several of the venereal diseases, especially syphilis, can enter the body through the skin at any point whatsoever. The condom thus affords little protection against syphilis. In its favor, however, it should be noted that the condom is the only commonly used device that is effective both as a prophylactic against gonorrhea and as a contraceptive against pregnancy. Carefully and consistently used, it can be reasonably effective for both purposes. While the condom is worn by the male, and it has traditionally been a male responsibility to make sure of its availability for coitus, it would seem that the enlightened female would want to keep a supply of condoms available to protect herself against VD and, if she is not otherwise protected, against pregnancy as well.

Antibiotics have been used on a prophylactic basis, administered either before or after possible exposure to VD. This practice cannot be recommended for routine use because it tends to breed antibiotic resistant strains of pathogens, including but not limited to those which cause the venereal diseases, and because it tends to build allergies to the antibiotics in those who receive them.

The ideal personal preventive for the venereal diseases would, of course, be a vaccine for each disease. Few communicable diseases have been controlled until effective vaccines have been developed. Some progress has been made toward the development of an effective vaccine against syphilis, but has not yet reached a useful stage of development. The prospects of an effective vaccine against gonorrhea seem especially dim, since no natural immunity to this disease develops, even after repeated infections.

### Public Health Measures

Many methods are used by public health agencies in their fight against the venereal diseases and, while these diseases are still rampant, it seems certain that their incidence would be even greater than it is but for the efforts of dedicated public health workers.

Most public health departments carry out programs of education as to the prevention and symptoms of venereal diseases and the importance of prompt treatment. The media used often include newspapers, billboards, radio, TV, and posters in public places. Some public health departments assist local schools in their VD education programs, providing classroom materials and/or teacher training for effective VD instruction.

Clinics for the diagnosis and treatment of VD are also common functions of the public health departments. The services of clinics are usually offered at little or no cost to the individual. The laws in most states have been revised to allow the treatment of minors, often as young as 12 years of age, without obtaining permission from their parents or otherwise notifying them. It has been found that when parental permission must be obtained prior to treatment, many young people will avoid treatment out of fear of reprisals from parents, increasing the chance of permanent damage from the diseases.

Another important public health function in VD control is case-finding. In many localities, each patient treated for a venereal disease, especially for syphilis, is interviewed to determine from whom he might have caught the disease and to whom he might have transmitted it. Then these people can be contacted, notified that they may be infected, and asked to visit the public health department or their private physician for VD testing. Since so many cases of VD are symptomless, this is the only way in which many infected people can learn of their disease before serious damage is done. Sometimes a patient is asked to name not only his sexual partners, but any of his friends who he feels might be infected as well.

One of the real barriers to effective case-finding is that, while by law every case of VD a physician treats must be reported to the local health department, in reality the majority of cases are not reported. The reporting rate for privately treated gonorrhea is especially low, though the reporting of gonorrhea is essentially just for statistical purposes, rather than for case-finding. Many public health departments lack adequate funds for thorough case-finding for even the more serious syphilis, let alone gonorrhea.

While it might seem overly obvious, the VD patient should be warned to refrain from sexual contact with his previous partners until they have been tested and, if necessary, treated for VD. It is common (and frustrating) in VD clinics to find that a newly cured patient has gone back to the same partner who infected him before and becomes infected again and again.

A technique that has revealed thousands of cases of syphilis is compulsory blood testing for certain groups such as applicants for marriage licenses, pregnant women, military personnel, hospital patients, and new employees of many corporations. Most of the cases so detected are in the symptomless *latent period* and, without detection and treatment, many would progress into *late syphilis* with its irreversible damage to vital organs and even death.

In summary, while public health departments are making great efforts to control VD, syphilis and gonorrhea remain as epidemic diseases, and it is imperative for the individual to take reasonable precautions against

his own infection, to have blood tests once or twice a year if there is the possibility of exposure to syphilis, to know the symptoms of these diseases, and to seek prompt treatment if their symptoms develop.

## OTHER INFECTIONS OF THE REPRODUCTIVE AND URINARY ORGANS

In addition to the true venereal diseases, the reproductive organs are susceptible to several other kinds of infections. These infections are not usually classified as venereal diseases because they are very commonly transmitted through nonsexual means, although each of these infections may also be contracted through sexual contact.

In recent years there has been a great increase in these infections. This may be related to an increase in casual sexual contacts and definitely is related to modern birth control methods. Birth control pills change the vaginal environment, creating a more moist, alkaline condition, favoring infection by *Candida, Trichomonas,* and Herpes viruses, as well as gonorrhea. At the same time, pills and IUDs have somewhat replaced birth control methods such as condoms and vaginal foams which actively help prevent the transmission of infections.

### Candida

One of the more troublesome infections of the sexual organs, and especially the vagina, is caused by a yeastlike organism called *Candida albicans.* This organism is a normal inhabitant of the mouth, digestive tract, and vagina, but it is usually held in check by the other organisms present and by the body's natural defenses.

Various factors can act to reduce normal defenses against *Candida* (also called a "yeast" infection), allowing it to erupt into a serious infection. One of these factors is intensive antibiotic therapy for some other infection. During such therapy the normal bacterial "flora" of the intestine and vagina may be reduced in numbers, allowing *Candida* to flourish instead. Poor nutrition may also lead to *Candida* eruption, as may any general weakening of one's health. Diabetes, which impairs the body defenses against most kinds of infections, is frequently associated with severe *Candida* infections. Hormone therapy, including use of birth control pills, as well as pregnancy may alter the vaginal environment to favor growth of *Candida*. A moist environment also encourages the organism; spending many hours in a wet swim suit or in clothing that does not "breathe" freely sometimes leads to severe *Candida* infections, especially of the vagina and labia.

Vaginal candidiasis (the medical name for *Candida* infection) is most troublesome of the *Candida* infections. The characteristic symptoms of vaginal candidiasis include burning and itching and a whitish discharge, which can be quite abundant. There may be patches of white *pseudomembrane* (false membrane) on the vaginal lining. In treating vaginal candidiasis, there are several considerations. First is keeping the vaginal area dry and correcting any contributing conditions such as poor nutrition. A variety of effective oral and vaginal medications are available by prescription. It is important that male sex partners use condoms during the period of infection to avoid "ping-pong" infections in which the male is infected and later reinfects the female.

Other sites of *Candida* infection include the penis, vulva, and mouth cavity. Infection of the mouth cavity is called "thrush" and occurs most commonly among infants, elderly persons, or patients on intensive antibiotic therapy over long periods of time. *Candida*

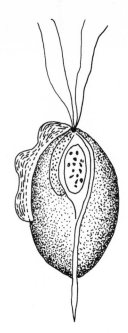

*Trichomonas vaginalis* of humans.

rarely enters the blood, but once within blood plasma it may cause serious or even fatal kidney or heart damage.

### *Trichomonas*

Another common cause of vaginitis is infection by the protozoan (or one-cell animal) *Trichomonas vaginalis*. *Trichomonas* lives in the vaginas of many women without producing noticeable symptoms. Symptomless infections of the male prostate gland, urethra, and seminal vesicles are also common. Under certain conditions, however, *Trichomonas* can multiply enormously in either the male or female reproductive organs. Symptoms in the female can include intense itching and burning of the vagina, small rashlike spots on its lining, and a profuse discharge of a thin, foamy, yellowish discharge which may have a foul odor. Symptoms in the male, though they rarely occur, include urethritis or, even more rarely, inflammation of the prostate or seminal vesicles.

*Trichomonas* is a common infection among adult females throughout the world. The organism is transmitted from person to person by contact with vaginal and urethral discharges of infected persons during sexual contact, during birth, and possibly by contact with infected articles. Symptomless vaginal infections are often converted into troublesome vaginitis through modification of the vaginal environment produced by the hormonal changes associated with birth control pills or pregnancy.

Trichomoniasis can be successfully treated by medically prescribed oral or vaginal medications. Simultaneous treatment of sexual partners is important in preventing reinfection. Even though a partner may be symptomless, he may well carry the organism.

### Genital Herpes Virus

Some of the most troublesome and persistent genital infections are caused by viruses from the *herpes simplex* group. Herpes simplex viruses are apparently carried by most people at all times, though usually in a state of latency (dormancy). Some 70 to 90 percent of adults carry antibodies against herpes simplex, but these antibodies do not prevent occasional activation of the virus. In addition to genital sores, herpes viruses are associated with cold sores, fever blisters, eczema, corneal infection, meningitis, encephalitis, and possibly uterine and other cancers.

Most people receive their initial infection with herpes virus during childhood. The antibodies carried by most adults are transferred across the placenta to the fetus during pregnancy so most infants are protected from infection during the first few months after their birth. If the mother acquires her first infection during pregnancy, however, and the child is born before sufficient maternal antibodies can be transferred across the placenta, severe infection of the newborn may occur, often with fatal consequences. The virus may be widely distributed in infant tissues, producing severe lesions in skin, mucous membranes, liver, and brain.

Much more typically, infection occurs during childhood and without serious complications. Children are usually infected through contact with the virus in the saliva of other children or adults or through contact with the eczema or other lesions in infected persons. About 90 percent of initial childhood infections are symptomless; about 10 percent of children suffer a mild illness of fever and general discomfort (malaise) lasting only a few days. Following initial infection, herpes virus usually is carried in the body cells in a latent state, being periodically reactivated by various stimuli such as fever, mechanical irritation, and certain foods.

Genital herpes simplex sores in adults may result from either the reactivation of latent herpes infections or from newly acquired virus transmitted through genital or orogenital sexual contact. These sores may occur on the labia or within the vagina in females or on the penis or within the urethra in males. Herpes simplex sores may appear either as blisters over a red base or as red, eroded lesions. In either case, genital herpes may be quite painful, especially during coitus.

Unlike *Candida* and *Trichomonas,* there is no specific treatment for herpes simplex virus. Viruses in general are not susceptible to control by antibiotics or other drugs.

### Uterine Cancer as a Venereal Disease

A possible although still unproven association has been suggested between a herpes simplex virus (type II) and cancer of the cervix or the uterus. The virus is often found within cancerous cells, but no cause-and-effect relationship has been established.

A possibly correlative statistical association has been proposed by some cancer researchers (and disputed by others) in which the incidence of cervical cancer may be statistically related to a patient's sexual history. According to those who accept this association, the incidence of cervical cancer is higher among women who begin sexual intercourse at younger ages and among those with a history of many sexual partners. Conversely, the incidence of uterine cancer has been reported to be low among virgins, women experiencing intercourse at a later date, and women with a history of few sexual partners.

Assuming the statistical relationship between early coitus and uterine cancer is valid, such a relationship would be compatible with the role of a sexually transmitted herpes simplex virus as a causal agent for such cancer, since the herpes viruses are noted for their ability to lie dormant for many years. The incidence of uterine cancer increases with age, although it is possible that the cells of some particular younger woman might be more susceptible to infection by a virus.

Other factors might also account for an association between early intercourse or multiple sexual partners and cervical cancer, again assuming that such an association exists. Genetic mutation of the cervical cells is one such possibility. The cause of such mutation might be repeated mechanical trauma during coitus or perhaps some carcinogenic (cancer-causing) chemical in semen, although the latter seems extremely unlikely. Still another possibility is that the stimulus for cancer production might be irritation and weakening of the cervical tissues by chronic infection with one or more of the many sexually transmitted pathogens.

## Cystitis

Cystitis is infection of the urinary bladder. Any of a variety of bacteria and other organisms may cause this problem. The symptoms include frequent, burning, or painful urination, chills, fever, fatigue, and, infrequently, blood in the urine. Bladder infections occur more often in females than in males, because the shorter urethra of the female makes it easier for bacteria to reach the bladder.

Cystitis should be treated promptly with medically prescribed drugs. Untreated it may become a chronic problem or spread to the kidneys. Cleanliness, frequent urination, and drinking adequate water helps prevent this infection.

## Nonspecific Urethritis

Nonspecific urethritis (NSU), also called nongonorrheal urethritis (NGU), is a term often applied to any infection of the urethra other than by gonorrhea. Numerous pathogens have been associated with urethral infections. In many specific cases, the infecting agent is never definitely identified.

NSU is often transmitted through sexual contact and is more common among people having a variety of sexual partners. Most cases can be cleared up with the combination of prescribed medication, avoidance of alcohol and caffeine, and abstention from sex until the infection is healed.

## Pubic Lice

Pubic lice, commonly called "crab lice" or "crabs" because of their crablike appearance, are small, gray insects (1/16 inch long) that live as external parasites on the body. They live in body hair, holding onto the shaft of the hair with their crablike pincers. They prefer pubic hair but will also live in the hair under arms and in eyebrows and beards, but never scalp hair (which is too fine in texture). Crab lice do not really pinch with their claws, but they do feed on human blood, causing an intense itching and discoloration of the skin. They often remain attached for days, with their sucking mouthparts inserted into the skin of an unfortunate host. Female lice attach eggs, called nits, to the body hair. These eggs hatch in 6 to 8 days. Since sexual maturity is reached in only 14 to 21 days and each female lays up to 50 eggs, a crab louse infection can grow to alarming proportions in just a short time. Heavy infestations may result in fever and other disorders caused by toxins injected by the feeding lice.

Pubic lice may be transmitted through sexual intercourse, but they can also be spread through less intimate physical contact with infested people or by use of contaminated clothing, toilet seats, bedding, or other materials.

Crabs can usually be killed by washing the affected body parts with a special shampoo, such as Kwell, available at most pharmacies. Several applications are required. Contrary to popular belief, infested hair need *not* be shaved, and exposed clothing need not be

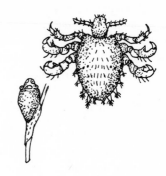

The pubic louse, *Phthirus pubis*. Egg attached to hair, lower left.

thrown away. However, it should not be worn until it is cleaned or thoroughly washed in hot water.

# 18
# The Noncommunicable Diseases

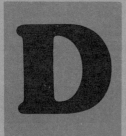

During the first half of the twentieth century, advances in preventive medicine vastly altered the pattern of disease in the United States and many other countries. The table of the leading causes of death in the United States shows the shift in importance from communicable to noncommunicable diseases.

Improvements in diagnosis, treatment, sanitation, nutrition, housing, and working conditions, as well as more specific preventive measures, such as immunizations, have played important roles in the conquest of the communicable diseases. Drugs, such as antibiotics and sulfas, have greatly reduced communicable diseases, even as other public hazards, such as those in the lower economic areas of our cities, have remained.

The increase in noncommunicable diseases has been due in large part to the increased average lifespan. Many of these diseases are cumulative and degenerative in nature; they require relatively long periods of time to develop and some of them are apparently related to the general aging processes. In just one hundred years—from 1860 to 1960—the proportion of persons in the United States over 45 years of age climbed from 13 percent to 29 percent of the population. This increase in older-age groups is currently changing the whole field of preventive medicine. Whereas previous efforts were directed largely toward the control of communicable diseases of early life, efforts are now being directed increasingly toward the noncommunicable diseases—those common in middle and later life.

## CANCER

Throughout a person's life the cells in many parts of his body are constantly dividing to provide replacements for worn out or damaged cells. In cancer the normal, orderly division and growth of the cells is replaced by rapid, uncontrolled division and growth. In most cases cancer seems to start when a single cell goes "wild."

The general term cancer includes a group of related diseases that are characterized by

## LEADING CAUSES OF DEATH IN THE UNITED STATES—1900 AND 1970

| 1900 (LIFE EXPECTANCY 46.1 YEARS FOR MALES, 49.5 YEARS FOR FEMALES) | | 1974 ESTIMATE (LIFE EXPECTANCY 67.8 YEARS FOR MALES, 74.6 YEARS FOR FEMALES) | | |
|---|---|---|---|---|
| RANK | CAUSE | RANK | CAUSE | PERCENT OF ALL DEATHS |
| 1 | Tuberculosis | 1 | Heart and circulatory disorders | 53% |
| 2 | Pneumonia | 2 | Cancer | 18% |
| 3 | Intestinal infections | 3 | Accidents | 6% |
| 4 | Heart diseases | 4 | Pneumonia and influenza | 3% |
| 5 | Diseases of infancy | 5 | Diabetes | 2% |

the abnormal growth and spread of body cells. Considered as a group, the various types of cancer are the *number two* cause of death in the United States today. Approximately one in every four Americans will develop cancer sometime during his life. Currently, approximately 16 percent of all deaths in this country are attributed to some form of cancer.

Generally, a cancer cell can be distinguished from a normal cell principally by its nucleus. The nucleus of a cancer cell is usually larger than that of a normal cell, and differs in the number and appearance of its chromosomes, and in the number of nucleoli present (see figure of a cancer and normal cell). The earliest detectable sign of cancer is an increase in the number of chromosomes in a cell. Not only are these numbers odd and irregular, but also the chromosomes may be abnormally shaped.

An outstanding characteristic of cancer cells is their invasive ability. Normal cells are slowed in dividing by close contact with surrounding cells. But cancer cells do not show such a response. They continue to divide and push into and invade the surrounding normal tissue.

Another important characteristic of cancer is metastasis, the transfer of disease from one organ to another. Cancerous growths tend to shed living cancer cells. These cells can be picked up by the blood or lymph and be carried to remote parts of the body. Wherever these cells happen to lodge, they begin to grow, divide, and invade. Thus, through the process of metastasis, the body of the cancer victim may become riddled with dozens of growths at many locations.

Any mass of new tissue that persists and grows without serving any useful purpose is called a tumor or neoplasm ("new tissue"). The growth of tumors is characteristic of many, but not all, kinds of cancer. Tumors are divided into two classes—benign (noncancerous) and malignant (cancerous).

Benign tumors tend to grow more slowly than malignant tumors and are usually surrounded by a fibrous membrane that prevents them from invading surrounding tissues. They may, however, reach such an enormous size that they exert dangerous pressure on the surrounding organs. Benign tumors commonly occur on the skin as warts or birthmarks, inside the body as fibrous tumors or cysts, or on the skeleton as growths of bone tissue. Some benign tumors, if exposed to certain harmful irritations, may become malignant.

Malignant tumors are cancerous growths. Kinds of cancers may be recognized by their names, which often end in *oma*. Some examples: carcinomas are malignancies of epithelial tissues; melanomas, of pigment cells; lymphomas, of lymph tissues; sarcomas, of connective tissues, and so forth.

Although cancer can kill in many ways, three conditions most often lead to the death of the cancer victim—anemia, infections, and debility.

Anemia is the inability of the blood to carry sufficient oxygen in the body. In some types of anemia there is an insufficient production of red blood cells, or red blood cells

are produced but do not survive long enough. In other cancers there is internal bleeding that results in a dangerous loss of red blood cells.

Infection often results from the inability of the white blood cells to destroy infection germs. In some types of cancer few white blood cells are produced. In other cancers, such as leukemia, vast numbers of white cells are produced, but they are malformed and unable to fight germs.

Debility, the lack or loss of strength, is common in almost all forms of cancer. It may result from simple undernutrition, such as might occur when there has been damage to some part of the digestive system. Debility may also be a side effect of treatments such as surgery, drugs, or radiation.

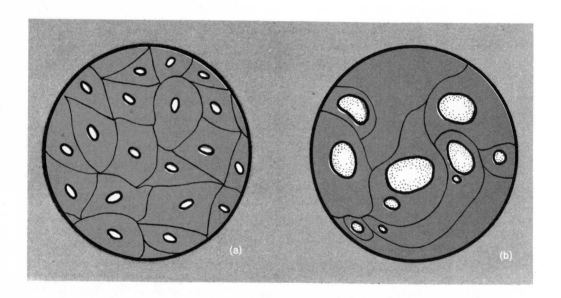

Cancer cells and normal cells as they might appear under the microscope. Cancer cells have large irregular nuclei, and the cells often take strange shapes. (a) Microscopic view of "Pap" smear to detect cervical cancer showing normal cells. (b) Microscopic view of "Pap" smear to detect cervical cancer showing cancer cells.

### Symptoms of Cancer (see Table on Some Major Cancer Sites)

The degree of success in treating cancer depends largely upon how early the disease is detected and treatment is begun. It is extremely important for everyone to recognize the early symptoms of cancer. They are:

1. Any sore that does not heal, regardless of its appearance or location.
2. Any lump or thickening anywhere on or in the body.
3. Any unusual bleeding or discharge from any body opening.
4. Any change in a wart, mole, or birthmark, such as a change in its color or size.
5. Persistent indigestion or difficulty in swallowing.
6. Persistent hoarseness or cough.
7. Any change in bowel or urination habits.
8. Any unusual pain—seldom a symptom of early cancer, but not to be ignored.

If any of these symptoms appear, either singly or in combination, a physician should be seen as soon as possible. Any of these symptoms can be produced by many conditions other than cancer, but prompt treatment of cancer is so essential that it is foolish to take a "wait and see" attitude. If cancer is found, it can be promptly treated; if cancer is ruled out as a cause of the symptom, needless worry can be avoided.

### Diagnosis of Cancer

A physician can definitely confirm the presence of cancer in several ways. Some of these methods are applied when a patient notices one of the early symptoms of cancer. Others are used on a routine, periodic basis to detect generally symptomless forms of the disease.

*X-rays.* Certain cancers, such as lung cancer, may be detected through x-rays. It is important that smokers have chest x-rays frequently. Some authorities recommend chest x-rays every six months for smokers.

*Smear Tests.* Since many kinds of malignant tumors shed cancer cells from their surface, it is often possible to detect cancer through a microscopic examination of certain body fluids. This is accomplished by smearing the fluid onto a glass microscopic slide, staining it, and examining the slide under the microscope.

The most commonly used smear test is the Papanicolaou ("Pap") smear test for cancer of the uterus. In this simple procedure, a microscope slide is prepared from the secretions of the upper vagina. Since most uterine cancer begins on the cervix, which extends into the vagina, cancerous cells may be present in the vagina while the uterine cancer is still in its early development.

Uterine cancer usually remains on the cervix for one to two years before it begins its devastating spread through the entire uterus and the surrounding organs. If the cancer is detected through a Pap smear during this early period, the chances of a successful cure are excellent. It is strongly recommended that every woman have a Pap test every year, without fail, starting in her late teens. After age forty-five, the test should be made every six months.

*Blood Tests.* Leukemia and other cancers of the blood-forming organs are normally diagnosed through a count of the blood cells on a stained microscope slide. Some progress has been made toward the development of blood tests for other forms of cancer, but it must be emphasized that there is currently no way of detecting many forms of cancer through blood tests.

*Rectal Examinations.* The lower portion of the large intestine is a common place for cancer to develop. Cancers in this area are usually symptomless in their early stages. But a physician often can detect rectal cancers through a visual inspection of the inner walls of the lower large intestine.

*Biopsy.* A biopsy is the microscopic examination of cells removed from a living organ for the purpose of diagnosis. This procedure is normally applied when an organ or tumor is suspected of being cancerous. A small slice of the suspected tissue is removed and examined, often while the patient waits in the operating room. If the tumor is cancerous, extra care is taken to ensure the complete removal of all accessible cancerous tissue.

### Theories of Causation

Several important factors distinguish research into the causes of cancer from analogous research on other diseases. First, dominating much of this research is the basic premise that underlying the answer to the riddle of cancer causation is the understanding of the functioning of the normal cell. By studying the chemistry and physiology of normal tissues, scientists hope to eventually learn by comparison between normal growth patterns and abnormal, cancerous ones.

Second, there is the as yet poorly understood relationship between causes and "triggers" of cancer. Certain external stimuli are apparently related to the development of the disease, but more basic "causes" also appear to be involved.

And third, further complicating all this is the fact that there are indications that some animal cancers are caused by viruses; as yet, no human cancers have been connected with a specific pathogen.

### The Basic Causes

*Heredity.* Only a few uncommon forms of cancer are definitely hereditary. One type of cancer of the eye follows a predictable hereditary pattern. Several other forms of cancer, while not yet proven to be hereditary, do seem common in certain family lines, suggesting that the tendency toward these cancers may be inherited. Examples of these cancers include colon cancer and breast cancer.

*Mutations.* In addition to the possibility that some cancers are hereditary in nature, scientists are looking at another aspect of the genetic causation of the disease. When a cell becomes cancerous, definite changes occur in the chromosomes. It is possible the effect of certain chemicals is to alter the hereditary material and "dictate" a new, cancerous growth pattern.

*Viruses.* In recent years, considerable evidence has accumulated associating at least some forms of human cancer with viruses. While a definite cause-and-effect relationship is yet to be proved, the presumptive evidence is strong enough to warrant an intensive research effort to determine the role, if any, that viruses play in causing cancers.

It seems likely that cancer-causing viruses (if they exist) have long periods of latency during which they are present in the human body cells in an inactive state. Perhaps certain irritants, such as chemicals or radiation, act to "trigger" cancer by activating these viruses.

If cancer-producing viruses can be isolated and cultured (grown in tissue culture) this might open the door to the production of anticancer vaccines, which would seem to be the ideal solution to the cancer problem.

It is logical to wonder whether cancers are contagious, if viruses do cause cancer. The only current evidence of communicability is in the case of cervical cancer, which is rather strongly associated with the presence of a form of herpes simplex (type II), presumed to be transmitted through sexual intercourse (see discussion on page 395). While males rarely suffer cancer of the penis, they apparently do carry the herpes simplex type II virus.

There is no definite evidence that any other form of human cancer is ever "caught" from another person.

### Cancer Triggers

Several factors are known to produce cancer with prolonged exposure to human tissues. These forces are often referred to as "causes" of cancer ("Does smoking cause cancer?"), but the term "triggers" better relates these factors to the influences mentioned above.

*Chemical Carcinogens.* Hundreds of chemicals have been definitely proved to be carcinogenic (cancer causing), either to man or to experimental animals. Some of these carcinogens are contained in tobacco smoke and the smoke from other burning vegetation. Others are carried by various petroleum derivatives such as tars, asphalts, and oil; coal derivatives; and soot.

*Sunlight.* The factor in sunlight that causes skin cancer is its ultraviolet radiation. Since ultraviolet has little penetrating power, it is not associated with cancers of the deeper tissues.

*External Irritation.* Some cases of cancer seem to be the result of a prolonged irritation such as the constant rubbing of a tight belt or brassiere strap over a wart, mole, or birthmark or the rubbing of loose dentures and bridges against the jaw.

*Extreme Heat.* Prolonged exposure to very hot objects seems to be an occasional cause of cancer. The high temperature of a pipe stem may be a factor contributing to lip cancer which often develops in pipe smokers.

*Radiation.* It has been well established that exposure to excessive x-rays and other forms of radiation increases the chances of cancer. It has been found that either a single exposure to a high level of radiation or the repeated exposure to more moderate levels increases the risk of leukemia. It must be stressed that medical and dental x-rays present very little risk. The risk involved in these x-rays (which may be used to detect tuberculosis, fractured bones, dangerously infected teeth, and so on) is far less than the risk in not taking them.

### Treatment of Cancer

Many people have the mistaken idea that a cancer diagnosis is the same as a death sentence. In fact, this notion keeps many people away from doctors altogether when they fear they have cancer. Actually, with prompt medical treatment the chances of survival are good with many types of cancer. Even when the disease cannot be completely cured, proper treatment often can extend a patient's life.

We already discussed the relationship between pathogens and the treatment and cure of communicable diseases. Until the pioneering work of Robert Koch and Louis Pasteur in the nineteenth century, doctors treating a communicable-disease patient could only try to make the patient comfortable, for the ability to cure depended on understanding of the cause.

Thus, in comparison with the history of the treatment of communicable disease, we have the paradoxically fortunate situation of cancer cures and treatment despite our lack of knowledge of the disease's cause. The methods of treatment of cancer deal not with eliminating the (unknown) causative agent, but rather with eliminating the cancerous cells and/or interrupting their growth pattern. There is no absolute standard for evaluating the success of a cancer cure; a cancer

# INCIDENCE, DEATHS, AND ADDITIONAL INFORMATION
## FOR SOME MAJOR CANCER SITES

| SITE | NO. OF NEW CASES PER YEAR BY SITE AND SEX | | NO. OF CANCER DEATHS BY SITE AND SEX | | WARNING SIGNAL—WHEN LASTING LONGER THAN TWO WEEKS—SEE YOUR DOCTOR |
|---|---|---|---|---|---|
| | MALE | FEMALE | MALE | FEMALE | |
| LUNG | 64,000 | 15,000 | 57,900 | 14,100 | Persistent cough or lingering respiratory ailment |
| BREAST | 600 | 73,000 | 250 | 32,400 | Lump or thickening in the breast |
| COLON AND RECTUM | 38,000 | 41,000 | 22,900 | 24,500 | Change in bowel habits; bleeding from the rectum; blood in the stools |
| PROSTATE | 38,000 | | 17,800 | | Difficulty in urinating |
| UTERUS | | 46,000 | | 11,800 | Unusual bleeding or discharge from vagina |
| PANCREAS | 11,000 | 8,400 | 10,900 | 8,300 | Nausea, feeling of fullness, abdominal discomfort |
| LYMPHOMAS (cancers of lymph tissues) | 14,200 | 11,300 | 11,100 | 9,200 | Painless enlargement of lymph nodes; pain in abdomen and back; persistent sore throat; trouble in swallowing |
| OVARY | | 14,000 | | 10,500 | Abdominal discomfort and pain; pressure, constipation, swelling of abdomen |
| STOMACH | 9,700 | 6,700 | 8,700 | 6,000 | Persistent chronic indigestion; aversion to rich food and meat; decreasing appetite; dark, tarry stools |

# INCIDENCE, DEATHS, AND ADDITIONAL INFORMATION
## FOR SOME MAJOR CANCER SITES (Continued)

| SAFEGUARDS | ADDITIONAL INFORMATION |
|---|---|
| Best safeguard is prevention by not smoking; annual physical checkup and chest x-ray series for smokers | The leading cause of deaths among males and is increasing in females as more females smoke—is preventable by not smoking. Commonly metastases to the brain, bones or liver. |
| Annual checkup; monthly self-examination | Uncommon in males. Develops most frequently in females who have not lactated. This is the leading cause of cancer death in women. |
| Annual checkup, including protoscopy | Considered a highly curable disease when annual physical checkups include proctoscopic examination for early detection. |
| Annual checkup including palpation of prostate gland and urinalysis | One of the most common types of cancer in males. Usually develops in males past age 60. |
| Annual checkup including pelvic examination and Papanicolaou (''Pap'') smear; avoid casual sexual contacts (?) | Uterine cancer deaths have declined 50 percent during the last 25 years, with wider application of the ''Pap'' smear; many thousands more lives could be saved. This cancer is increasingly being linked to a virus causation which may be spread to the female by the male. Most often develops in women who have had children. |
| Annual checkup including urinalysis | Only detected by physical checkup. Is usually fatal when it develops. |
| None known | These diseases arise in the lymph system and affected individuals often lead normal lives for years. *Lymphosarcoma* is frequently found in children. These diseases are found throughout the body in the lymph system including lymph nodes. |
| Annual checkup and notification of a physician when swelling in abdominal area is noticed | The growth may become quite large before producing any pain or discomfort. Woman often feels a necessity to urinate when there is no need. |
| Often is thought to be a peptic ulcer at first. Any persistent chronic indigestion should be brought to attention of a physician | Most wait too long for treatment; has been decreasing in last few years but is still a major cause of death in the United States. |

*405*

| SITE | NO. OF NEW CASES PER YEAR BY SITE AND SEX | | NO. OF CANCER DEATHS BY SITE AND SEX | | WARNING SIGNAL—WHEN LASTING LONGER THAN TWO WEEKS—SEE YOUR DOCTOR |
|---|---|---|---|---|---|
| | MALE | FEMALE | MALE | FEMALE | |
| LEUKEMIA (cancer of the blood-forming tissues) | 11,000 | 8,000 | 8,600 | 6,700 | Weakness; loss of weight; fatigue; bleeding from mucous membranes; enlarged liver and spleen |
| BLADDER AND URETHRA | 15,000 | 5,800 | 6,300 | 2,900 | Blood in urine; frequent painful urination |
| ORAL (including pharynx and larynx) | 10,500 | 4,900 | 5,550 | 2,050 | Sore that does not heal; difficulty in swallowing; hoarseness |
| SKIN | 76,000 | 39,000 | 3,100 | 2,100 | Sore that does not heal, or change in wart or mole |

patient is generally considered "cured" only after he has shown no sign of the disease for at least five years after treatment.

In a sense, a doctor treating a cancer patient works "backwards." He studies the location, pattern, size, effects and symptoms of the cancerous growth and plans his treatment accordingly. He might use a single method of treatment, or might combine a few different methods to effect a cure. The three basic methods of cancer treatment in use today are surgery, radiation, and chemotherapy.

*Surgery.* The key to successful treatment of cancer is to diagnose it at a stage when the cancer can be removed entirely from the body. The major use of surgery in the treatment of cancer is to attempt to remove completely all of the cancerous tissue in the involved area. Because of the spreading nature of cancer, varying amounts of normal tissue

| SAFEGUARDS | ADDITIONAL INFORMATION |
|---|---|
| | *Acute leukemia* mainly strikes children and is treated by drugs which have extended life from a few months to apparent cures. *Chronic leukemia* strikes usually after age 25 and progresses slowly. Cancer experts believe that if drugs or vaccines are found which can cure or prevent cancers they will be successful first for leukemia and lymphomas. |
| Annual checkup with urinalysis; do not smoke tobacco | There is some linkage with cigarette smoking. Consequently, not too common in females except in smoking females. One urination may be bloody while the next is entirely clear, or the bloody urine may slowly change to a normal color over a period of days; blood may not reappear for several months—any blood in the urine (except during menstrual flow in females) should be brought to the attention of a physician. |
| Annual checkup, including mirror laryngoscopy; do not smoke tobacco | Many more lives should be saved because the mouth is easily accessible to visual examination by physicians and dentists. |
| Annual checkup, avoidance of overexposure to the sun | Skin cancer is readily detected by observation, and diagnosed by simple biopsy; there are few deaths considering the large number of cases each year. It is not considered one of the 10 major causes of cancer deaths in either men or women. |

SOURCE: Adapted from *1973 Cancer Facts and Figures,* American Cancer Society, Inc., 1973.

are often removed along with the malignant growth. Surgery may be used to remove certain endocrine glands (ovaries, pituitary, or adrenal glands) in an effort to check the spread of cancer in organs that depend on the hormones produced by these glands for growth. It is also used to relieve pain in cases of incurable cancer by severing nerves serving the area of pain.

Surgery, radiation, and chemotherapy are being combined in an effort to find the most effective cancer cures possible. Chemicals are now being fed directly into surgical wounds to prevent the spread of any remaining cancer cells into the blood or lymph. Preoperative radiation to prevent implantation and growth of tumors in tissue surrounding the surgical area is also being used.

*Radiation.* Radiation has been used as a cancer treatment for about fifty years. Amounts of radiation that seem to have no

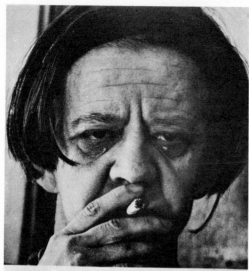

internal organs. Low-energy x-rays are used for superficial cancers such as skin growths.

*Radioactive cobalt.* Radioactive cobalt releases a much more penetrating beam than does x-ray. Used in a procedure similar to that used with x-rays, cobalt therapy involves a placement of the patient in such a position that he or the cobalt can be rotated during his exposure to the radiation beam so that the tumor is at the center of rotation. This placement and rotation permit a maximum amount of radiation without unnecessary damage to nearby healthy tissue.

*Radioisotopes.* The advantage of radioisotopes is that they are picked up by the body through the digestive system, like many other chemicals. A physician may select the appropriate radioactive isotope on the basis of the area or organ he wishes to reach. Certain glands and organs tend to collect specific chemicals. As small, harmless doses of a radioisotope are introduced into the body, they accumulate at the area of the tumor. The thyroid gland, for instance, tends to collect and accumulate iodine. Consequently, in the treatment of cancer of the thyroid, a radioisotope of iodine ($I^{131}$) is introduced into the body and accumulated by the thyroid gland. Its destructive energy is thus concentrated in a strategic spot to attack the tumor.

*Laser radiation.* Laser radiation is a relatively new type of light energy that was first made available for biomedical research in the late 1950s and early 1960s. In cancer therapy beams of laser light are focused on a tumor. (They may be focused internally through special glass rods). This radiation has produced death in certain types of cancerous cells. After laser radiation the cells have also shown chromosomal changes. This indicates that the cellular changes induced by lasers may be more than just heat reactions.

effect on normal cells cause considerable damage to cancerous cells, and sometimes even destroy the cancer completely. Some types of cancer, however, are not affected by doses of radiation that are safe for normal tissue. Three sources of radiation are used in cancer treatment—high-voltage x-ray machines, radioisotopes (elements such as cobalt that release energy and nuclear particles as they change to other elements at a predictable rate), and laser radiation.

*X-rays.* X-rays are controlled beams of electrons at variable high-energy levels. X-rays of extremely high-energy levels readily penetrate tissues and can be used to arrest the growth of or kill cancerous cells in deep

Chemical compounds are now being used in conjunction with radiation. These drugs markedly increase the radiosensitivity of cancer cells. Under some conditions doses of radiation in combination with drugs are much smaller than those required when radiation is used alone.

*Chemotherapy.* Although surgery or radiation can often remove or arrest localized cancers, rarely can they cure cancers that have spread beyond their point of origin. They cannot be used to cure cancers of the blood or blood-forming tissues which are widespread from the beginning. For many years scientists felt that the only way to treat such cancers would be with drugs or chemicals that would destroy cancer cells and yet not harm normal tissues. Prior to the 1940s, however, there was no evidence that such drugs could be produced.

Today approximately twenty drugs are being used in the treatment of cancer. These drugs are of three main types—hormones, cell poisons (alkylic agents), and metabolic antagonists.

Hormones are chemicals that are produced and secreted by the endocrine glands of the body. They influence or control many of the body's activities such as growth and reproduction. Many cancers occur in hormone-controlled tissues such as the breasts, prostate gland, and uterus. Cancer tends to appear in these areas at a time of life when the body hormones are changing. These changes seem to produce an environment which the cancers depend on for growth.

Cell poisons, or alkylic agents, interfere with the division of cancer cells and stop their growth. But since they also damage normal cells in the same manner, they have had limited use.

Metabolic antagonists are drugs that are

The unsung hero of cancer research — the guinea pig. *Photo by Ewing Galloway.*

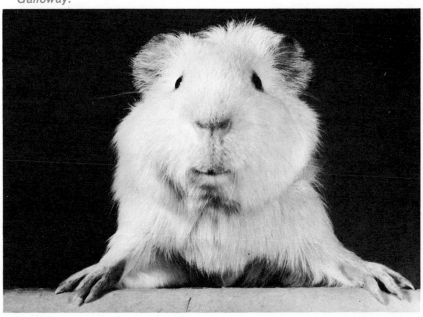

## MOST FREQUENT TYPES OF CANCER BY AGE GROUPS

| AGE | MOST FREQUENT TYPES OF CANCER[a] |
|---|---|
| 0–15 | Leukemia, cancer of brain, lymphosarcomas, cancer of bone, kidney |
| 15–34 | |
| male | Leukemia, Hodgkin's disease, cancer of brain, testis, lymphosarcomas |
| female | Cancer of breast, leukemia, uterus, Hodgkin's disease, cancer of brain |
| 35–54 | |
| male | Cancer of lung, colon and rectum, pancreas, brain, stomach |
| female | Cancer of breast, uterus, lung, colon and rectum, ovary |
| 55–74 | |
| male | Cancer of lung, colon and rectum, prostate, pancreas, stomach |
| female | Cancer of breast, colon and rectum, uterus, lung, ovary |
| 75 & over | |
| male | Cancer of prostate gland, lung, colon and rectum, stomach, pancreas |
| female | Cancer of colon and rectum, breast, stomach, uterus, pancreas |

[a]Cancer of the skin is omitted from this table since there is seldom adequate reason for failure to diagnose it correctly and early.

SOURCE: Adapted from *1973 Cancer Facts and Figures,* American Cancer Society, Inc., 1973.

very similar in their chemical structure to food materials (such as vitamins) needed by cancer cells. These drugs are taken into the cells but do not fulfill their needs, thus slowing or even stopping the growth of the cancer. The metabolic antagonists have been most effective in producing remissions (temporary improvements) in leukemia. These remissions may last for months or even years, but the symptoms of leukemia often return eventually, and the disease may become resistant to drugs that have worked previously. But in many cases, combinations of drugs have produced remissions that have lasted long enough to be classified as possible "cured" cases of leukemia.

### Survival Prospects for Cancer Patients

The survival of cancer patients depends on many factors. One of the most important is the location of the tumor. Other factors include the degree to which the tumor had spread when treatment was begun, the age and general health of the patient, and the method of treatment. (See figure on cancer survival rates and types of cancer by age groups.) Because of the larger number of men who have lung cancer, the survival of males in general is somewhat below the survival rate of females.

Chances for survival are also closely related to the size of the tumor and how much tissue is involved. Patients with strictly localized tumors generally have the best survival rates. The rates usually decrease in direct relation to the advancing tumor stage. Some people, however, with extremely small and localized cancers, die quickly despite apparently adequate treatment while a very few people with widespread metastasis live for many years with no treatment at all. This phenomenon, like many in cancer research, is unexplainable as yet.

## OTHER MAJOR NON-COMMUNICABLE DISEASES

### Arthritis

Arthritis is a general term for any inflammation of the joints. Many different types of arthritis are known to medical science today. But the causes of only a few of these types and the cure for even fewer are known.

This disease is the number one crippler in the United States today. It is estimated that more than thirteen million Americans suffer from some form of arthritis. For more than three million of these people, the symptoms are severe enough to limit their activity. The measurable cost of arthritis in this country, including treatment and loss of earning power, is well over a billion dollars per year.

Arthritis becomes more common and more severe as people grow older. Its symptoms commonly include a stiffness in the joints and mild to extreme pain. With certain types of arthritis, the joints become twisted and deformed.

The best available treatment methods for many types of arthritis do not actually cure the disease, although they may help to relieve pain and minimize the crippling effect. Heat treatments, physical therapy, and pain-relieving drugs are among the standard treatments. Simple aspirin is one of the most important arthritis remedies. For certain specific types of arthritis, physicians may prescribe other treatments.

Experts emphasize that although a definite cure for most forms of arthritis is not yet available, severe crippling often can be prevented if diagnosis is made early and proper medical care is begun promptly.

### Diabetes

Diabetes is a disturbance of the metabolism (body chemistry), resulting from a deficiency of the hormone insulin. Insulin is produced in the pancreas by special clusters of cells called the islets of Langerhans. Insulin has the important function of increasing the rate of movement of glucose (blood sugar) through the membranes of most of the cells of the body. In diabetes, the blood sugar is unable to enter the cells in adequate amounts.

Diabetes is a hereditary disease that is transmitted through recessive genes. Not everyone who inherits the genes for diabetes will actually develop the disease, however. Diabetes is most common among older people, especially among older people who are overweight. It less commonly becomes a problem during youth. Many persons who carry the hereditary makeup for diabetes can

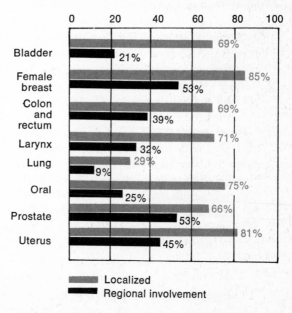

SOURCE: 1973 *Cancer Facts and Figures,* American Cancer Society, 1973, p. 6.

411

avoid the disease entirely by merely controlling their food consumption.

Between 1 and 2 percent of the population of the United States is definitely known to suffer from diabetes, but surveys in which large numbers of persons have been tested for diabetes have shown that its true incidence may be closer to 4 percent of the population. This indicates that many people have this dangerous disease without even knowing it. Periodic testing for diabetes is important for everyone, especially for relatives of known diabetics.

There may or may not be noticeable symptoms of diabetes. The most common symptoms that do appear include frequent urination, excessive thirst, craving for sweets and starches, and weakness. The most common medical test for diabetes is analysis of the urine for the presence of sugar. If sugar is present, a test is made for the level of sugar in the blood. The blood-sugar level is abnormally high in diabetics.

Some cases of diabetes can be controlled with modification of the diet or increased exercise. The diet should be lower than average in carbohydrates (sugars and starches). Exercise increases the movement of blood sugar into muscle cells, thus helping to control the disease.

Many cases of diabetes, however, require treatment with insulin or other drugs. For many years insulin was the only effective drug for the treatment of this disease. If the dosage of insulin is properly balanced with the intake of carbohydrates, most of the consequences of diabetes can be prevented. This is not a cure for the disease, merely a control. The drug must be taken indefinitely.

Until recently, insulin in oral doses could not be used because, being a protein, it was digested. Several other drugs are available which can be taken by mouth. These drugs stimulate the cells of the pancreas to produce insulin. Such drugs are effective only in diabetics whose cells have retained some ability to produce insulin. If this ability has been totally lost, as in many severe cases, insulin dosage by injection is still the only effective treatment.

If diabetes is not adequately controlled, severe dehydration and acidity of the body fluids may occur. The result may be diabetic coma (unconsciousness), which is almost always fatal unless the patient receives immediate medical treatment. The breath smells of acetone and breathing is rapid. Another situation that requires immediate medical treatment is insulin shock, the result of an overdose of insulin. In insulin shock, the blood-sugar level is too low for proper functioning of the central nervous system. As the blood-sugar level drops progressively lower, the person first trembles and seems nervous, then goes into convulsions, and finally drops into a state of coma. This coma can be distinguished from the diabetic coma by the absence of acetone breath and rapid breathing. If an overdose of insulin has been administered to a diabetic and he is still conscious, sugar or some product containing sugar, such as candy or orange juice, should be given to him. If he is already unconscious, he should receive immediate medical attention.

In addition to diabetic coma, untreated diabetes may lead to early death from heart disease or infection; or to blindness, kidney disease, stillbirth, or infant death of babies born to diabetic women.

The key steps in preventing such damaging results of diabetes are, in summary:

1. Avoid becoming overweight. This alone will prevent many potential cases of diabetes from ever developing.
2. Have periodic medical examinations that include tests for diabetes.
3. Seek medically supervised treatment of a diagnosed case, including proper diet, exercise, and drugs.

### Asthma

Asthma is a disease in which there are periodic attacks of difficulty in breathing. During an attack, wheezing and shortness of breath may be mild or so severe as to require medical treatment in order to prevent death.

The choked breathing that accompanies an asthma attack is caused by a narrowing of the bronchioles, small tubes inside the lungs. This narrowing can be the result of a swelling of the membrane that lines the bronchioles, a spasm (constriction) of the tubes, or a mucus blockage of the tubes.

There are many causes of asthma, among which allergic reactions are prominent. About 75 percent of the people who have asthma are allergic to one or more substances. Many cases of asthma are associated with bacterial infections of the sinuses, throat, and nose. Most of these cases improve if the infection clears up. In some asthmatic patients, attacks are brought on or made worse by emotional stress that may lead to constriction of the bronchioles.

It is important that asthma sufferers receive the best available medical treatment, since prolonged or repeated attacks can cause permanent damage to the lungs and heart. Forced breathing can stretch the lung tissue and lead to the very serious condition known as emphysema. In emphysema, it is impossible to exhale completely, so shortness of breath follows even slight exertion. An extra load is also placed on the heart which must work harder to force blood through the damaged lungs. With proper treatment, such serious effects can be greatly reduced or eliminated entirely in many cases.

The treatment of asthma must be under the supervision of a physician. No one should try to diagnose or treat himself. The exact cause of the attacks must be determined in order to decide the proper type of treatment. If an allergy is involved, the substance causing the allergy can sometimes be avoided or,

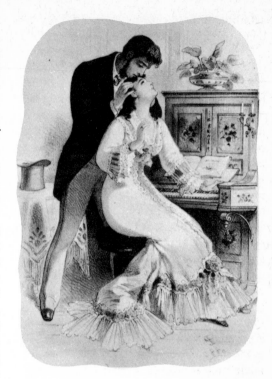

Modern drugs and the general improvement of living conditions have almost eliminated tuberculosis from the current scene, but it was once a leading cause of death. The famous tragedy of Marguerite *(La Dame aux Camélias* by Alexandre Dumas) centered on her early death from tuberculosis. *Photo courtesy of Archivo Fotográfica Internacional.*

in some cases, the patient can be desensitized by a series of injections. If an infection is involved, it should be promptly treated. Ways may have to be found to reduce emotional stress, if this is the cause of the attacks. A change of climate may or may not be useful. The decision to move to another area should be made only after consultation with a physician. Various drugs are prescribed to provide relief from asthma attacks.

### Chronic Bronchitis

The inside of the bronchioles is lined with a highly specialized membrane. This mem-

413

brane secretes a layer of mucus to trap the foreign matter that enters the lungs. Millions of hairlike cilia constantly sweep the layer of mucus with its trapped foreign particles upward to the throat where it is swallowed.

Repeated irritation of this ciliated mucous membrane can paralyze the action of the cilia, eventually destroy them, and stimulate an excessive production of mucus. This is the condition known as chronic bronchitis. Since the cilia can no longer clear the lungs of mucus, it accumulates until the flow of air through the bronchioles is obstructed. This obstruction then triggers a spell of coughing that helps clear the lungs. Frequent coughing is the most important, prominent symptom of chronic bronchitis. Other symptoms may include shortness of breath and wheezing.

The main treatment of chronic bronchitis consists of eliminating the irritation that causes it. The source of irritation is often smoking tobacco. The so-called "smoker's cough" is in reality a symptom of chronic bronchitis. The first step in treating any lung disorder is to stop smoking. If the source of irritation is an infection, this should receive prompt treatment. Coughing itself can contribute to the irritation of the bronchioles, thus creating a self-perpetuating condition. Coughing should be avoided unless absolutely necessary, and then it should be as gentle as possible. Above all, chronic bronchitis should receive the treatment of a physician.

### Emphysema

Emphysema is a deterioration of the lungs that develops gradually over a period of years. It is therefore more common among older persons, although it may begin to develop during youth. In emphysema, the thin walls of the tiny air sacs lose their elasticity and tear. This reduces the ability of the lungs to exhale.

The lungs swell up permanently, creating a "barrel chest" appearance in the victim. Exhaling becomes extremely slow and difficult. The blood circulates with difficulty through the damaged lung tissue, creating a great burden on the heart, which must pump blood through the lungs before it can circulate to the body. Emphysema is an extremely disabling disease and often leads to fatal heart failure.

The development of emphysema often can be traced to prolonged asthma or chronic bronchitis. The most common link between emphysema victims is a history of heavy smoking. The disease is far more common among smokers than among nonsmokers.

There is no real cure for emphysema. A physician may prescribe certain measures, such as mild exercise, drugs, and special breathing techniques, but these mainly help the patient live with his condition; they do not cure it.

## HEART AND ARTERY DISEASES

Heart and artery diseases are presently the number one health problem in the United States. Almost 25 percent of the adult population of this country has definite or suspected heart diseases. Cardiovascular ailments are by far the chief causes of illness, disability, and death among both middle-aged and elderly people in this country. Among these, coronary heart disease, illness of the blood vessels supplying the heart, is responsible for the greatest number of deaths (over 50 percent of all cardiovascular diseases). Causes of other cardiovascular disease deaths, in order of decreasing importance, are stroke and hypertension. These three diseases are responsible for more than 80 percent of all cardiovascular disease deaths.

Like cancer and emphysema, heart diseases appear to be related to the extension of the average life span, which permits degenerative diseases the decades they may require to develop. However, certain other factors are definitely involved in the high incidence of heart disease—the stresses of personal accomplishment, diets high in saturated fats, the tendency toward obesity with age, lack of sufficient physical exercise, and the incidence of smoking. These factors appear to relate to a higher incidence of heart disease in this country than in societies lacking these characteristics.

The severity and danger of heart and artery diseases cannot be minimized; a disease in an arm or leg may cripple a person, but a disease of the heart may lead to his death.

### Congenital Diseases

Abnormalities in the development of the heart often occur during the first three months of fetal life. Although the specific causes of many congenital malformations of the heart are unknown, some of the causes are known to include certain maternal illnesses or bodily upsets during the first three months of pregnancy. These include German measles, mumps, or influenza. Ionizing radiation, such as x-rays, and certain drugs, such as thalidomide, have many similar effects.

Some congenital heart defects result from the failure of the infant's heart to properly make the shift from fetal circulation to infant circulation. Before birth, the fetal circulatory system simply pumps the blood supplied by the mother's heart and lungs. It does not oxygenate blood itself and the fetus' lungs are inoperative. Two openings in the fetal heart provide for a natural "short circuit": the foramen ovale is an opening in the septum (major dividing panel) of the heart; the ductus arteriosus is a connection between the pulmonary artery and the aorta (see figure on fetal circulation). At birth the child's lungs become functional and the placental circula-tion is broken. Normally, during the first year a septum closes over the foramen ovale. This closure is incomplete in about 20 percent of all individuals. The ductus arteriosus normally closes during the first month of life.

Many congenital heart ailments can be treated surgically. The development of artificial valves has greatly contributed to the success of surgical treatment.

### Degenerative Disorders

Although the heart is very resistant to many disorders, certain conditions can seriously reduce its efficiency. The total effects are cumulative, becoming more and more serious as they go without correction or treatment. Heart disease may be the result of infections, toxins (poisons), injuries, poor nutrition, inactivity, emotional problems, or other disturbances which weaken the heart.

*Rheumatic Heart Disease.* Much heart disease in childhood is the result of rheumatic fever, which usually first attacks the individual when he is between the ages of five and fifteen.

A small percentage of persons suffering from certain streptococcal infections develop the symptoms of rheumatic fever (a swelling and pain in the joints, accompanied by fever). The original infection may be in any part of the body, but it will likely be strep throat, scarlet fever, or middle-ear infection. Rheumatic fever is actually an allergic response to a streptococcal infection. In about 60 percent of the cases the heart is inflamed, and in about 25 percent of the cases it may be permanently damaged.

Although other layers of the heart may be infected, the most common damage is done to the endocardium (the inner lining of the heart). Inflammation of this lining causes the heart valves to become scarred. Blood deposits on such scarred valves; they thicken and either lose their flexibility or stick together.

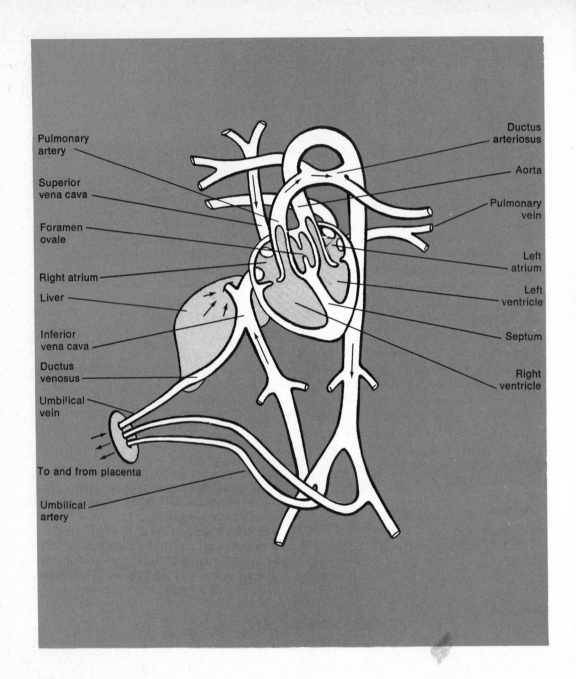

Pulmonary
artery

Superior
vena cava

Foramen
ovale

Right atrium

Liver

Inferior
vena cava

Ductus
venosus

Umbilical
vein

To and from placenta

Umbilical
artery

Ductus
arteriosus

Aorta

Pulmonary
vein

Left
atrium

Left
ventricle

Septum

Right
ventricle

Fetal circulation.

Open-heart surgery has been increasingly effective in relieving such damage. Antibiotics have lowered the incidence of rheumatic fever and reduced the death rate. As a preventive measure, all streptococcal infections should be promptly brought to the attention of a physician. A person with a history of rheumatic fever must be particularly prompt in seeking treatment for infections, as one attack leaves him highly susceptible to repeated attacks.

*Heart Murmurs.* Heart murmurs are abnormal sounds produced by vibrations that result from improperly working heart valves. They may be due to the endocarditis of rheumatic fever. The "murmur" sound heard through a physician's stethoscope results from an incompletely closing valve; blood flows back across a valve into a heart chamber as it relaxes, producing the characteristic sound.

Murmurs are occasionally heard in hearts that are actually normal. A young person may engage in such strenuous exercise that the flow of blood through the valves creates a temporary turbulence, or murmur.

*Atherosclerosis.* Atherosclerosis is an artery disease. The walls of the arteries become thickened and hardened. A mixture of cholesterol and other fatlike materials is deposited along the arterial walls. This deposit is called *plaque*. The arteries gradually become hardened with deposits of calcium and other minerals. The end result of atherosclerosis is that the inside diameter of the artery is reduced and the inner lining of the artery is rough and irregular.

One of the major dangers of atherosclerosis is that of blood clotting. The roughness of the inner surface of the artery may cause a clot (thrombus) to develop. Such a thrombus may cause the partial or complete obstruction (occlusion) of the blood vessel at this particular spot and shut off the blood flow. On occasion such blood clots may break loose in the bloodstream, and be carried to another point in the circulatory system.

Although such damage may occur in any blood vessel, it is more serious in certain places than in others. If it blocks an artery in the heart, the individual will have a heart attack; if it is in the brain, a stroke; if in the foot, gangrene; if in the kidney, high blood pressure; if in the eye, blindness.

The consequences of hardening of the arteries usually appear during old age, but there is growing evidence of it in young adults. The full-blown disease in older people is probably the result of a lifetime of fat deposition within the arteries.

Cholesterol, a major component of animal fats, appears to be one factor causing this condition. A certain amount of cholesterol is necessary for certain body functions, but an excess is usually deposited in the walls of arteries, resulting in a hardened condition.

Some authorities now suspect that large quantities of table sugar (sucrose) in the diet may be a factor in the development of atherosclerosis, perhaps even more important than animal-fat intake.

*Hypertension.* Hypertension simply means high blood pressure. As a normal heart pumps blood through the body, a certain degree of pressure is exerted against the blood vessels. With each beat of the left ventricle, a wave of pressure starts at the heart and travels along the arteries. This wave is called the pulse. The pulse can be felt on any arteries that are close to the surface of the body, such as on the wrist, the sides of the throat and the temple. The pulse results from the blood pressure. The blood pressure at the moment of contraction is the systolic pressure; it should normally be sufficient to displace about 120 mm of mercury in a glass tube. The blood pressure at the moment of relaxation of the heart is the diastolic pressure; it normally displaces about 80 mm of mercury. Blood pressure readings, frequently taken during a general physical examination, are presented as a ratio of the first figure over the second.

Most physiologists consider a blood pressure reading of 150/90 as excessive. This can be considered a useful definition of high blood pressure.

Hypertension is very common. It is believed that about one out of every five Americans suffers from it at some time in his life, and that about 13 percent of all deaths are a direct result of it. Hypertension becomes more common with increasing age and affects men about twice as often as women.

In about 90 percent of the known cases, it is described as essential hypertension, a hereditary condition. In other cases it may be due to the removal of a kidney, kidney disease, excessive narrowing of the arteries, hormone imbalance, or excessive salt in the diet.

Hypertension is damaging for two reasons: (1) it puts an excess work load on the heart and the left ventricle in particular; (2) the arteries may be damaged by excessive pressure. A hypertensive patient tends to develop cardiovascular ailments much sooner than a person not suffering from hypertension. This high blood pressure in the arteries causes a hardening (sclerosis) of blood vessels all over the body. The vessels become weakened; clots tend to form in them much more easily; some vessels rupture and hemorrhage. Hemorrhages in the vessels of the brain (cerebral hemorrhages) and vessels of the kidneys are particularly destructive.

*Cerebrovascular Accidents (Strokes).* The brain receives over one-fifth of all the blood pumped by the heart. As with the heart, any interruption in the normal flow of blood to the brain can have serious consequences. Such interruptions, commonly called strokes, may come about in several ways (see table for ways strokes occur). Three-fourths of these accidents result from arterial hemorrhage and one-fourth from clots forming in the cerebral arteries. Depending on which part of the brain is destroyed, either of these kinds of accidents may cause speech impediments, loss of memory or mental confusion, some degree of paralysis, blindness, or even death.

Considerable progress has been made both in the treatment and rehabilitation of stroke patients. While some individuals lead a restricted life because of the permanent loss of some essential brain function, others recover quickly, depending on the site and extent of the brain damage.

*Varicose Veins.* In the previous discussion of veins, it was mentioned that some of the veins of the body, such as those in the limbs, are provided with valves to prevent the backflow of blood as it is raised to the heart. These valves may be destroyed when veins are overstretched by an excess amount of blood for a prolonged period of time. This sometimes occurs in pregnancy or when a person stands on his feet much of the time. Stretched veins become larger in cross section, but the valves do not stretch accordingly. Such valves fail to prevent the backflow of blood. The result is increased blood pressure in these veins. Circulation in surrounding muscles is inadequate, and nutrients fail to diffuse into such tissues properly. Muscles often become painful and weak, and the skin may become ulcerated.

Therapy for varicose veins includes elevating the legs to heart level, or binding them tightly. The legs may also be injected with certain agents that harden and plug the most protruding veins. The weakened sections of veins may be removed surgically. The blood then will be carried by other veins.

### Coronary Heart Disease

The coronary blood vessels surrounding the heart derive their name from the fact that

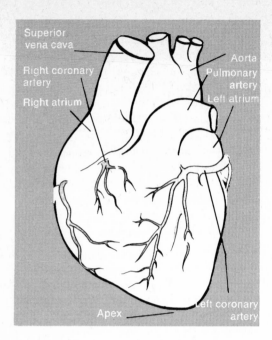

The heart, showing the coronary arteries.

they encircle the heart like a crown, or corona (see figure showing coronary vessels). These vessels transport almost a half pint of blood every minute over the surface of the heart. Any sudden blockage of one of the coronary arteries deprives that section of the heart of its blood supply; cardiac cells die, heart contractions may cease, and circulation may come to a standstill. If a coronary artery is completely plugged, the condition is called a coronary occlusion or heart attack. If the obstruction is only partial or is in one of the smaller coronary tributaries, prompt treatment often leads to the individual's recovery. An occlusion in a main coronary artery is very serious and may cause sudden death. Other causes of the coronary diseases include heavy physical exercise, aging, dietetic habits, obesity, smoking, or hypertension.

Pain from the heart may be due to a blood-flow deficiency in the coronary vessels. This is referred to (actually felt in) the left arm and shoulder. Such pain from the heart is called angina pectoris. Angina pectoris may not actually be noticed until the work load is too great in relation to the blood flow in the coronary vessels. People who experience it repeatedly often do not feel pain unless they exercise or experience strong emotion; others experience it much of the time.

Fortunately, the great majority of coronary disease patients recover and are able to lead active, useful lives, providing they receive proper treatment under good medical supervision. Approximately one-fourth of all deaths in the United States, however, still result from coronary artery diseases. Also, it is estimated that more than one out of every ten Americans suffers some degree of insufficiency of blood supply to the heart.

### Factors Relating to Heart Disease

Increased understanding of American lifestyles and their influence on heart disease has contributed to some reduction in the death rate from these illnesses. (See table on factors relating to heart disease.)

### Symptoms of Heart Disease

Symptoms vary according to the exact illness. Even though they may be absent, heart disease itself can be present. When symptoms are present, they can sometimes be mistaken for those of other body disorders. For example, dizziness and indigestion are common to many conditions. Legitimate symptoms of coronary heart disease are often overlooked. Breathlessness, for example, may be mistakenly attributed to bronchitis, or coughing to smoking. Generally, however, there are certain important symptoms that should be looked for and referred to a physician. (See table on symptoms of heart disease.)

### Treatment of Heart Disease

The treatment selected for a heart patient will depend on the nature of his disease and

## WAYS IN WHICH STROKES OCCUR

| CAUSE | EXPLANATION |
|---|---|
| Hemorrhage (bleeding) | The wall of an artery of the brain may break, permitting blood to escape and thus damage surrounding brain tissue; such escape reduces the flow of blood to other brain parts. |
| Thrombosis (clot formation) | A clot of blood may form in an artery of the brain and may stop the flow of blood to the part of the brain supplied by the clot-plugged artery. |
| Embolism (blocking of a vessel by a clot floating in the bloodstream) | A clot from a diseased blood vessel may be pumped to the brain and stop up one of the brain's arteries. |
| Compression (pressure) | A tumor, swollen brain tissue, or a large clot from another vessel may press upon a vessel of the brain and stop its flow of blood. |
| Spasm (tightening and closing down of the walls of an artery) | An artery of the brain may constrict and thus reduce the flow of blood to an area of the brain. If the spasm is of short duration permanent damage may not occur. |

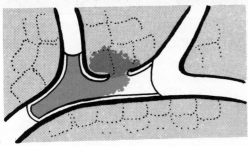

HEMORRHAGE (Bleeding)

The wall of an artery of the brain may break, permitting blood to escape and thus damage surrounding brain tissue; such escape reduces the flow of blood to other brain parts

THROMBOSIS (Clot formation)

A clot of blood may form in an artery of the brain and may stop the flow of blood to the part of the brain supplied by the clot-plugged artery

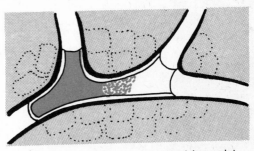

EMBOLISM (Blocking of a vessel by a clot floating in the bloodstream)

A clot from a diseased blood vessel may be pumped to the brain and stop up one of the brain's arteries

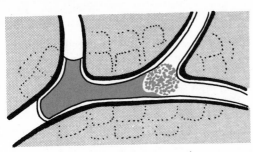

COMPRESSION (Pressure)

A tumor, swollen brain tissue, or a large clot from another vessel may press upon a vessel of the brain and stop its flow of blood

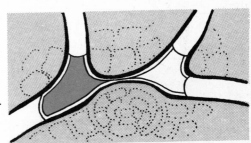

SPASM (Tightening and closing down of the walls of an artery)

An artery of the brain may constrict and thus reduce the flow of blood to an area of the brain. If the spasm is of short duration permanent damage may not occur

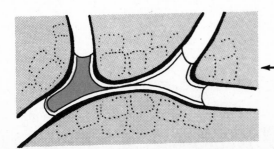

## FACTORS RELATING TO HEART DISEASE[a]

| FACTOR | EXPLANATION | RISK INVOLVED |
|---|---|---|
| Serum cholesterol | Refers to cholesterol carried in liquid portion of blood. The amount of cholesterol in the blood is believed to relate to diet and heredity | A person with serum cholesterol over 240 mg. % has more than three times the risk of a person with less than 200 mg. % |
| Age | | A man in his 50s has four times the risk of attack as a man in his 30s |
| Blood pressure | Refers to elevated levels of blood pressure, or hypertension | A person with systolic blood pressure greater than 160 has four times the risk of an individual with SBP of less than 120 |
| Cigarette smoking | Although referring to any cigarette smoker, the greater the amount and the longer the smoking history the greater the risk. Pipe and cigar smoking do not appear related | A cigarette smoker has nearly twice the risk of the nonsmoker |
| Vital capacity | Refers to amount of air a person can forcefully inhale and exhale | An individual with low vital capacity has about twice the risk of an individual with high vital capacity |
| ECG abnormalities | Refers to recording of electrical activity related to the contraction of cardiac muscle | An individual with an ECG abnormality has two and a half times the risk of an individual with normal ECG |

[a]Miscellaneous suspected factors include gross obesity, insufficient physical activity, and inheritance.

## POSSIBLE SYMPTOMS OF HEART DISEASE

| SYMPTOM | EXPLANATION |
|---|---|
| Breathlessness | Unusual shortness of breath associated with moderate exertion might be an early symptom of a weakened heart muscle. It signals a marked oxygen shortage somewhere in the body. If, for instance, a person is out of breath after climbing one flight of stairs, he should see his physician |
| Chest pains | Pain or a tight feeling in the chest during or after exertion or excitement may be due to oxygen deficiency. Cardiac pain is often in the center of the chest, very pressing, and may move to the shoulders and arms. Chest pains may also result from other causes, but it is best to be safe and consult a physician when such pains occur |
| Swelling of feet and ankles | If the heart fails to pump with usual vigor, the blood flow slows down and fluid may gather in the tissues (edema). This may be noticed first in the feet and ankles. It also may occur from other causes |
| Persistent fatigue | Frequent tiredness without apparent reason may be a sign of heart difficulty or hypertension. Other possible symptoms of heart disease may include a heavy feeling in the limbs, a weakness, and a lack of vigor during or following exertion |
| Miscellaneous symptoms | Other symptoms that may occur in some cardiac patients include cyanosis (blueness of skin due to insufficient oxygen in blood), loss of consciousness, recurrent bronchitis, and heart palpitations |

how critical his case is. A chronic illness (one slowly affecting the individual) usually permits time for a more deliberate diagnosis and treatment. Surgery for the repair of congenital conditions, for example, may be planned some time in advance. In a critical, sudden heart attack case, however, prompt diagnosis and treatment are needed.

*Emergency Care.* The person who has just had a heart attack is in need of immediate emergency care. He should be taken to a hospital at once. His first medical treatment is usually to provide the oxygen that the weakened heart is unable to supply. This may involve the use of oxygen, drugs (such as nitroglycerin) to dilate the obstructed blood vessels, or electric or drug stimulators to revive his faltering heart. Next, measurements are needed for pulse and blood pressure, electrocardiograms to record the electric impulses of his heart, or x-ray and fluoroscopic examinations to measure the size and outline of the heart. All efforts must be made as soon as possible to reduce the blood-pumping load placed on the heart by reducing the patient's physical exertion and emotional excitement.

The first week (and especially the first 48 hours) after a heart attack is the most critical period. The largest number of deaths from heart attacks occur during this time. The danger of death is reduced as time goes on. With coronary patients, new blood vessels gradually form around the obstructed vessels, setting up new circulation, and an adequate oxygen-food supply is slowly restored to the deprived cells. Scar tissue forms over the affected area, and slowly, as the heart returns to normal, the patient can resume many normal activities.

*Long-term Care.* The cardinal rule of all treatment for heart patients is to prevent anginal discomfort. Absence of such pain is a good indication that the heart muscle is receiving adequate circulation. To help circulation, drugs are often used: digitalis for a fuller heartbeat; nitrates, such as nitroglycerin, to dilate coronary blood vessels and reduce pressure; anticoagulants to reduce the possibility of clotting; sedative drugs to quiet the body; and other drugs to cause certain actions to take place in the kidneys to help relieve pressure on the heart. A diet is planned which includes all essential foods in adequate amounts. The person must learn to rest and limit his activity, if necessary. Schedules of moderate exercises must be established. Physicians usually insist that their patients lose any excess weight and stop smoking.

Through careful treatment by a physician, a patient is often able to resume much or all of his previous routine and may expect to live a nearly normal life. His longevity will depend, however, upon his properly understanding his condition, faithfully using all medicines prescribed, and preventing situations that might cause another attack.

### Prevention of Cardiovascular Diseases

Whether or not cardiovascular disorders are preventable largely depends upon their causes. Diseases due to infection or malnutrition are often preventable. Heart damage caused by rheumatic fever can be prevented by reducing the incidence and severity of rheumatic fever with proper and prompt use of antibiotics in treating streptococcal infections. On the other hand, we are unable to predict or prevent many of the congenital malformations of the heart and blood vessels.

Circulatory problems can be greatly reduced by a reduction in cigarette smoking. The prevention of atherosclerosis appears to depend upon a reduction of cholesterol in the blood. Excessive blood pressure, underlying many cardiovascular problems, can often be reduced by regular physical exercise.

### Smoking and Cardiovascular Diseases

It has been suggested for years that smoking has adverse effects on the cardiovascular system. Studies of large groups of people reinforce this suggestion by showing that cigarette smokers, in particular, are prone to die earlier (in middle age rather than old age) of certain cardiovascular disorders than are nonsmokers. Chief among these disorders is coronary artery disease.

The cardiovascular effects of smoking are caused by nicotine alone. Low concentrations of nicotine, as obtained from the smoking of one or two cigarettes, cause in most persons an increase in the resting heart rate of 15 to 25 beats per minute (30,000 extra beats per day), a rise in blood pressure, and an increase in the heart output. As the number of cigarettes smoked increases, there is also a dangerous decrease in blood flow to both the coronary arteries and the arteries of the rest of the body. Such a decrease is easily noted in the fingers after smoking (temperature drops because of a lack of blood). Such decreased blood flow accounts for the association of cigarette smoking and the increased incidence of coronary disease.

If as few as eight cigarettes are smoked within a period of one day, there may be an impairment of the oxygen-carrying mechanism of the blood. Such oxygen reduction in the body reduces the body's ability to produce adequate energy. This affects the total performance of the individual.

### Physical Exercise

Endurance fitness is a term used to describe the ability of the body to engage in prolonged physical activity without undue fatigue or overexertion. Such fitness is some indication of the overall health of the heart and the lungs (in fact, of the entire cardiovascular-respiratory system)—not simply an indicator of the person's muscular strength or agility.

It takes two things to create energy for physical activity—food and oxygen. The body stores nutrients, but it cannot store oxygen. During physical activity much of the oxygen of the blood is used up by the contracting muscles. This increases the amount of carbon dioxide ($CO_2$) in the blood and decreases the available oxygen ($O_2$). The result of such activity is increased respiration in the lungs, an increased heart rate, and an increased flow of blood throughout the body. During severe strenuous exercise, however, the $CO_2$ concentration accumulates quickly and the body's supply of $O_2$ dwindles rapidly. After such exertion has stopped, it takes the body some time to get rid of the $CO_2$ and restore its $O_2$ supply.

Consequently, a person's fitness may be judged by the efficiency of this oxygen-delivery system. The factors in the blood which affect oxygen-carrying capacity include the number of red blood cells (normally about 4.5 to 5.5 million per cubic millimeter of blood) and the amount of hemoglobin in these cells. Even if the lungs can process large amounts of oxygen, the body tissues can receive only limited amounts if the red cells or hemoglobin which deliver the oxygen are in short supply. A totally fit individual has more blood than one who is not fit. Because he has more hemoglobin and more blood plasma (the fluid portion of the blood), which contain the red blood cells, his total volume of blood is greater. Tests show that men in good physical condition invariably have a larger blood supply than average men of comparable size.

The heart takes the oxygen-filled blood from the lungs and pumps it throughout the body. It also takes carbon dioxide-filled blood from the body and pumps it into the lungs. The heart works harder, faster, and less efficiently in a nonexerciser than in a totally fit individual. Someone who is in condition and is active on a regular basis may have a resting heart rate of between 55 and 60 beats per minute. An inactive nonexerciser may have a resting heart rate of 70 or more. If the heart rate of a fit individual is 60 beats per minute, his heart beats 3,600 beats per hour, or 86,400 beats per 24 hours. If the heart rate of a nonexerciser is 80 beats per minute, his heart rate is 4,800 beats per hour, or 115,200 beats per day. The nonexerciser, then, forces his heart to beat nearly 30,000 more times each day.

The heart of a totally fit person can beat less because the decreased heart rate is more than compensated for by increased blood volume. In other words, each pump of the heart moves a greater volume of blood. Also, as the volume of blood increases, the body builds more blood vessels, especially in the muscles. Called *increased tissue vasculariza-*

*tion*, this is a remarkable phenomenon which delays aging by keeping tissues alive and healthy.

In the totally fit individual, blood pressure is usually lower than in the nonexerciser, because blood vessels are more pliable and have less resistance to blood flow. Exercise improves existing blood vessels and, thus, reduces blood pressure. However, a person retains reduced blood pressure only as long as he remains in condition. Reduced heart rate, vascularization, and reduced blood pressure are essential to building endurance and in combating fatigue. They contribute to an increased blood supply which saturates tissues, such as cardiac muscles, with oxygen and carries away more wastes. Oxygen saturation is extremely vital to the health of the heart, the most important muscle in the body.

Regular exercise can help prevent heart disease. It is uncommon for an athlete who has maintained a vigorous exercise program throughout life to develop coronary heart disease. Furthermore, studies of former athletes who have had coronary heart disease (any destructive process involving blood vessels conducting blood to the heart muscle) show that these athletes engaged in less vigorous exercise than did other athletes. If a person does have a heart attack, his chances of survival are greatly increased if his blood vessels are healthy enough to supply the heart tissue with large amounts of energy-producing oxygen.

The National Heart Institute and the American Heart Association agree that one of the major causes of *atherosclerosis,* a major cardiovascular disease, is lack of exercise. Many studies indicate that the chemical cholesterol is greatly responsible for atherosclerosis. Exercise helps the body to maintain normal levels of cholesterol despite relatively high intakes of fat. Vigorous physical activity three days per week for five weeks produces significant decreases in plasma cholesterol. Such decreases are linked to the reduced blood pressure attained through exercise. High blood pressure stimulates the production of cholesterol in the liver. This, in turn, increases cholesterol levels in the blood which accelerate the formation of cholesterol plaques and lead to atherosclerosis.

There are many factors (diet, heredity, smoking, obesity, lack of physical activity) linked to the enormously widespread incidence of degenerative cardiovascular conditions. It is difficult to single out any one factor and say that it is the major cause of such conditions. However, the individual who seems to have a good chance of suffering a heart attack is one who eats too much, smokes too much, worries too much, and gets insufficient exercise. Such a person, especially if he comes from a family with a history of heart conditions, is "a heart attack waiting for a place to happen."

Physicians, physiologists, and, recently, the general public have begun to accept the idea that lifetime muscular activity will lead to a decrease in the incidence of degenerative cardiovascular conditions. Dr. Paul Dudley White, the well-known cardiologist who has long been an advocate of exercise, said, "I believe that the physiological effect of regular exercise throughout one's life will probably, in time, be proved one of the best antidotes against the alarming development of the epidemic of coronary thrombosis and high blood pressure in this country." He added, "One of the faults of our current civilization is that our young adults at about the age of twenty-five become 'too busy' to exercise. Yet, for the next two decades of their lives, they probably need it even more than when they were children."

Exercise that makes a person breathe quickly and deeply develops his oxygen-delivery system. By the time he begins to puff, he has reached his maximum rate of oxygen delivery. Regular exercise routines enable us to lengthen the period of time we can exercise before we begin to puff. Jogging, swimming, cycling, walking, stationary running, and handball are particularly useful.

As a person ages, his oxygen delivery becomes less effective and his blood pressure rises. Eventually the weakened circulatory system cannot match the work load and the cardiovascular system breaks down. Then a person is more likely to have a heart attack or stroke and is increasingly vulnerable to many other illnesses.

### Other Ways of Preventing Cardiovascular Illnesses

The incidence of cardiovascular disease could be substantially reduced if more people followed these simple guidelines:

1. Eat the proper foods in reasonable amounts.
2. Avoid infections or secure adequate treatment of infections.
3. Avoid excessive emotional stress and upsets.
4. Get adequate and regular rest.
5. Exercise regularly and in keeping with your general level of fitness.
6. Have regular physical examinations.
7. Do not smoke, or at least cut down your daily use of tobacco.

## FOR FURTHER READING

Benenson, Abram S. (ed.), *Control of Communicable Diseases in Man* (11th ed.). New York: The American Public Health Association, 1970. *Comprehensive reference on infectious diseases in compact paperback form.*

*Cancer Facts and Figures.* New York: American Cancer Society. *An annual publication of the ACS containing the most pertinent cancer statistics from the previous year; available from the ACS local offices.*

Jones, Kenneth L., Louis W. Shainberg, and Curtis O. Byer, *Total Fitness.* San Francisco, Canfield Press, 1972. *Gives thorough background on fitness and specific activity programs.*

Jones, Kenneth L., Louis W. Shainberg, and Curtis O. Byer, *VD.* New York, Harper & Row, Publishers, 1973. *Includes other common genital infections as well as the venereal diseases.*

Morton, R.S., *Venereal Diseases.* Baltimore: Penguin Books, 1969. *A very good reference explaining the venereal diseases and their signs, symptoms, and implications.*

Podair, S., *Venereal Disease: Man Against a Plague.* Palo Alto, California: Fearon Press, 1969. *Selected information concerning venereal diseases and their impact on society.*

Shimkin, Michael, *Science and Cancer.* Washington, D.C.: Department of Health, Education, and Welfare, 1969. *An excellent layman's explanation of the nature of cancer and the efforts being made to understand and control it.*

Vermes, Jean C., *Pot is Rot: & Other Horrible Facts About Bad Things.* New York: Association Press, 1969. *Goes into many of the problems of modern society and youth; the best section is the one on venereal disease.*

Wood, Paul, *Diseases of the Heart and Circulation.* Philadelphia: Lippincott, 1968. *An authoritative medical text on the ailments common to the circulatory system and its organs.*

# Glossary Index

Antagonist drugs, **134**
Antibiotics, **380**–381; use of with colds, 256, 381
Antibodies, **379**
Antidepressants, **96**
Antigen, **379**
Antihistamines, **256,** 258
Antioxidants, **186**–187; hazards of, 187
Antipsychotic drugs, **96**
Anxiety, **83**
Appendicitis, **197**–198
Appestat, **200**–201
Arteriosclerosis, 86–87, 213, **417**
Arthritis, **261**
Artificial insemination, **351**
Artificial sweeteners, **187**
Asexual reproduction, **286**–287
Aspirin, **254**–255
Asthma, **413**
Atherosclerosis, fats and, **182,** 206, 426
Attrition, **5**
Ausubel, D. P., 140
Aversion therapy, **95;** for alcoholism, 156–157
Avoidance, **73**

Bacteria, as pathogens, 374
"Bad trips," **125**
Bannister, Roger, 209
Barbiturates, **118**–120; action of, with other drugs, 109, 111, 119; effects of, 119; medical uses of, 118; symptoms of use of, 119; withdrawal from, 119–120
Basal body temperature, **341**
Basal metabolic rates, **180**
Beauty, appreciation of, 65
Behavior therapy, **94**–96
Beriberi, **190,** 192
Berne, Eric, 94
Bestiality, **286**
"Binge" pattern, **154**
Biological age, **212**
Biological oxygen demand (BOD), **11**
Biopsy, **402**
Birth control (*See* Contraception; Fertility control)
Birth rate: in developing nations, 34–35; fluctuation of, 32–33; role of women in society and, 50–51; in United States, 36–39; by race, 36, by income, 37, by education, 37–38
"Blackout," **154**
Blastocyst, **354**
Blood sugar, **181;** level of and: appetite, 200, insulin shock, 412
"Blue baby," **337**

Blue Cross, 239
Blue Shield, 239
Boom babies, 39
Breast feeding, 365
Bronchial tubes: effect of smoking on, 164–165
Bronchitis, chronic, 413–**414;** and smoking, 167, 414
Butylated hydroxytoluene (BHT), 187

Caffeine, 258–259
California: Civil Addict Program in, 132; drug abuse laws in, 144; Mental Health Act (1969), 133; urbanization rate in, 25
Calisthenics, **217,** 222, 228
Calories (kcal), **180;** average world-wide distribution of, 44–45; content of some foods and drinks, 207; quantity needed, 199, 200, 204; sources of, 199–200; storage of and obesity, 205
Cancer, **398**–411; cell structure of, 399; cure for, 403, 406; diagnosis of, 401–402; as fatal disease, 400; as major killer, 233–234; metastasis of, 399; and smoking, 166–167; survival prospects, 410; symptoms of, 401; theories of causation, 402–403; treatment of, 403, 406–410; uterine, 288, 395–396
Candida, **393**–394
Cannabis drug family, **120**–125; compulsive use of, 125; relative effects of potency and dosage, 120, 122, 123
Carbohydrates, **181**–182; diets of low, 205–206
Carcinogens, **164**
Carotene, **190**
Carson, Rachel, 18
Castration, **274**
Cell, **325**–328; division of, 330–332; genetic code in, 328–330; parts of, 326–328
Cellulose, **181**
Cervix, **288**
Cesarean section, **363**
Chancre, **389**
"Change of life," **289**
Chemical substances, rate of invention of, 4
Chemotherapy, **96;** for cancer, 409–410; for disease, 380–381; for mental illness, 96; precautions, 381
Childbirth, 358–364; care of newborn after, 362; changes in mother after, 364–365; complications of, 362–364; estimated date of, 359; fetal position at, 358–359; labor of, 359–360; natural, 361; reducing pain of, 361–362
"Childhood" diseases, **381**
Chiropractic, **249**

Cholesterol, 192, 417, **420,** 426
Chromosomes, **326**–328 (*See also* Genes)
Cigarette advertising industry, 159, 160
Cilia, **378**–379; effect of smoking on, 164, 165
Circuit training, 227–229
Circulation, fetal, 337; diagram of, 416
Circulatory endurance exercises, **217,** 224, 227
Circumcision, **295**
Civil commitment procedure, **132**
Clinical psychologists, **97**
Clinics, 250
Clitoris, **299,** 300
Cocaine, 126, **128**
Codeine, **116**
Co-enzymes (*See* Vitamins)
"Cold turkey," **134**
Color-blindness, 335
Combustion, **6**
Common cold: remedies for, 255–256
Communicable diseases, 237, **373**–397 (*See also* Venereal diseases), control of, 212; major, 381–387; protection against, 377–379; stages of, 376–377; theories of, 374–376; treating with drugs, 379–381
"Community life," addiction to, 137
Compensating acts, **81**
Comprehensive Drug Abuse Prevention and Control Act (1970), 142; schedules and penalties for violation of, 141–142
Compulsive cannabis use, **125**
Conditioning, physical, **217**
Condom, **342;** use of for venereal disease prevention, 391–392
Congeners, **151**
Congenital defects, **336**–338; causes of, 337; heart disease, 337; kinds of, 336; prevention of, 337–338
Constipation, **198;** as cause of indigestion, 195
Contact lenses, **257**
Contraception, 276, **341**–346; chemical, 343–344; hormonal, 344–346; mechanical, 342–343; for sexual intercourse outside marriage, 278; and world population problem, 47, 49–51
Cooper, Kenneth H., 215, 227
Coping devices, 76–77
Coronary heart disease, **415,** 420–421
Coronary thrombosis, 213, **418**
Corpus fibrosum, **287**
Corpus luteum, **287**
Cosmetics, false claims of, 264
Coughs and cold remedies, 255–256
Counterconditioning, **95**
Cowper's glands, **295**

Cross-tolerance effect, **135**
Cryptorchidism, **294**
Cunnilingus, **301,** 302
Cyanosis, **337**
Cyclamates, **187**
Cyclazocine, **134**
Cystitis, **396**
Cytoplasm, **326**

Daytop House, 136
Death: causes of in United States, 233–234; premature, 212
Death rate: in developing nations, 34–35; reduction of, 32
Debility, **400**
Decibel scale, 26–27
Defense mechanisms, 72–76
Deficiency diseases, **189**–193; mineral, 183–184, 192; vitamin, 184, 185–186, 190–192
Degenerative conditions, **212**–213
Delirium tremens, **156**
Delusions, 82, **88**
Denatured alcohol, **147**
Denial, **73**–74
Dentist, **249**–250
Dependency, drug (*See* Drug dependency)
Depressant drugs, **108**–109; alcohol as, 148
Depression, **83**
Dermatology, **245**
Desensitization, **95**
Deserts, uses of, 42
Deviancy (*See* Sexuality, deviate)
Diabetes, **411**–412
Diaphragm, **342**
Diet, **188;** American patterns of, 44–45, 183; balanced, 44–45; disease and, 189–193; measuring adequacy of, 188–193; practical, 206, 209; pregnancy and, 338, 358; recommendations for healthy, 198–200; reducing, 205–208; substances needed in, 180–186
Digestion, **194**
Digestive system, 194–198; disorders of, 195–198; functions of, 196; structure of, 195
Dionne quintuplets, 364
Diploid number, **326**
Disease: communicable, 237, **373**–397; degenerative, 212–213; diet and, 189–193; noncommunicable, 398–427 (*See also* specific kinds)
Divorce, 320–323; effects of, 322; grounds for, 320–321; incidence of, 321–322; infidelity as cause of, 278; prevention of, 322
DNA (deoxyribonucleic acid), **328**–330
Dole, Vincent, 134

Illegitimacy, **276**
Illinois Narcotic Advisory Council, 133
Illness, frequency of in United States, 232–233
Illness period, **377**
Immaturity, causes of, 68–69
Immunity, **379;** schedule for, 380
Implantation, **354**
Impotency, **306**–307
Incest, **284**–285
Incubation period, **377**
Indigestion, **195**
Infant mortality: in substandard housing, 27; in United States, 212, 232, 233
Infection, **376**–377; cause of cancer, 402–403; result of cancer, 400
Infertility, **349**–352; causes of, 349–351; emotional factors in, 350; in men, 349; treatment of, 350–351; in women, 350
Infidelity, **320;** divorce and, 278
Influenza, **378**
Insulin, 104, 106, **411**–412
Insulin shock, **412**
Interferon, **379**
Internal medicine, **244**
Interstitial cells, **296**
Intrauterine devices (IUD), **342**–343
Inversion layers, **5, 7**
Iodine deficiency, **192,** 261
Iron deficiency, **192**
Isometric contractions, **216**
Isopropyl alcohol, **147**
Isotonic contractions, **216**–217

Jogging, **224**–226
Johnson, Virginia, 273, 296
Joint Commission on Accreditation of Hospitals, 251

Ketones, **206**
Kinsey, Alfred, 273, 296
Koch, Robert, 403
Kwashiorkor, **189**–190

Labia, **288**
Labor, **359**–362; false, 359; induction of, 364; reducing pain of, 361–362
Laxatives, **198**
Lead poisoning, 27–28
Leucocytes, **379**
LH (*See* luteinizing hormone)
Lice, pubic, 396–397
Life expectancy, 32, 212–213, 234
"Living together," **324**

Lobeline, **172**
Lobotomy, **96**
Love: marriage and, 310–311; maturity and, 68
LSD (lysergic acid diethylamide), 88, **126,** 144
LTH (*See* luteotrophin hormone)
Lungs: effect of smoking on, 166
Luteinizing hormone, **290**–291, 294
Luteotrophin hormone, **290**–291, 294
Lysine, **193**
Lysozymes (in tears), **379**

Major medical insurance, 240
Malnutrition, **189**–192
Malthus, Thomas, 39
Marijuana, 120–125; dosage and effects of, 123–124; legalization of, 138–139; penalties for possession of (1970), 144; percent THC in, 120–121; sales in United States of, 121; use of, 122, 123–125
Marijuana Tax Act (1937), 142
Marriage, 308–323; adjusting to, 318–320; alternatives to, 323–324; because of pregnancy, 276; counseling before, 317–318; and divorce, 320–323; engagement for, 315–317; financial resources and, 309; following divorce, 322–323; frequency of in United States, 308; group, 324; laws regulating, 314–315; secret, 318; selecting a partner for, 309–314; sexual adjustment to, 319; social regulation of, 314–315; successful, 308–314
Maslow, A. H., 60, 61, 62, 64
Masochism, **286;** homosexuality and, 280
Masters, William, 273, 296
Masturbation, **274**–275
Maturity, developing, 68–69; and marriage, 309
Medicaid, 236
Medical care: choosing, 243–252; financing, 236–242; high cost of, 235
Medical personnel, 243–252; percent of in population, 245 (*See also* specific types)
Medicare, 236–237, 238
Meiosis, **331**–332
Menarche, **289**
Menninger, Karl, 76
Menopause, **289**
Menstrual cycle, **289**
Menstruation, **288**–289; after pregnancy, 365
Mental health aide, **97**
Mental hygiene legislation: drug abuse treatment and, 131–133
Mescaline, 88, **125**–126
Metabolism, **179**–180
Metastasis, **399**

Tacoma Narcotics Center, 136
"Talkdown" phase (drug abuse treatment), **133**
Tampon, **288**
Terry, Luther, 165
Testicles, **294**
Testosterone, **296**
Tetrahydrocannabinol (THC), **120**–122
T-groups, **93**–94
Thalidomide, 337
Therapeutic communities, 136–138; criticisms, of, 137
Thiamin (B₁) deficiency, 190
Thyroxin, 180, **192**
Tobacco (*See* Smoking)
Tolerance, drug, 109–111, **113;** levels of heroin use, 115; to residue in food, 21; reverse, **111;** to solvents, 117
Toxemia, **358**
Toxicity, **21**
Toxin, **374**
Trace elements, **181**
Traits, inherited vs. acquired, 332; sex-linked, 334–336
Tranquilizers, 96, 107, **120**
Transactional analysis, **94**
Transmission (of disease), **376**–377
Transsexuality, **285**–286
Transvestism, **285**
Trichomonas, **394**–395
Triplets, **363**–364
Tubal ligation, **346**–347
Tumor, **399**–440; benign, 399; malignant, 400
Twins, 363

Ulcer, peptic, **195,** 197
Undernutrition, **189**
Underweight, **208**
Urban environment, 25–30; future of, 28–30; growth of, 25; noise pollution in, 26–27; stress in, 28; substandard housing in, 27–28
Urethritis, **396**
Urinary organs: infections of, 396–397
Urology, **245**–246
User (drug), **106**
Uterine cancer, **395**–396
Uterus, **288**

Vagina, **288;** diameter of and penis size, 303–304; infections of, 393–395; lubrication of, 299

Values, development of, 69–71
Vaporization, **5**–6
Varicose veins, **420**
Vas deferens, **295**
Vasectomy, **347**
Vectors, **374,** 376
Venereal diseases, **381**–397; frequency of in United States, 381–383; kinds of, 382; prevention of, 391–393; risk of, 276–277; telling children about, 383–384; transmission of, 383–384; uterine cancer and, 395–396
Viruses: as pathogens, 374; cancer and, 402–403
Vitamin deficiency diseases, 184, 185–186, 190, 192
Vitamins, 181, **184,** 185–186; as co-enzymes, 184; dangers of excess, 256; as food additives, 187; natural versus chemical, 262
Volatile solvents, **116**–117; toxic effects of, 117
Voyeurism, **284**

Walking (as exercise), 224
Water, importance of, 184, 186
Water pollution, **10**–13; effects of, 11; measurement of, 10–11; purification processes, 11–13
Weight: amphetamines and, 128; control of and diet, 200–209; desirable adult, 199; during pregnancy, 358; general health and, 201
Weight training, 222–224
White blood cells, role of in immunity, 379
Willis, J. H., 114
Withdrawal (coitus interruptus), **339**
Withdrawal illness, **113;** alcohol, 119–120, 156; amphetamine, 129; barbiturate, 119–120, 134; clinics for smoking, 172; narcotic-solvent, 113, 134; opium, 113
Women: exercise and, 213; status of and birth rate, 50–51; suicide rate of, 84–85
"Wonder drug," 104

Xerophthalmia, **190**
X-rays, and cancer diagnosis, 401

"Yeast" infection, **393**–394

Zygote, **354**